Political Corruption
In and Beyond the Nation State

Robert Harris

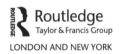
Routledge
Taylor & Francis Group

LONDON AND NEW YORK

First published 2003
by Routledge
11 New Fetter Lane, London EC4P 4EE

Simultaneously published in the USA and Canada
by Routledge
29 West 35th Street, New York, NW 10001

Routledge is an imprint of the Taylor & Francis Group

© 2003 Robert Harris

Typeset in Times by
BC Typesetting, Bristol
Printed and bound in Great Britain by
TJ International Ltd, Padstow, Cornwall

British Library Cataloguing in Publication Data
A catalogue record for this book is available from the British Library

Library of Congress Cataloging in Publication Data
Harris, Robert, 1947–
    Political corruption: in and beyond the nation state/Robert Harris.
        p.   cm.
    Includes bibliographical references and index.
    ISBN 0-415-23555-3 – ISBN 0-415-23446-1 (pbk.)
    1. Political corruption. 2. Transnational crime. I. Title.

JF1081.H37 2003
364.1′323–dc21   2003046536

ISBN 0-415-23556-1 (pbk)
ISBN 0-415-23555-3 (hbk)

Political Corruption

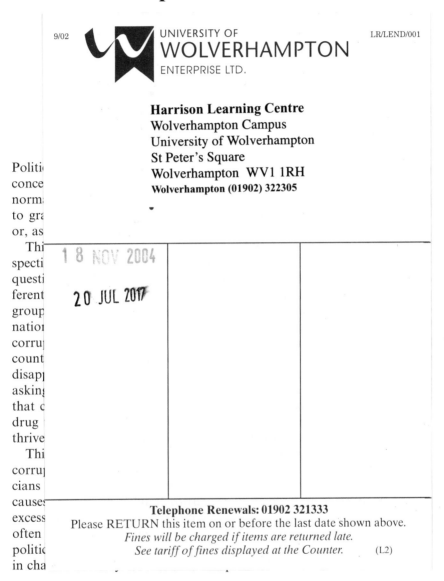

Politi
conce
norm;
to gr;
or, as
    Thi
specti
questi
ferent
group
natioı
corruị
count
disapị
askinɡ
that c
drug
thrive
    Thi
corruị
cians
cause:
excess
often
politiᴄ
in cha

Robert Harris is Professor in the Department of Politics and International
Studies, University of Hull. He has taught and researched in Hong Kong,
Japan and Malaysia and has published widely in criminology.

In memoriam

Lucy Dorothea Emily Harris (1914–2000)

Who knew exactly what political corruption was without having to write a book about it, and whose wisdom, kindness and undying love of the two generations following her will live on long after this book has been forgotten.

Contents

Preface

Why has not man a microscopic eye?
For this plain reason, man is not a fly.

(Alexander Pope, *Essay on Man*, I, 193–194)

The literature of political corruption is remarkable in terms of subject matter, disciplinary background and the ambitions (normative or analytic) of the writers. This does rather mean, however, that while the smorgasbord is a glittering feast of contrasting foods from all round the world, the price one pays for this variety is the absence of a wholly satisfying home-cooked meal. We cannot examine the literature of political corruption as we can that of Doric architecture or fibre optics because its very nature means that its study cannot operate within a single set of disciplinary boundaries.

Understandably given the nature of the topic, most texts are edited collections. These range from the vast compendia associated with Heidenheimer (most recently Heidenheimer and Johnston 2002) and, at much higher cost, Williams (Williams 2000a; Williams and Theobald 2000; Williams *et al.* 2000; and Williams and Doig 2000) to more modest multi-disciplinary collections, normally clustered round a sub-theme. These collections are without exception valuable, and though inevitably some of them, for example Levi and Nelken (1996a), Heywood (1997) and Doig and Theobald (2000), contain contributions of mixed quality, in all cases the best is very good indeed. Among these collected editions Heyman (1999) contains especially valuable material, both in terms of the overall quality of scholarship and for a rigorous editorial selection policy which, by combining conceptual consistency with substantive diversity, offers genuine scope for identifying likeness in things unlike. As such, it constitutes a step towards the elusive goal of a comparative approach. Other studies offer tentative comparisons, typically of countries geographically contiguous or with cultural, racial or historical similarities, though few develop a systematic comparison of specified variables. Certainly there is as yet insufficient agreement on how best Lancaster and Montinola's stringent conditions to meet:

the most central goal of all comparative analyses [is] the assessment of rival explanations. The advancement of logical explanations, grounded in systematic empirical testing of theoretically-derived hypotheses, facilitates healthy debate about the primacy of one explanation over another.

(Lancaster and Montinola 1997: 186)

For example, Lo's excellent study of political corruption in China and pre-retrocession Hong Kong, while offering a coherent theoretical explanation based on the Gramscian version of hegemony, is predominantly an account of corruption in two countries which, for well-rehearsed reasons, took different political and economic paths (Lo 1993). On the other hand a three-pronged study of political corruption in Spain, Italy and Malta (Heywood *et al.* 1994) is not comparative at all, and while it provides interesting in-country perspectives from which tentative comparisons can be constructed, a synthesizing chapter would not have come amiss.

Other studies explore political corruption in the context of policing, organized crime and drugs. Studies of the international and transnational policing of corruption cover activities including organizational liaison, front-line technologies and jurisdictional ambiguities. The last of these is especially important in the USA, where turf wars are characteristically fought out not just by gangsters but by law enforcement agencies at federal, state and township levels (Caputo 1976). Bayart *et al.* (1999) offer a sophisticated study of the criminalization of various weak states in Africa. In the field of transnational policing Sheptycki (2000a) contains outstanding chapters (though see also Anderson and den Boer 1994; Fijnaut 1993), as does Fiorentini and Peltzman (1995) in that of the economics of organized crime.

In addition to such collections, the literature contains some outstanding attempts at synthesis, but not, for the most part, of recent vintage. Scott's early book (Scott 1972), though now substantively of mainly historical interest, and which, in spite of its title, *Comparative Political Corruption*, is not primarily a comparative study, was among the first to offer a coherent political anthropology of corruption, advancing hypotheses still worthy of scholarly attention thirty years on. The present book, self-evidently, is also not a collected edition (though more than once in the course of its preparation the author wished it were). The rationale for the book was that there already existed more collected editions than any scholar could digest, that in spite of their excellent scholarship it was scholarship of a microscopic kind, and that there was less justification for more of the same than for a synthesis of what already existed. This book was conceived of as such a synthesis, though the Promethean character of this ambition quickly became apparent.

Fortunately, however, in spite of suffering from all too obvious draw-backs (not least an unavoidable dependence on secondary sources, not all of them susceptible to cross-checking), single authorship also brings potential benefits, though it must be for readers to judge whether this generalization applies to the present effort. For example, while one has to sacrifice primary research and depth of knowledge in a single area, one should gain both analytic consistency and the chance to sustain a coherent conceptual framework within which to encapsulate the object of study. Though collection editors also try to offer such a framework, often in a synthesizing chapter, the vagaries of contributing authors combined with the need for editors to avoid being so discourteous as to criticize any of them make it rare for such chapters to be especially illuminating.

This book's conceptual framework entails locating political corruption in the context both of nation state politics and international relations. Its concern is hardly at all with individual scandals but with the ways in which political systems facilitate (or do not facilitate) them and react (or do not react) to them. The book falls into three main parts, each comprising two complementary chapters. Chapters 1–2 debate aspects of the nature of political corruption, proposing that it is best regarded not as an aberration from, but as an aspect or extension of, normal politics. It is, after all, normal politics which permits it to occur; many of the skills and characteristics of political corruption are similar to those of normal politics; and it is not always clear where the line is to be drawn between the rough-and-tumble of normal politics and political corruption. We also argue that political corruption thrives in the interstices between different parts of the polity, and, on the international stage, in the interstices between nations, particularly where ambiguity or manipulation creates grey areas between different functions of government. Chapter 1 is primarily conceptual and definitional, while Chapter 2 introduces relevant aspects of the political economy of corruption.

Chapters 3–4 address the problem by examining national political corruption in two contrasting countries, the People's Republic of China (PRC) and the United Kingdom. PRC is what we define as a high-corruption state – where corruption has so infiltrated the organs of government as to make corruption the norm and honesty the sometimes dangerous exception. The United Kingdom on the other hand is now (but has not always been) a low-corruption country where political corruption is the exception, not the rule. There we trace briefly both the country's mid-nineteenth-century transition from high corruption and the manner in which the system today deals with corrupt individuals.

Chapters 5–6 apply these notions to the international and transnational dimensions of political corruption. The role of nation states in an international system, little changed in basic structure since the Treaty of Westphalia of 1648, has had to adapt to vast transformations, but never at greater speed than over the last quarter of the twentieth century. Globalization, particularly since the end of the Cold War, has opened ever more markets to ever more illegitimate activity, and the nation state system has been challenged by this explosion in transnational crime. Money laundering, people trafficking, the drugs trade, weapon smuggling and so on are now firmly embedded in global transactions, and involve breathtaking sums of money. The manner in which, and the extent to which, the international system has adjusted to such challenges are the main themes of these chapters.

As ever in such an enterprise, my debts to family, friends and colleagues are considerable, even to the several people who, hearing the topic, helpfully warned me that writing the book might put my life in danger. Douglas and Muriel Hague have been especially solicitous in this respect. Many colleagues at the University of Hull and Hong Kong Baptist University have done all and more than fellow scholars should to advise, assist and befriend me. Naming individuals is usually invidious and sometimes causes resentment, since those who are not named may believe they should have been and some who are may wish they had not been, fearing an apportionment of blame for the book's deficiencies. As always, however, that particular buck rightly stops with the author. Nonetheless, particular thanks are due to my University of Hull colleagues Dr Xiudian Dai and Professors Philip Norton (the Lord Norton of Louth) and Noël O'Sullivan of the Politics Department, as well as to my former colleague Professor Guharpal Singh, now of the Theology Department at the University of Birmingham. In addition my friend and one time fellow pro-vice-chancellor Professor Howell Lloyd of the History Department was characteristically thought provoking on many topics, including political corruption, over many years, many dinners and many bottles of wine. Certainly he gave me a better understanding of how corruption operated in the Jacobean Court than I have been able to convey in the few paragraphs that space has permitted me to devote to it in this book.

Part of the book was prepared when I was working in Hong Kong, and my colleagues at Hong Kong Baptist University, particularly Dr Sammy Chiu, Dr Marcus Chiu and Dr Victor Wong, gave help, support and above all friendship. In addition my good friend and collaborator Dr Lo Tit Wing, associate professor at City University, Hong Kong, an expert in this and several other areas, also deserves thanks for his invaluable help and advice, as do staff of the Independent Commission Against Corruption. Back in England more friends, including Jenny Harvey of the University of Hull and Professors David Webb and Noel Timms, gave me helpful ideas and stimulated my thoughts. David in particular prodded me firmly on one occasion when the scale of the endeavour was proving daunting, rightly advising me to tell myself exactly what I would tell a Ph.D. student in a similar situation. On the subject of Ph.D. students, the experiences of supervising the thesis of Dr Amirzada Asad of Peshawar University and subsequently collaborating with him on the book of the thesis proved pleasingly relevant to this book too. I am also grateful to Edwina Welham, my editor

at Routledge, for her support throughout, and in particular for her understanding over the unavoidably late delivery of the manuscript. Finally the
three women and one man in my life – my wife, Josephine, and my children –
alas, the English language lacks, so far as I know, an acceptable alternative
word to describe adult offspring – Ruth, Amelia and George – have always
been generous and often amazing, in very different ways.

1   The idea of political corruption (I): conceptual and definitional issues

> *Meno:*   But how will you look for something when you don't in the least know what it is? . . .
> *Socrates:*   . . . Do you realize that what you are bringing up is the trick argument that a man cannot try to discover either what he knows or what he does not know? He would not seek what he knows, for since he knows it there is no need of the inquiry, nor what he does not know, for in that case he does not even know what he is to look for.
> *Meno:*   Well, do you think it is a good argument?
> *Socrates:*   No.
>
> (Plato, *Meno*, 80D–E)

Political corruption is a multifaceted and mutable concept, defiant of precise or comprehensive definition. Although in an interconnected world almost all areas of social and political science present definitional or conceptual problems at the margins, in political corruption these margins are especially wide. Domestically, because political corruption is often so intimately interconnected with business enterprises, legitimate as well as shady, the term is sometimes used in situations better understood as simple fraud or embezzlement. Globally the fractures in the international system arising from national sovereignty, jurisdictional disputes and lack of coordination among international organizations give political corruption many forms to take and many cracks in which to hide. Hence we shall argue that political corruption can no longer be plausibly analysed only within a nation state framework.

In addition, the line between what is and is not corrupt can be so fine as to be indiscernible even to those involved. Where this is not so and corruption is manifest it is often impossible to disentangle political from other forms of corruption. A kleptocracy[1] like Mobutu's Zaïre, for example, could not have functioned without corrupting the civil servants, judiciary and generals who together constituted an interdependent and secretive power elite; the same applies in high-corruption countries from the Philippines and Indonesia to Moldova and Georgia.

Many problems, analytic, conceptual and investigative, face students of political corruption. For example, in the United States it is clearly the formal duty of elected representatives to serve the people without fear or favour; equally clearly, in practice the political system works on rather different principles. Party discipline is weak and interest groups strong, and, in the absence of a Burkean representational system, Congressmen can effectively become advocates for powerful interests within their own electorates. Hence emerge both 'fixers', those descendants of old-fashioned party bosses who ensure that the vacuum created by weak parties is filled by strong interest groups (Rogow and Lasswell 1963: 22), and 'iron triangles' of congressional committees, civil servants and private interest groups (Smith 1988; Tullock 1993). In such situations the symbiotic nature of political, bureaucratic and interest-group relations creates a collusive structure impermeable to external influence and largely invisible to electors:

> Bureaux are adept at responding to threatened budget cuts with promises to eliminate services most valued by voters, thus marshalling the vote motive in favour of their bloated budgets. . . . The major armament manufacturers together with individuals who live around and service military installations ally themselves with congressmen dependent on defence military contracts for their constituents and with bureaucrats from the Department of Defense whose budgets are dependent on high military appropriations from the US Congress. Such iron triangles are very resistant to voter attacks even in circumstances that clearly call for budgetary retrenchment.
>
> (Tullock 1993: 56–57)

In politics a gap almost inevitably exists between public discourse and private reality. In most western democracies the only acceptable rhetorical justification for entering politics is to serve the people. But since the reality of politics is no less self-seeking than that of any commercial organization politicians juggle an altruistic public discourse with a private one in which, as with any job, their motives are geared primarily to personal ambitions such as self-advancement or securing a comfortable lifestyle. This dissonance between appearance and reality sets the scene for the theatre of deception which democratic politics can easily become. The cognoscenti – Washington insiders, Westminster villagers and trusted members of the press corps – know what is going on, but the reality presented to the public, except on the exciting occasions when a scandal breaks, is normally a carefully spun tapestry.

This dissonance between appearance and reality also means that when minor scandals, which would be dealt with quietly if at all by most corporations, become public they are a source of fascination. Miscreant politicians in competitive democracies, whether corrupt or not, therefore risk being dealt with firmly once their conduct has come to public notice and been negatively received.[2] This is especially so if the conduct in question threatens the party's electoral prospects and therefore their colleagues' career interests. It is even more so if the politicians concerned lack a strong enough power base to be able to raise the stakes by heightening the risk attached to any action against them.

Most major scandals are events beyond the equilibrating capacity of the system to manage, events which cause it to spin out of control like a heating system with a faulty thermostat, until, at least in a mature state, adjustments to existing regulatory mechanisms or new ones bring it back into equilibrium. Such scandals should almost never be analysed individualistically. In Watergate,[3] for example, only at *one level* did the corruption stem from Nixon the man – his paranoia, his resentment at the conspiracy of 'insiders' to keep him outside the magic circle, his self-imposed mission to save the United States from the subversive forces of permissiveness, and so on. At a *second level* it stemmed from the fact that all societies contain people like Nixon but not all states make them president.[4] Hence whatever Nixon the man may have done, the presidency which enabled him to do it was a product of the US political system. While manipulating state agencies and his opponents' decision-making,[5] controlling information flows, heavy-handedly calling in political debts, pressurizing companies for contributions and conspiring with FBI Director J. Edgar Hoover to engage in illegal phone-tapping were certainly disgraceful, disgraceful presidential behaviour is not exactly unique. In fact Nixon was almost obsessively aware of the corruption, criminal associations and cover-ups perpetrated by his predecessors, not least the popular hero Kennedy whose legacy he so resented; and the White House tapes several times show that Nixon saw himself as acting no differently from his opponents. At a *third level* Nixon's concern was to maximize his freedom to govern, an ambition which led him to try to centralize the bureaucracy, control public opinion and equate dissenting views about his 'secret war' in Cambodia and Laos with un-American activity. This in turn was a response to the fact that though, famously, the buck stops with the President, the President's freedom to govern is inhibited by Madisonian checks and balances designed to keep him in semi-permanent tension with Congress. Hence Nixon is better understood not as a uniquely evil man, which he certainly was not, though as a driven and tormented one he may have been a risky president. Rather he was the product of a political system which, if similar problems were not to recur, required a step-change rather than fine tuning.

Of course both a very corrupt politician and a very honest one are easy to spot independently of culture; it is the shades of grey that give us pause. This applies both in less-developed countries (LDCs) with low literacy levels, immature or inadequate constitutional safeguards and poor communications, and in developed ones with an informed electorate, strong civil society and free press. Within the grey area political corruption for the most part involves a range of understood practices which give cause for concern only when some boundary is overstepped or when political, commercial or criminal purpose is served by exposure. The distinction between lobbying, the very stuff of democratic politics, and rent-seeking (putting one's personal interests above those of the electorate) often has little practical meaning. That such a distinction exists, however, is probably a product of the myth, prevalent in the United States with its cultural adulation of the Founding Fathers, of a binary divide between the altruistic and the self-seeking politician. Once this binary divide is questioned, conventional views of political corruption require reconsideration.

These observations suggest three main points, all to be developed in this book. *First*, political corruption is, for the most part, best understood not as a discrete phenomenon but as an extension of normal political behaviour, presenting problems of quantity, where corruption is taken to excess, or quality, where it involves activities deemed unacceptable by local or international law or significant opinion formers. *Second*, it is a transnational and international activity, and analyses based on a nation state framework have been overtaken by events on the world stage. *Third*, it is an interstitial activity, operating in the cracks between different sectors in one state, or, transnationally, in those between the political frameworks of different states.

Following signposts: the impossibility of adequate definition

> 'You know that it is much easier to ask questions than to answer them. But answer yourself, and . . . make your answer precise and accurate . . .' . . . 'Thrasymachus,' I said trembling, 'don't be hard on us, for if Polemarchus and I have gone astray in our scrutiny of the argument, our sin has assuredly not been deliberate . . . We are in earnest, my friend, believe me, but the task, I fancy, is beyond our powers; and, therefore, you clever people should rather pity than scold us.'
>
> (Plato, *The Republic*)

> *Boswell:*   Then, Sir, What is poetry?
> *Johnson:*   Why, Sir, it is much easier to say what it is not. We all *know* what light is; but it is not easy to *tell* what it is.
>
> (James Boswell, *The Life of Samuel Johnson*)

The literature on political corruption contains many attempts at definition, none of them entirely satisfactory. Heywood, for example, perfectly sensibly suggests that in liberal democracies it is best understood as 'an abuse of trust and an attempt to control the political arena through an undemocratic use of power and influence' (Heywood 1994: 3). This definition, however, excludes corruption in political systems where political leadership is not conceived of as a trust, where the head of state is above the law, or where democracy is not the norm. It is understandable that the chimera of a unified definition has preoccupied generations of scholars, for scholars are trained to follow the common sense proposition that it is hard to discuss something unless one knows what it is. But:

> Definitions of corruption generally focus on one of several aspects of the phenomenon . . . 'public-interest-centred', regarding corruption to be in some way injurious to or destructive of the public interest . . . 'market-centred', suggesting that the norms governing the exercise of public office have shifted from a 'mandatory-pricing model to a free-market model', especially in circumstances where such governing norms are unclear or nonexistent – as in new states . . . 'public-office-centred', stressing the public office has been misused . . . 'public-opinion-centred' . . . legal criteria . . . difficulties surrounding the criteria . . . are clear. . . . Yet to narrow corruption to purely legal criteria in order to escape from these difficulties seems equally problematic.
>
> (Szeftel 1983: 164)

Nonetheless it is hard to find an acceptable alternative. One approach is to analyse the numerous anthropological case studies which exist for areas of commonality, construct a grid of corruption-friendly and unfriendly circumstances and apply it to the available ethnographies. But this also only takes us so far: case studies are *sui generis* and rarely permit precise comparison. Another approach is to construct elaborate schemata intended to encapsulate the full range of corrupt activities. To Alatas, for example:

> corruption may be divided into seven distinct types: transactive, extortive, investive, defensive, nepotistic, autogenic and supportive. . . . Failure to make the distinction between the different types of corruption and to place them in their proper evaluative context only leads to confusion and time wasting.
>
> (Alatas 1990: 3)

This is a logical approach, and one need not share Alatas's confidence in the clarity, exclusivity or applicability of his categories, or indeed his passionate anti-corruption ethic, to see that it could offer a basis for development. It has, however, still to be determined how fruitful such a development would be, and though further testing of the typology is necessary the possibility that it could lead to conceptual progress should certainly not be dismissed. Padhy, on the other hand, suggests a tripartite distinction involving *nonfeasance* (failing to perform a required duty), *malfeasance* (committing an unlawful act) and *misfeasance* (the improper performance of a legitimate action) (Padhy 1986: 3). This is an interesting approach, but by defining as corrupt all failures to do one's duty it offers such a counsel of perfection that only the most saintly could claim to be other than intermittently corrupt.

Many single-sentence definitions characterize political corruption as the exploitation of elected public office for private gain; but these simply describe normal political behaviour which is only perceived as corrupt when it becomes quantitatively unacceptable (people become greedy), or qualitatively so, extending into areas deemed sacrosanct by significant opinion formers. *Most* politicians exploit public office for private gain when given legitimate opportunity to do so just as most individuals exploit such opportunities as their circumstances yield them. What political system does not make use of patronage? How many politicians fail to reward their supporters once in office? (One of patronage's cruder manifestations, the spoils system, has a long pedigree in US politics: see Summers 1987: 23 *et seq.*) How many decline to benefit personally from office by generous interpretation of the perquisites available to them? Or, on demitting office, by parachuting into directorships, consultancies, after-dinner speaking engagements or book contracts?

To claim that most political corruption is better regarded as an extension of political activity than as a radical departure from it is not to retreat into a culturally pluralist, but ultimately nihilistic, cul-de-sac: the charms of such an approach have seduced too many scholars already. Neild, for example, defines political corruption, on the face of it perfectly reasonably, as 'The breaking, for the sake of financial or political gain, of the rules of conduct in public affairs prevailing in a society in the period under consideration' (Neild 2001: 1). Definitions such as this, however, present several difficulties. *First*, in that they are predicated on the assumption that there is, or can be, agreement in a given society as to what is and is not corrupt, they anticipate unrealistic levels of intra-societal consensus, not least among both the predatory classes and their victims. The negative public response to the dubious use of presidential pardons or immunities in countries ranging from the United States to Indonesia illustrates this point. *Second*, they assume all interest groups will have a view on the matter, whereas some may not. We cannot assume training in constitutionalism, the existence of a European-style scepticism towards politicians or even high levels of literacy in many countries whose occupants most regularly encounter corruption. More often in such countries the propaganda of corrupt leaders themselves shapes popular views on the subject, usually through media control or the influence of local placemen. *Third*, whether an act is corrupt may be unclear and necessitous of judicial determination. Entrepreneurs, political as well as commercial, by definition test the boundaries of legitimacy by operating in innovative and creative, not to say morally and legally ambiguous, ways. But such ambiguity is not synonymous with corruption, and the rules of politics and business are not always so clear as the legal divide between, say, stealing and not stealing a chocolate bar. *Fourth*, the logic of this kind of definition leads to the conclusion that in a kleptocracy, where no effective rules of political conduct exist, there can be no political corruption. This creates the self-evidently illogical proposition that, the rules being themselves the products of corruption, corruption is capable of abolishing itself. It would seem particularly absurd to deem non-corrupt an act that most international scholars, jurisdictions and inter-governmental organizations, to say nothing of educated people around the world, would consider such but which avoids the designation for reasons that are themselves corrupt. *Fifth*, such an approach is based on the assumption that rules concerning corruption are matters of national policy and legislation. This no longer suffices in the international and transnational world. If potential inward investors believe a country is corrupt they will either exacerbate whatever corruption exists by exploiting it or inflict collateral economic damage by declining to invest. Either way the country's vulnerability is increased. *Sixth*, in a world fuelled by international trade and commerce the explanatory potential of cultural peculiarities is considerably diminished. While such peculiarities certainly exist, as any westerner who has traded in the Middle East, the Indian sub-continent or South-East Asia will testify, wise LDC traders are increasingly adapting to western norms. So while one should not be naive about the sweeteners paid by western companies, often in contravention of their own laws, a degree of cultural convergence is both discernible and inevitable.

A further problem exists with attempts to define political corruption by reference to criminal law. The efforts of virtually all criminologists or statisticians of crime are impeded by the problem of clandestinity, which creates a large dark figure of unknown criminal activity. The student of political corruption faces both this problem and a further one stemming from the fact that many transgressors lie (usually in both senses of the word) at the heart of their country's power elite. Not surprisingly when the objects of suspicion may themselves be responsible for framing, interpreting or implementing constitutional and criminal law, numerous examples exist of powerful rulers being above those same laws. But are laws drafted on the instructions of those engaged in nefarious activity any more helpful to the task of defining corruption than a statute prohibiting housebreaking designed by a burglar so as to omit all reference to his or her preferred modus operandi?[6]

> after President Trujillo, the 'benefactor' of the Dominican Republic (1930–61), took over the country's only shoe factory there was no secret about the ensuing decree forbidding anyone in the capital from going barefoot. . . . Likewise President Zayas of Cuba (1921–5) made no secret of his attitude towards the National Lottery: 'his wife notoriously always drew the first prize and his daughter the second – both without shame'.
>
> (Whitehead 1983: 148)

But the problem is not restricted to tin-pot dictatorships. Democratic governments may also, especially when long in power, become arrogant in attitude, blurring constitutional distinctions between party and government and between government and state. For example, in an effectively unaccountable legislature in Campania, Southern Italy, 'the mayor demanded that 323 items be voted on as one block . . . most of these items concerned ratification of contracts awarded . . . as a result of private negotiation rather than public tendering' (Behan 1996: 139). Prior to the 1990s it would have been hard to find a supposedly communist country in Eastern Europe where corruption was other than endemic. While in most such countries capitalist transformations have changed the character of corruption they have by no means inevitably diminished its extent: on the contrary, in a number of former 'second world' countries they have led to increases, as well as exposing what was previously concealed. In Russia, host at the time to some 3,000 criminal gangs, and in some cities ungovernable:

> members of the Duma complained in July 1994 that their proposed law on corruption had its provisions concerning corruption in banking deleted at the presidential level. The legislative framework needed to combat organized crime . . . had been impeded by corrupt legislators and individuals at the executive level. . . . As a consequence of the corruption of the law enforcement apparatus and the lack of a specific organized crime statute in the criminal code there has been no major organized crime trial in the past three years in the former Soviet Union . . . large-scale organized crime enjoys impunity in the successor states.
>
> (Shelley 1994: 344; see also Beare 2000a)

Factors such as this render any analysis of political corruption based solely on criminal law very problematic. The student of corruption has to accept that the law itself may have been subject to partial formulation, interpretation or implementation, and is as much a product of corruption and an instrument for its achievement as a reference point for its definition. So, like Neild's definition discussed above, Scott's belief that corruption involves 'breaching the formal norms of office' (Scott 1972: 5) not only begs two questions – who determines the formal norms? and who decides when they have been breached? – but also presupposes that we can abolish corruption by abolishing the rule proscribing it:

> When a Thai cabinet member joins a Chinese business board, an act that does not violate any law, he substitutes a board member's salary and perquisites for what previously would have taken the form of illegal bribes. In this way the process of influence is moved from corrupt to legal channels.
>
> (Scott 1972: 74)

In the face of such imponderables, therefore, we can only share Socrates' embarrassment at being attacked by Thrasymachus for having more questions than answers, and despair of the possibility of finding a satisfactory *definition* of political corruption. Nonetheless we do need a *signpost* to point us in the right general direction, even though we may have to exercise judgement at future crossroads where no such signpost exists. We take as such a signpost Summers's definition of political corruption as a two-limbed phenomenon involving '*the use of public position for private advantage or exceptional party profit, and the subversion of the political process for personal ends*' (Summers 1987: 14; italics added). Even this, however, demands a gloss. *First*, we ascribe to the adjective 'private' the dual definition of 'personal' and 'secret' (a deconstructive reading unlikely to be what Summers had in mind). *Second*, Summers's emphasis on the whole *process* being subverted is of central importance since this book is more concerned with systemic corruption than with individual predation in predominantly non-corrupt systems. *Third*, 'subversion' does not imply that to be politically corrupt one must do the subverting oneself: one may equally well continue to exploit a system already subverted by one's predecessor, as has occurred in states ranging from Haiti to Indonesia. We proceed with this signpost in mind, but stress again that it is not perfect, simply the best that can be offered for the moment.

Political corruption and globalization

> OPEC countries on average retain some 75 per cent of their oil revenues for the state budget, allowing for operating expenses. But, in the case of African oil producers, this proportion is closer, even in the best cases, to the range of 55–70 per cent. The difference represents a supplementary profit shared by the oil companies and African elites. . . . Similar practices may be identified in the management of the uranium mines of Niger, phosphates in Togo, and bauxite and aluminium in Guinea. Only a meagre revenue reaches the state treasury, or even none at all, while the real royalties are paid directly to politicians in foreign bank accounts.
>
> (Hibou 1999: 84–85)

The idea that the international system contains characteristics of both a civil society and an anarchic state is not new (Bull 1977), but it remains apposite in spite of the great changes that have occurred since it was formulated. The international system contains sufficient shared understandings and interests to be recognizably a 'society', and this enables most things to proceed reasonably smoothly most of the time. On the other hand the limited and partial nature of international law and law enforcement makes that society vulnerable to the ineffectively policed illegalities, ranging from aggression to trade embargoes, of individual states. Such elements of political anarchy make it, in Hedley Bull's (1977) classic formulation, an 'anarchical society'.

If we are right to argue that political corruption today is increasingly an international and transnational problem requiring international and transnational solutions this is not especially encouraging. Nonetheless, it need not lead us to defeatism or an excess of relativism. *First*, it would be wrong to exaggerate the importance of disputes at the margins as though no agreement existed as to either what corruption is or what to do about it. There are numerous disputes about who should act against corruption, who should pay, how it should be balanced against such conflicting considerations as national sovereignty, privacy, human rights and so on. These, though, are comfortingly familiar *political* arguments, in the company of which we may feel reasonably at home. *Second*, the Organization for Economic Cooperation and Development's (OECD) Convention on Combating Bribery of Foreign Public Officials came into force in 1999, committing its thirty-four signatories, who include all the world's largest economies, to adopting common rules on the punishment of companies and individuals who bribe foreign public officials for business purposes. A related text prohibits regarding bribes to foreign officials as tax deductible. Other international organizations, including both the World Bank and the International Monetary Fund, since the late 1990s, have been taking the issue increasingly seriously, and several international banking organizations, in particular the Bank for International Settlements, have for some time been doing the same. Supranational organizations such as the European Union are moving in the same direction. The consistency of developments such as these, combined with the status and influence of the organizations concerned, should be sufficient to persuade even the least idealistic international relations analyst that something is beginning to stir. *Third*, the trend towards jurisdictional extension started by the United States with the Foreign Corrupt Practices Act (FCPA) 1977, which criminalized the bribery of foreign officials,[7] seems likely to continue. While jurisdictional extensions of this kind are currently straws in the wind, the trend towards the gradual integration of national and supranational law seems unlikely to be reversed. And it is within a framework for the transnational regulation of transnational illegality that a way forward probably needs to lie.

Nonetheless, political support for treaties and codes of practice, for example in money laundering, may be easier to secure than operational cooperation among enforcement personnel. In areas such as transnational policing such cooperation is certainly patchy (Sheptycki 2000b), transnational cops being some years behind transnational robbers.[8] This is not surprising: *first*, the politics of crime control driven by domestic not global imperatives, and street crime and burglary are of greater concern to most voters and interest groups than bribery and corruption in far-off lands. Hence, *second*, funding and organizational support for such bodies as Europol are often unsatisfactory, seconded individuals can find themselves in a career cul-de-sac, and seldom are the cooperating agencies free of rivalry with and suspicion of each other. *Third*, at the end of the Cold War the United States scaled back its overt and covert international policing operations, subsequently refocusing them on specific Middle Eastern targets for anti-terrorist purposes at the expense of, particularly, East Asia, Latin America and sub-Saharan Africa. The consequent loss of the covert infrastructure is proving particularly hard to make good. *Fourth*, neo-liberal trends in criminal justice have led to a softening of both laws and law enforcement in respect of what John Stuart Mill called self-regarding acts – soft drug use, pornography, Sabbath trading, homosexual behaviour and so on. In fact political corruption is no more a self-regarding act than insider trading, but rather 'a crime with victims who may never know they are victims' (Fennell 1983: 18). Their victimization ranges from paying speed money for a minor service or bearing the costs of politicians' refusal to adopt reforms which would reduce the scope for bribery to tolerating the negative impact of corruption on inward investment, customs duties and international aid. Nonetheless, if corruption is generally perceived as a consensual activity between briber and bribed its pursuit sits uncomfortably with any trend in the direction of deregulation and is unlikely to attract reliable or widespread support. *Fifth*, domestic companies, in bribing foreign politicians or officials, are widely perceived as taking necessary steps to secure contracts in the face of unscrupulous foreign competition, and few western governments are likely to show excessive zeal in pursuing their own successful exporters. In addition, since the contracts benefit the economy of the exporting country, the moral outrage of voters, as inadvertent beneficiaries of corruption, is always liable to be muted. *Sixth*, the unproductive political capital costs involved in corruption (notably bribe money, unproductive for all purposes except the tautologous one of facilitating corruption) need not fall wholly or even mainly on western suppliers. Because contracts are awarded not to the lowest bidder but to the highest briber, corruption relegates price competition to a marginal role in the tendering process, and corruption costs can be factored into tenders with only limited commercial risk. Hence the paradoxical situation arises that in many corrupt transactions populations unwittingly fund the bribery of their own leaders.

This, naturally, is not the whole story, and all parties do incur real costs in competitions whose rules are not transparent, where enforcement is difficult and the involvement of local criminals likely. Such costs include not only loss of inward investment for customer countries ranking high on Transparency International's Perceptions of Corruption Index[9] but also other losses for developed world countries and blue-chip international companies. Time and expense are incurred in tendering, the volume of international trade is reduced in the event of a company's decision not to proceed and the company faces potentially damaging reputational costs if it does go ahead. In addition, because corruption constitutes a market imperfection it opens the door for unscrupulous companies to provide inferior services at high prices, denying both sides mutually advantageous trading relationships and potentially causing law enforcement problems for supplier countries. Accordingly, while at least some hidden corruption costs accrue to countries on both sides, corruption benefits accrue solely to the corrupt parties themselves.

So in an increasingly interconnected world in which domestic political activity is heavily influenced by international, including inter-governmental, organizations, regional trading blocs, superpower leverage and the policy preferences of multi-national corporations, analysing political corruption as solely or mainly a product of nation state politics is no longer tenable. If, for example, we take disaster relief as an instance of the relationship between the international system and political corruption we find that for four main reasons it is especially vulnerable to depredation. *First*, disaster relief attracts large but uncoordinated sums of money without a mature structure for coordinating and processing them. *Second*, the intense public sympathy which disasters provoke fades quickly, and subsequent interest diminishes within weeks, so monitoring reconstruction is costly to the media and of little popular interest. *Third*, disaster relief is normally directed at a single sovereign state, though intermediary bodies may be responsible for distribution. Hence the capacity of donor countries (or supranational groupings such as the European Union) to ensure it is not diverted by corrupt elements in the recipient country is characteristically limited. And *fourth*, reconstruction involves the speedy allocation of contracts which are hard to police and often associated with conflicts of interest, the involvement of organized criminals, for whom fraud against the European Union and other funding bodies is now big business, and local quid pro quo arrangements.

For all these reasons the auditing of aid expenditure is seldom comprehensive. For example in Italy following the 1980 Irpinian earthquake, billions of lire intended for reconstruction disappeared as kickbacks or into party coffers (Behan 1996: 68), with numerous reconstruction contracts awarded to politicians' key clients. Investigations into this expenditure were conducted by carefully selected magistrates, paid some L100 million[10] for each one, in defiance of a prohibition imposed by their self-regulating body, the Consiglio Superiore della Magistratura (della Porta 1998). In Taiwan following the 1999 volcanic eruption the provincial governor, Pang Pai-hsien, was arrested for corruption, influence-peddling and destruction of evidence (Blatt 2000). In Nicaragua following the 1972 earthquake President Anastasio Somoza Debayle pocketed much of the aid, helping swell his personal fortune to some $400 to $500 million by the time of his overthrow by the Sandinistas in 1979 (Merrill 1993). In parts of sub-Saharan Africa fictitious NGOs set up to channel disaster aid (or indeed any aid) into the pockets of corrupt ruling elites and their supporters, aided by a corrupt banking sector, represent not civil society but the privatization of the state (Hibou 1999: 99).

Modern communication systems and the neo-liberal economic principles accompanying them have transformed the global market, which overwhelmingly means the developed world. Nation states remain key players in the international system, but today their interactions are accompanied, sometimes dominated, by multi-national trading and financial corporations, some of them richer and more powerful than medium-sized states, and able to influence domestic and employment policies even in stable and affluent democracies. So far as the developed world is concerned, military conflicts are characterized less by war between nations than by attempts to combat the unwanted by-products of a globalized world – the interlinked phenomena of drugs, prostitution, money laundering, people trafficking, international organized crime and state-sponsored terrorism. Transnational problems require transnational solutions, and the inevitable concomitant of this is the future prospect of the gradual erosion of the role of the nation state, or at least most nation states other than the United States, as key players in international relations.

Inevitably in an international system characterized by unipolar superpower dominance, US influence on international relations is immense. The USA's economic, military and cultural influence, not least on such intergovernmental organizations as the World Bank, International Monetary Fund and World Trade Organization, has helped transform the world order since the early 1990s, and today's international relations cannot be understood in terms appropriate to the Cold War. Equally, many nation states are experiencing the pincer movement of 'glocalization' created by, on the one hand, the emergence of supranational regional groupings and, on the other, that of sub-national (tribal, ethnic or regional) pressure groups (see Held 1991), many of them funded by corrupt or violent means. These latter pressures reflect the emerging concept of 'umbrella states' with pooled or diminished sovereignty, increasingly centrifugal and mobile in character, containing a variety of races, cultures, tastes and lifestyles, and enjoying more diffuse modes of affiliation and identification than hitherto (Harris 2003). Hence, increasingly, the nation state is beginning to appear too small to deal with the big challenges of international politics and too big to deal with small community issues affecting its own people.

Corrupt politics, business and organized crime: indistinguishable or interchangeable?

the essential glue binding together the legitimate sectors of the community and the underworld criminal organization . . . the organized criminal group has opportunities to cloak itself in a patina of legitimacy as it interacts with the upperworld, and as it amasses resources (capital, information,

> organizational skills) and extends its networks into the legitimate business and economic sectors of society.
>
> (Lupsha 1996: 31)

The interrelatedness of corrupt and legitimate political and business activities increases the problem of identifying and analysing corruption. Many parts of the world are characterized by the interrelatedness of corrupt and legitimate organizations. In a successful criminal business the symbiosis of corruption and legitimacy is created, sustained and developed by the political configurations that mark out some countries as especially propitious for criminal enterprise. For example, the conjunction of weak central banks and strong private ones presents major regulatory challenges in parts of Africa and Asia. For this configuration to exist the subordination of banking to political interests is necessary. This requires a strong and unaccountable executive in a position to neutralize the legal system, privatize the banking system and use it, as Soeharto and his family did in Indonesia, effectively as a bottomless personal current account. One result is repeated high-risk loans, including those

> uncollectable due to the theft of relevant documents or arson; large sums withdrawn over the counter by senior bank officials; loans made to leading politicians which will never be repaid; loans made under cover of forged documents; the creation of companies purely as a means of gaining access to loans and which rapidly go bankrupt; the forging of details of accounts and of the operating capital of banks; the diversion of funds intended to improve a bank's liquidity.
>
> (Hibou 1999: 74)

In sub-Saharan Africa these characteristics are further enhanced by the region's status as one of the world's few remaining cash economies. This makes it especially vulnerable to tax evasion (often jocularly designated the second biggest sport after soccer) and money laundering, both effectively part-time services offered by the banking system. Not surprisingly, major international banks such as the Banque Nationale de Paris and Crédit Lyonnais have withdrawn from the financially anarchic franc (now Euro) zone, and the banking systems in Congo-Brazzaville, Chad and the Central African Republic are reportedly in their death throes.

Naturally, few corrupt politicians ignore the public good, because buying popularity, albeit with the money of others, is essential to their maintenance of power. So the genuine social and economic achievements of President Soeharto in Indonesia help explain the support his regime continued to receive from the rural poor in particular. During his thirty-two-year rule poverty declined, rice yields doubled, per capita calorie intakes increased by 50 per cent, infant mortality halved and the proportion of the population with no schooling fell from over 50 per cent to around 15 per cent (Hill 1998: 94). Nonetheless, few if any politicians or officials in LDCs possess a strong public service perspective, and many hold a proprietary view of office. Public officials may well have bought their office from politicians for the express purpose of creating a maximizing unit; politicians may openly use their power to obtain unimaginable wealth for themselves, their families and their actual or potential supporters. In the Sudan it has been claimed that 'corruption can be viewed as a principal mode of financial accumulation for a particular social class or classes' (Kameir and Kursany 1985: 8). In Ethiopia, Emperor Haile Selassie was estimated to have possessed over $15 billion in foreign assets on his death in 1975 (Walter 1985: 46). In Indonesia, at the time of his fall in 1999 President Soeharto had acquired such a huge sum for himself and his family that he was offered an amnesty if he returned $25 billion held mainly in overseas accounts. In South Korea, on his retirement President Chun Doo Hwan (1980–1988) was, with his family, required to return 13.9 billion won ($20 million) to the government (Quah 1999). In Zaïre, Mobutu was regarded as a role model by many ordinary people for having risen to great heights from the depths of poverty (Wrong 2000) and, like Robert, Lord Clive, before him, appears to have stood 'astonished at [his] own moderation'.[11] Independent estimates of Mobutu's wealth vary between $5 and $6 billion, and in 1982 he himself once admitted to having assets of over $4 billion (Agbese 1998: 11). However, his estimates varied wildly:

> 'I only have 325 million dollars, and that is not much for a leader of such a large country,' declared Mobutu. . . . His palace in the jungle town of Gbadolite has dumbfounded visitors. The runway . . . the luxurious marble palace with faucets of solid gold and the fresh flowers flown in from Johannesburg in South Africa, are just some of the curious details.
>
> (Heilbuth and Bülow 1997)

Mobutu's possessions included eleven chateaux in Belgium and France, estates in Spain, Italy and Switzerland (each with up to twenty-six resident servants), mansions in each of Zaïre's eight provinces and a palace in his home province. Apparently he owned several ships and Boeing aircraft, fifty-one Mercedes cars and shares in every foreign company in the country. He took 5 per cent commission on mineral exports, owned the third largest employing company in Zaïre (George 1988: 106–107) and claimed 40 per cent of gross proceeds of the 1974 Ali–Frazier world heavyweight championship fight in Kinshasa (Korner *et al.* 1986). He requisitioned US transport planes delivered as part of a military aid programme for criminal purposes and was accused by the Central Intelligence Agency (CIA) of stealing $1.4 million of funding destined for the FNLA (Front National de Libération de l'Angola) during the Angolan Civil War. Ultimately his legacy to the Democratic Republic of Congo was a $13 billion debt.[12]

As we have stressed, it would be a mistake to analyse such predation individualistically. Corrupt politicians cannot operate alone and must exploit their access to resources by developing client systems (less powerful people dependent on them) and, except in the case of presidential corruption, patron systems (more powerful people on whom they are dependent). In most LDCs, political corruption entails vote buying; in some this is a routine political activity. At an obvious level vote buying is akin to drug taking in competitive sports in that once one side embarks on it with impunity the choice facing others is between possibly winning corruptly and certainly losing honestly. In addition, because the resources required to buy the votes must themselves be acquired, one form of corruption seldom stands alone. The corrupt politician takes bribes, reinvesting part of them in vote buying (della Porta and Vannucci 1997: 118), thereby creating a vicious circle wherein the necessity of vote buying creates the necessity for bribe taking.

The existence of political corruption may also be used to justify political reactions which, though in fact further manifestations of power politics, are capable of representation as a clean-up campaign. So political corruption can be used, particularly by the military, to justify a coup (Scott 1972; George 1988: 148; Pasuk and Sungsidh 1994; Agbese 1998; Dynes 2000). Alternatively the targeted deployment of anti-corruption legislation, otherwise honoured in the breach, to remove powerful enemies was a particular tactic of Mao Zedong in China. Mao used his 'Four Cleans' (*Szu-ching*) campaign immediately before the Cultural Revolution to weaken the power base of his opponent Liu Shaoqi and to discipline dissidents in order to prepare the ground for their arrests (Lo 1993: Chapter 2).

Corruptly raised funds may go directly to politicians or be invested in party funds to maximize their chance of re-election and hence ensure continued rent-seeking opportunities. Though there are a few national exceptions to this (notably France, where rent-seeking opportunities have traditionally been available to senior politicians, and Italy, where Silvio Berlusconi entered politics mainly to defend his commercial interests), in few developed countries is power *systematically* deployed corruptly for direct predatory reasons. More often wealth is deployed to secure power, fame or status, usually by successful professionals and businessmen making financial sacrifices in pursuit of office.

In such situations party funding takes on major significance since the projected costs of political promotion and advertising always outstrip available funds. In the USA in the 1970s secret contributions to President Nixon's re-election fund, aggressively solicited by his campaign committee from corporations such as Braniff International, American Airlines and Gulf Oil, contravened both federal electoral law and Inland Revenue Service rules (Clarke and Tigue 1976: 14, 107–109).[13] In Germany in the 1990s the Christian Democrats maintained a network of secret bank accounts to hold illegal anonymous donations from home and abroad. At home the local party in Hesse used a Swiss bank account to funnel millions of Deutschmarks into party funds; internationally President Mitterrand of France is said to have made corrupt donations totalling £23.6 million through the oil group Elf-Aquitaine. Although in its final days in power the German Christian Democrat party destroyed two-thirds of its computer files the German Parliament demanded repayment of US $21 million and fined the party some $3 million.

As the epigraph to this section makes plain, however, it is organized crime that binds together the corrupt (or corruptible) politician and businessman. In Russia, for example, organized criminals are involved not only in intrinsically criminal activities such as drug supply but in large transnational corporations which exploit their reputation and political connections to secure contracts. There corrupt politicians and organized criminals cooperate in the oil and gas industries (whose internationalism offers great scope for money laundering), aluminium (a centralized and therefore relatively penetrable industry) and gem smuggling. In southern Italy the success of organized crime, which, though the influence of mafiosi in Sicily and the Camorra in Naples, stretches back to unification (Catanzaro 1992), accelerated dramatically following the Second World War, creating a situation in which politicians, bureaucrats and organized criminals became largely indistinguishable. In Naples:

> The classic business figure has always been that of the *mafioso imprenditore*, i.e. the gangster who moves into legitimate business. Today, given the power of the Camorra in some areas, one can see the emergence of an *imprenditore mafioso* – an individual who previously worked within the law by and large, acting as a banker or consultant to a firm known to have Camorra connections, advising on areas of investment, profit distribution and a whole host of legitimate financial problems. Once this *imprenditore mafioso* learns the tricks of the criminal trade, he or she is in an excellent position to strike out independently.
>
> (Behan 1996: 90)

By such means laws may be preferentially framed and interpreted, jurisdictional inconsistencies and privacy rules exploited and technical arguments made and countered; but still it may not always ultimately be clear even to those involved whether they have been corrupt. The extraordinary case of the Bank of Credit and Commerce International (BCCI) is a well-researched instance of the near seamless merging of legitimate and illegitimate capital for the purpose of corruption on a global scale (Adams and Frantz 1992; Passas 1993; Lupsha 1996). Though when examined in retrospect and in its entirety the corruption of BCCI is not only manifest but breathtaking in conception and execution, determining the point at which it became corrupt and the precise ways in which it meshed its corrupt and legitimate banking activities has proved well-nigh impossible.

Thus far we have queried the meaningfulness of any binary divide between corruption and non-corruption. At a deeper level, however, lies the more general question of whether other such divides – between law and lawlessness, or order and disorder, say – continue to have meaning. Of course we may take it for granted that most politicians periodically use a long spoon to sup with the devil: this is an unavoidable part of their business. Nonetheless, the pattern of criminal gangs taking over the functions of failing states (Lupsha 1996: 27), to some scholars the defining characteristic of a Mafia as opposed to an organized crime gang (Anderson 1995), is indicative of a more fundamental political realignment. In some countries the power of transnational criminal organizations can rival or exceed that of the state (Williams 1994), and the existence of a vacuum at the heart of the polity is a strong predictor of the rise of organized crime (Anderson 1995). In the former Soviet Union there is widespread acknowledgement not only of endemic corruption (Varese 1997) but also of the existence of a parallel paramilitary controlling structure managed by criminal gangs, combining predatory banditry with normal policing functions (Altman 1989; Humphrey 1999: 199).

Elsewhere the status quo is maintained by deploying criminal elements such as the Tonton-makout in François Duvalier's Haiti (Scott 1972: 85; Trouillot 1990: 189–190) as secret police accountable only to the corrupt leader. In Italy, at unification the state utilized the expertise of organized crime in regulating criminality rather than trying to eradicate the various *cosche* (Schneider and Schneider 1999). In Naples, for example, policing was effectively handed over to Camorra gangs by the new Prefect, Liborio Romano, as the most effective means of maintaining order against the threat of mass rebellion (Behan 1996: 17). Similarly, after the Second World War public order was the Allies' primary concern in Sicily. Accordingly they appointed mafiosi mayors, ensuring that Mafia, greatly weakened after 1924 by Mussolini's Prefect of Palermo, Cesare Mori, became integral to post-war political and administrative machinery locally and, through their links with the Christian Democrats, nationally. These links were only broken following the anti-Mafia investigations and the fall of Giulio Andreotti, who was said to have controlled a quarter of the Sicilian vote in the early 1990s. Still, however:

> organised crime functions as a vital, and perhaps even more efficient instrument of social control than the official representatives of law and order, as the fear it instils in the population, and the precarious or oppressive nature of employment in criminal enterprises, serve as useful shock absorbers for ruling politicians and powerful business interests.

> (Behan 1996: 194)

Organized crime, when it interacts with politics to maximum effect, can divert trading gains, particularly from arms sales, into offshore bank accounts, laundering them back into the national economy, sometimes through popular or philanthropic social investments such as schools, hospitals and sports facilities. In Naples, directly or indirectly, Camorra contributions provide work and subsistence for up to 500,000 people (Behan 1996: 134). In this sense organized crime funds and therefore controls social policy in countries where it has a political stronghold. Nonetheless, the cost of deploying criminal gangs as charity commissioners is high if it results in the country becoming locked into an unstable political and economic framework, buttressed by the bought popularity of criminals and the proceeds of crime. Once institutionalized, crime and criminals cease to be something to be shaken off, becoming instead an integral and expanding part of the machinery of state. For the symbiotic nature of the relation between political power and political corruption is such that the latter exists inside as well as outside the former, both a product *of* it and a transforming influence *on* it, simultaneously cause and effect.

In countries such as Russia, which have seen the collapse of the state's monopoly on armed force, the distinction between war and violent crime has become increasingly blurred. This is no less so when training overseas terrorist organizations becomes a legitimate or covert policy aim of states, as occurred with the USA in respect of the Contras in Nicaragua at the time of their conflict with the Sandinistas. In fact control of the security services can be a particular problem, and some activities of these services strongly resemble those of organized criminals:

> there seems a natural affinity between covert operatives and criminal syndicates. Both are practitioners of what one retired CIA operative has called the 'clandestine arts' – the basic skill of operating outside the normal channels of civil society. Among all the institutions of modern society, intelligence agencies and criminal syndicates alone maintain large organizations capable of carrying out covert operations without fear of detection. For example, when the CIA needed a legion of thugs to break the 1950 Community dock strike in Marseille, it turned to that city's Corsican milieu. When the agency attempted to assassinate Cuban leader Fidel Castro in the 1960s, it retained American Mafia syndicates who could not only kill on contract but ensure confidentiality . . . in the mountains of Asia, the CIA has allied itself with heroin merchants in Laos, Chinese opium dealers in Burma, and rebel opium armies in Afghanistan.
>
> (McCoy 1991: 15)

In parts of sub-Saharan Africa where the distinction between order and disorder seems especially opaque, Italian, Israeli, Russian, Ukrainian and

Asian (including Taiwanese) crime syndicates are ensconced and influential in up to fifteen countries (Hibou 1999: 83). In Taiwan the association between political leaders and organized criminals has traditionally been close, and their vote-buying capacity has enabled organized criminals to purchase power and influence. The Palestinian Authority derives some of its funding from the paramilitary extortion of its own citizens. In Colombia, when Pablo Escobar formed his private militia (Muerte e Secuestradores – Death to Kidnappers) in 1981, he created 'the rich and uniquely Colombian irony of a movement against criminal kidnappers funded and led by a long-time criminal kidnapper' (Bowden 2001: 44). In Turkey, as well as being actively involved in heroin distribution elsewhere in Europe, the terrorist Kurdistan Workers Party (PKK) levies taxes on drug traffickers passing through the lands it controls. In Northern Spain the separatist terrorist group ETA (Euzkadi Ta Askatasuna – Basque Fatherland and Liberty), dedicated to establishing an independent homeland based on Marxist principles in northern Spain, imposed a 'revolutionary tax' on businesses on pain of assassination (Woodworth 2001: 112). In short, where the forces of order – civil government, judiciary, bureaucracy, police, military – are corrupted, and those of disorder – paramilitaries, independent militia, organized criminals – deprive the state of its monopoly on the use of force and assume functions basic to the maintenance of order, 'order' and 'disorder' are on a highway to interchangeability. At this point corrupt and legitimate politics, corrupt and legitimate business and organized criminality become not merely indistinguishable, not even interchangeable, but for all practical purposes identical.

Political corruption as an interstitial activity

> Corruption and the response to it reveal the relative power of the executive, parliament, and the parties, and also illuminate the role of the criminal investigators, the judiciary, and the 'fourth estate' (the media).
>
> (Levi and Nelken 1996b: 2)

So political corruption must be viewed in terms of political behaviour, and is more an extension of such behaviour into unacceptable activities than a qualitatively distinct form of criminality. While individual heroes and individual villains certainly exist, to restrict our analysis to their morality or psychology would not suffice. When individual villains act corruptly in a low-corruption country, however traumatic it may be at the time, the system apprehends and punishes them, and then self-corrects by reviewing what went wrong and introducing new policies, procedures, regulations or legislation to minimize the likelihood of repetition. In high-corruption countries like Zaïre, the Philippines, Indonesia, Haiti, Paraguay and Nicaragua it is insufficient to focus solely on Mobutu, Marcos, Soeharto, Duvalier (*père et fils*), Stroessner or Somoza Debayle respectively, genuine villains though they doubtless were.[14] Like any other resourceful and successful entrepreneur they exploit the rent-seeking opportunities they inherited and create new ones by expansion and diversification, as well as by imposing any necessary new forms of coercion or terror. As both the products of prior corrupt opportunities and the causes of new ones their activities demand systemic (or political) explanation.

An example of this is electoral fraud. In simple societies this can involve simple bribe taking and vote buying, two sides of the same coin, as much as necessary of the fruits of the former being recycled into the latter. In such societies vote buying may be achieved by deploying positive incentives (money), negative ones (force or the threat of it) or both – a carrot-and-stick approach elegantly exemplified by Pablo Escobar's *plata o plomo* (silver or lead) policy: one either took Escobar's silver or received his bullet (Bowden 2001: 33). The scale of such activities can be considerable. For example in post-war Sicily, where an average mafioso could muster 40 to 50 votes, a politician could realistically hope to buy 75,000 to 100,000 votes in Palermo alone (Schneider and Schneider 1999: 178). In Thailand, Bo, a leading *kamnan* (village headman) and *jao pho* (influential businessman), arranged votes for his candidates in Chonburi by having his men repeatedly vote with their own identity cards with the collusion of poll officials (Pasuk and Sungsidh 1994: 63). In Cambodia, to buy the village headman is to buy the votes of the village he heads, a tactic widely deployed under the noses of UN observers of the July 1998 elections; the same applies in Melanesian communities in Papua New Guinea (Findlay 1999: 78). In India, the prolonged power of the National Congress Party was supported by their capacity to control the rural elites who in turn controlled the votes of their local clients.

The practice was, as we shall see in Chapter 4, common in Great Britain until successive extensions of the franchise in the nineteenth century made it impracticable; and in nineteenth-century USA, vote buying was institutionalized in the machine system:

> Because of the lack of voting machines and the party-made ballots . . . the briber could be sure that the floater would vote as directed. Indeed, practical politicians preferred to buy votes in bulk by negotiating with a 'striker', a man who could deliver a large supply of electors. . . . Where voter lists were compiled from assessment rolls, city officers added fictitious names to the roster weeks before the election to give newcomers and repeaters aliases enough under which to vote. Philadelphia's list included corpses and long-time nonresidents. . . . Corrupt officials were most useful when the votes were counted. It was a common saying that when San Francisco's polls closed 'the election had just commenced'. . . . In a rural Illinois county, officials assured their ally a one-vote majority by altering a precinct's total from a one to a nine,

and a notorious San Francisco county supervisor, acting as an election inspector, counted the votes to put himself into power – an act of remarkable audacity, since he had not even run for the job.

(Summers 1987: 57–61)

Such practices were not covert and exceptional but commonplace and widely accepted, and as such they were deployed as the tools of successful political entrepreneurs. As the conditions which promote and perpetuate them disappear, however, the character of politics changes: redundant practices are discarded, falling, as vote buying has in the industrialized west, into desuetude, and new tactics come to be deployed. Today votes continue to be available for purchase, whether by silver or lead, in Cambodia or Zimbabwe, but any attempt along these lines in the United Kingdom, where more sophisticated methods of securing political support exist, would clearly be not only unambiguously criminal but also vulgar and absurd.

So if political corruption is an extension of normal political behaviour, in order to understand it we must examine the processes which support and sustain it. We have referred to corruption's wide margins. These make it difficult to distinguish the roles of the different actors, normally politicians, bureaucrats, judicial officials, and police and military leaders. Their legitimate or constitutional activities may be distinguishable but their illegitimate or corrupt ones seldom are, since obfuscation, secrecy and interdependence are hallmarks of corruption networks. Outside the polity they interact, socially as well as professionally, with numerous social elites ranging from media celebrities, beauty queens and sports stars to legitimate and illegitimate businessmen and bankers, some of them most probably linked with organized criminals. The economic, social or sexual influence of such people on members of political elites blurs still further the relationship between the latter's professional and personal, as well as corrupt and non-corrupt, interactions. For this reason we see such interactions as marginal.

These margins we term *interstices*, and it is in interstices that political corruption thrives, slipping, as it were, through the cracks of the state. Where the bureau–political machinery is not mature, coherent or integrated, or where self-correcting mechanisms such as an independent judiciary or a free press are missing, the interstices are especially visible, enabling corrupt politicians and officials to exploit the resultant conflicts and ambiguities. Where civil society is weak, lacking the encouragement to probity and solidarity expressed by professional, trade and commerce associations, self-regulatory bodies and the like, corruption can emerge in low standards of professional conduct and minimal safeguards. Geopolitically, corruption thrives in the interstices created by national sovereignty, jurisdictional disputes, professional self-interest and the weakness of the judicial elements of the United Nations. Reforms to banking secrecy laws (to be discussed more fully later) have been slow and grudging; even now they are incomplete.

Resources allocated to transnational policing are substantially less than those allocated to transnational criminality; and new levels of ambiguity emerge when legitimate business enterprises are funded by laundered money.

Here we identify four forms of interstitial corruption: interstitial realignments following economic liberalization, political–bureaucratic interstices, political–judicial interstices and geopolitical interstices. We consider each briefly in turn.

Interstitial realignments following economic liberalization

Economic liberalization, though it is, as we shall argue later, normally necessary for long-term economic health and competitiveness, creates short-term rifts, ambiguities and disjunctions. It does this by overturning stable and routine relationships which, though usually inefficient and undesirable, previously produced a stable code of conduct in many areas of activity including corruption. Liberalization creates new rent-seeking opportunities and hence turbulence which can, if things go wrong (which they are almost certain to do in states lacking a strong civil society), develop into long-term dysfunctionality. For example, in South Africa a deregulated market was introduced in 1994 to replace a heavily controlled economy, solving one set of problems but creating another. The new constitution embraced the democratic and human rights discourses, instituting an executive accountable to the legislature, an independent judiciary, decentralized governance, and a Public Protector, Constitutional Court and Auditor-General (Heymans and Lipietz 1999: 28–29; Lodge 2002). But in such a politically and economically unstable country, lacking many of the structures of a civil society, democratization is vulnerable to replacing authoritarian constraints not with effective and accountable controls but with a power vacuum eagerly filled by organized criminals. Hence the *telos* of such a democratization process is not liberty, equality and fraternity but the Aristotelian one of tyranny. In the contemporary world this finds its commonest expression in criminal states under despotic rule. Liberalism and democracy are symptoms of reforming states rather than causes of reform itself, as neither can be imposed on an unreformed state without the danger of the worst aspects of its unreformed character being first accentuated and then strengthened. Hence the fate of liberalization and democratization is a litmus test for the underlying strengths and weaknesses of both the state in question and the society within it; but they will not of themselves produce reform unless other indicators are present.

In China, which we shall discuss in greater detail in Chapter 3, a qualified economic liberalism was superimposed on a political system intent on maintaining centralized control but decreasingly able to do so effectively. It hence fell between the stools of a command economy and a free market, lacking both the coercive controls necessary to sustain the former and the open competition essential to the latter. At the same time the absence of any popular collective sense of commitment or social responsibility meant that few people in a position to exploit the new opportunities were prevented from doing so by local or family pressure or internal restraint. Hence an early consequence of Deng Xiaoping's 'open door' policy of 1978 was rampant systemic corruption, as virtually everyone with the opportunity to do so threw themselves into the pursuit of material wealth, possession of which received, for the first time in living memory, enthusiastic official endorsement. And since the agents of control were as keen as anyone else to exploit this unique opportunity, the entire communist controlling structure was replaced by a national Klondike fever, with no means of assuaging it.

Political–bureaucratic interstices

It would be wrong to regard interstitial political corruption as unique to LDCs. In many western countries bureaucratic corruption, often in the form of bribery in contract procurement, is longstanding, and attempts to expunge it feature strongly in pan-European anti-corruption strategies (Council of Europe 1996, 1998). Bureaucratic corruption frequently illumines relationships between elected members and salaried officials as it can seldom thrive without at least the tacit support of politicians, whose relations with bureaucrats vary between the strong separation characteristic of the United Kingdom and the relative interchangeability found in the United States. In fact in the United States it was kickbacks from construction contracts in his former role of Governor of Maryland which began the process which culminated in the resignation of Vice-President Agnew in 1973 (Silverstein 1988: 20). In Greece, Spain and Italy complex administrative obstacles are frequently created in areas presenting such opportunities to administrators and politicians, for example issuing licences and permits (Krueger 1974; della Porta and Vannucci 1997: 114).

Among LDCs this relationship is likewise varied. In India, where politicians exercise direct power over bureaucrats, the system is widely abused through a 'transfer system' which permits politicians to reward corrupt officials with attractive postings or by permitting them to remain in their existing post, and to punish non-corrupt ones by frequent transfers and unattractive postings (Das 2001). In Thailand, where, in the provinces, senior appointed officials manage elected officials, securing election is seldom even rhetorically associated with public service, and elected positions are keenly sought by local 'big men' (*phu yai*) because of the rent-seeking opportunities they can yield:

> Local businessmen understand that if they are elected to the local political positions . . . they will have access to new contacts and new business opportunities. . . . Of the 2,046 provincial councils elected in October

1990, 61.6 percent reported their occupation as businessmen. One of the more popular businesses of these candidates was construction contracting.

(Pasuk and Sungsidh 1994: 81)

Banks can be crucial in supporting or inhibiting corruption, and their relationships with governments and the private sector deserve more specialized study than we can give them here. For example, in Europe the arrest in 1994 of his close friend Mariano Rubio, Governor of the Bank of Spain, for fraud, triggered a sequence of scandals highly damaging to Felipe González's corrupt ten-year government. In South-East Asia the Governor of the Bank of Indonesia was arrested in 2000 for illegally taking £53.3 million out of the small but corrupt Bank Bali to support former President Habibie's unsuccessful re-election campaign. Under Habibie's successor, the inept Abdurrahman Wahid, nepotistic appointments, bank withdrawals (including some in favour of Abdurrahman's masseur) and party donations continued, with reforming ministers dismissed under pressure from business interests (Kraar 2000).

Bureaucratic corruption in the form of speed money is common in many LDCs. This low-level corruption, however, often stems from the fact that senior politicians, having sold a position in the first place, factor the cost into salaries, which are normally maintained at imprudently low levels for administrators with discretionary powers. Practices such as this are naturally exacerbated where a necessary service is in the hands of a single individual, as is delivering car registration papers in Mozambique (Stasavage 2000). In situations where transfer systems exist, not only are rent-seeking opportunities time-limited but also, far from there being any reward for honesty, anyone who is honest is liable to be socially stigmatized as a fool:

A salary insufficient to support a family . . . certainly induces inspectors to accept or demand *mordidas* from individual violators. . . . An additional incentive for inspectors to accept bribes is that they know that they are on the job only temporarily . . . being an inspector is an opportunity not to be wasted, probably one of the few times in their lives when they will be able to make money. They know that when the regional fisheries delegation changes its executive at the end of every six-year presidential term, all the inspectors also change. . . . Being a conscientious and efficient inspector has nothing to do with keeping the job.

(Vásquez-León 1999: 249–250)

Political–judicial interstices

If you have honest magistrates instead of corrupt ones, the people will be obedient. If you have corrupt magistrates instead of honest ones, the people will be restless.

(Confucius, *Analects*)

It is very rare for LDCs to have a strong independent judiciary. In many cases judges lack even theoretical constitutional independence; sometimes their terms of appointment prohibit reforming activities (Williams 1987: 108). In many common law countries the Attorney General, simultaneously a member of the executive and Chief Law Officer, determines the initiation, prosecution and discontinuance of criminal proceedings. This role, an alternative to the separation-of-powers doctrine common in civil law jurisdictions, relies on the Attorney being guaranteed freedom from improper party influence on individual decisions. This in turn is dependent either on adherence to conventions reflecting high levels of self-restraint on the part of the executive or on checks and balances to guarantee independence. Such symptoms of stability are rare among the former African colonies to which Britain exported the role, many post-colonial constitutions giving primacy to security over freedom and confirming the dominance of the executive over the legislative and judicial branches. Where the judiciary is subordinate to the executive, the appointment of placemen judges to legitimate political corruption inquiries is common (Williams 1987: 108) though not invariable. Judge Warioba's report into rampant corruption in Tanzania, for example, attracted international praise for its range and frankness (Tanzania 1996) but was an exception to the general rule. Its domestic impact was slight.

In much of Latin America (Buscaglia 1997) and sub-Saharan Africa (Hibou 1999: 101) the judiciary is openly corrupt. In Indonesia the Attorney General himself conceded that most judges are corrupt, incompetent or both (Kraar 2000), while the pressure group Indonesia Corruption Watch claims only three out of thirty-one Supreme Court judges are non-corrupt and that 80 to 90 per cent of legal officials, including prosecutors, accept bribes. In Haiti, even before assuming formal power in October 1957 François Duvalier enacted the suspension by military decree of the civil justice system and the forcible retirement of the entire judiciary (Trouillot 1990: 151) to ensure judicial compliance with presidential diktat. In China there is widespread nepotism in judicial appointments and almost equally widespread judicial misconduct, including personal predation (Woo 2000). In 1998, for example, 2,512 judges and other court personnel were found to have acted illegally (Hao and Johnston 2002: 593).

The political–judicial interstice is not solely of concern in relation to LDCs. In parts of the United States, where judicial appointments have historically been 'the coin to recompense political service' (Summers 1987: 24), and where today Supreme Court appointments are the subject of intense political debate, judicial freedom from political interference remains, in practice, somewhat qualified. In northern Italy Antonio Di Pietro, leader of *Mani pulite*, faced criminal investigation, political and media pressure and death threats before resigning from the magistracy to begin a political career (della Porta 1998). In parts of southern Italy judges have theoretical independence but are compromised by social and family relations with politicians and by legal sweeteners offered as rewards for compliance (della Porta 1998). Corrupt senior judges marginalize uncooperative ones by measures including blocking promotions and transfers to low-status parts of the country. In Campania,

> the widespread toleration and practice of illegality by politicians . . . leads the judiciary to be selective in their application of the law, as any campaign for consistent judicial values would entail a head-on collision with the judiciary's political overseers. Consequently the administration of justice, too, is far from equal: an unemployed seller of contraband cigarettes is far more likely to spend time in jail than a gang leader accused of murder or drug trafficking.
>
> (Behan 1996: 170)

But whereas a dishonest judicial system facilitates high-level corruption, an honest one can be influential in resisting it. Three examples illustrate this point.

First, Italian magistrates, in asserting the rule of law against institutionalized corruption by initiating the *Mani pulite* ('clean hands') investigations in Milan in 1993, greatly assisted in attenuating the link between the Christian Democrats and the Mafia. Though its direct influence was not necessarily enduring (Ginsborg 2001), *Mani pulite* led to more than 7,000 arrests, including that of a former prime minister, Bettino Craxi, and 4,000 preventive custody orders (della Porta and Vannucci 1997: 100). *Second*, the Indian Supreme Court, in indicting Prime Minister Indira Gandhi on a charge of corrupt electoral practices, triggered the introduction of emergency powers in 1975, which in turn initiated the turn of events which led to the collapse of Mrs Gandhi's own increasingly corrupt Congress Party (Singh 1997). *Third*, the Spanish Supreme Court dealt determinedly with long-running scandals surrounding the Government, addressing, in addition to the dismissal of the Governor of the Bank of Spain already mentioned, the fraudulent activities of Government appointees and the Head of the Civil Guard. Most notoriously it brought to public attention the Grupos Antiterroristas de Liberación (GAL). These death squads were covertly resourced by the government's reserve funds to assassinate members of ETA (Heywood 1994; Woodworth 2001).

Geopolitical interstices

Geopolitically, too, political corruption is interstitial, this time globally, for many corrupt individuals and organizations operate most effectively by exploiting the gaps between sovereign states, mediated by increasing numbers of transnational and supranational bodies in both governance and commerce. These gaps are considerable: many national statistics designed to keep track of international payments for goods and services bear almost no relation to each other: although what is one country's export is another's import, as long ago as 1983 global payments exceeded receipts by $100 billion (Walter 1985: 19).

The existence of such interstices is by no means new, and a number of theories of state formation which are otherwise conflicting agree that criminality was at the core of the formative period (see Skaperdas and Syropolous 1995; Gallant 1999). The underlying structure of today's international system is little changed from the settlement deriving from the Treaty of Westphalia, which ended the ruinous Thirty Years War in 1648. Similarly, contemporary concepts of international law such as sovereignty, non-intervention and the balance of power are mainly seventeenth century in origin.

The Westphalian system operated reasonably successfully for around three hundred years, in good part on the basis of shared understandings as to the etiquette of international relations, mainly concerning diplomacy and the conduct of war, among mainly related European monarchical or aristocratic elites. It is, however, less obviously well suited to meet the challenges of globalization, which have as much, if not more, to do with the need for international or supranational oversight of commercial and financial transactions as with military activity. Currently the turbulence among nation states, regional supranational groupings, sub-state ethnic, religious or other affiliation groups demanding territoriality and self-determination, international organizations and multi-national corporations is considerable.

In the interstices between these various bodies there is scope for transnational crime such as money laundering, arms and people smuggling, the drug trade, state terrorism and international piracy to thrive. Such activities normally require political and bureaucratic acquiescence, and interstitial corruption of this kind may be undertaken by units ranging from rogue states (more cautiously dubbed 'states of concern' by former Secretary of State Madeleine Albright) such as Libya, Lebanon and Cuba, all of which have succoured terrorist organizations such as the IRA and ETA, to powerful individuals. Where the structures of central government are weak, powerful arms are often widely available and the scope for such individuals to transform themselves into warlords and form their own armies for political or financial purposes is considerable. Hence in Colombia in the 1980s Pablo Escobar justified terrorism as 'the atomic bomb for poor people . . . the only way for the poor to strike back' (cited in Bowden 2001: 146). In Burma in the same decade the warlord Khun Sa had a 40,000-strong private army armed with M16s and M60 machine guns. This enabled him both to control 60 per cent of the world's illicit opium supply, and to launch an abortive campaign for the presidency of the proposed breakaway state of Shan (McCoy 1991: 434).

In addition, the growth of regional supranational groupings has created major new geopolitical interstices, many of them offering new corrupt opportunities. In the European Union it has been claimed that 'waste and fraud are . . . natural effects of the way in which Member States have pooled sovereignty but not accountability' (Peterson 1997: 144).[15] Fraud accounts for up to 10 per cent of the multi-billion pound Common Agricultural Policy expenditure (Behan 1996: 133), while other programmes, including the educational Socrates and Leonardo schemes, are apparently run more as corrupt private fiefdoms than as accountable parts of a supranational political administration (van Buitenen 2000).

Conclusion

> The perplexing thing about life is the irresolubility of reality, of things and relations alike. Every wrong done has a certain justice in it, and every good deed has dregs of evil.
>
> (H.G. Wells, *Tono-Bungay*)

In this chapter we introduced three themes which will re-emerge later in the book. *First*, political corruption is an illegitimate extension of normal political activity. *Second*, it occurs transnationally and internationally as well as nationally and subnationally, and it is there that its greatest growth potential exists. *Third*, it operates interstitially – in the cracks within and between states, and between the public and the private spheres. The width and quantity of these interstices help us anticipate how common corruption will be: for example, where central control is weak, localized corruption will tend to be strong (LaPalombara 1994). None of this, however, is intended to excuse corruption, to deny the existence of extreme and sometimes horrific instances of it, or to question the fact that corruption is best regarded as a rational act deserving of punishment. In particular we shall show later that the weight of evidence is that political corruption is ultimately a damaging, not, as some have argued, a beneficial, activity.

Much of this chapter has been dedicated to considering definitional and conceptual problems surrounding corruption. In particular, popular definitions offer a certain resonance but fail the test of comprehensiveness. Because political corruption blurs with other activities, many of them legitimate, and normally involves collusive and complex networks, it is as hard to grasp conceptually as it is to prove forensically. Its proceeds may be well enough laundered to be available to set up legitimate businesses; by definition, corrupt politicians are business entrepreneurs; criminals may be more effective law enforcers than official agencies; they may attract more popular support than politicians; corrupt politicians and organized criminals may be the same people. In such situations the forces of order and disorder potentially become indistinguishable, if not interchangeable.

Part of the problem lies in the assumption, underlying many definitions, that political corruption deviates from a norm, that it is an individual problem, a metaphorical cancerous growth vulnerable to excision by the metaphorical surgeon's equally metaphorical knife. In both high- and low-corruption countries this proposition is, for different reasons, misleading. In high-corruption countries corruption is part of the fuel driving the economy, and anti-corruption campaigns become manifestations of the very corruption they are detailed to tackle, a weapon in a war between competing power groups. In low-corruption countries the temptation is to focus on individual sleaze and scandal. But though watching some high-profile politician toppled from his or her perch may make gripping television, noting how the political system deals with the fall-out is far more important, if rather less fun.

Prospective political entrepreneurs seldom lack opportunities to use their influence to extract wealth or, as the case may be, to use their wealth to extract influence, and why this is sometimes but not always deemed corrupt can also be instructive. For some of the ways of doing it – making party donations, utilizing royal, presidential or prime ministerial patronage, exploiting the honours system, offering membership of prestigious clubs, extending desirable party invitations and generous publicity – are perfectly normal political acts. Hence high-profile villains are spectacular distractions from the more intricate manifestations of corruption. They tempt us to the literature of scandal and invite us to forget that, however great their evil, they did not come from nowhere, that they could not have operated alone, and that in the absence of political change others will follow in their wake.

Political corruption is frequently indistinguishable from bureaucratic, judicial and military corruption: all are aspects of elite corruption, and if the corruption is systemic none can exist without the others. Nor is political corruption easily distinguished from business activity of any kind – indeed political corruption is itself a form of business activity – since corrupt politicians require partnerships with businesspeople to maximize the utility of their posts. Corrupt politicians may act as patrons of those below them or clients of those above them; most probably they will do both, operating in a chain of corruption wherein the strength of one link determines that of the next. After all, only if one is bribed adequately by one's patron does one have the wherewithal to bribe one's clients; and only thus can one achieve the conceptual integration of money and power so characteristic of political corruption.

The challenge of making sense of political corruption lies in part in its very normality. The skills of practical politics – networking, persuading, obfuscating, managing – are also the skills of corruption. But those designated corrupt have gone too far. They may have offended powerful individuals or states. They may have made enemies, had inadequate protective domestic and international support networks, become greedy or displayed lack of judgement, finesse or taste in the character or conduct of their corruption. Or they may just have been imprudent or unlucky. They may be monsters like Bokassa of the Central African Republic or Duvalier, but almost always they are not; and because their conduct is so seldom abnormal it is no more instructive or satisfactory to dub them evil than it is to designate every Nazi concentration camp guard a psychopathic monster.

We have distinguished throughout between high- and low-corruption countries. In the former, corruption being the norm, to be corrupt is simply to conform; and since the ablest individuals will always gravitate to activities which offer the best rate of return it will frequently be the ablest citizens who become criminals (Baumol 1990; Murphy *et al.* 1991). But even in low-corruption countries corrupt politicians will always exist, most probably characterized by overweening arrogance or vanity, the 'corner-cutting' instincts of the entrepreneur, or, as in the case of Nixon, those of a driven and haunted man believing wholly in the nature of his mission. Politicians can, perhaps, be more dangerous when trying to play God than when telling calculated professional half-truths.

Political corruption, as we have seen, is by no means the exclusive preserve of the less-developed world. Naturally, low-level bureaucratic corruption and flamboyant, grand political corruption are far commoner there than in the developed world where matters are normally conducted with greater finesse. Nonetheless, not only are there numerous instances of political corruption in the developed world but, particularly during the bipolar super-power era of the Cold War, the vulnerability of many LDC regimes to bribery was systematically exploited by both the Soviet Union and the United States.[16] Hence Mephistopheles as well as Faust, tempter as well as tempted, demand side as well as supply side, are implicated. Without the one there can never be the other.

Notes

1 A kleptocracy is defined here as a state viewed by its rulers solely as a maximizing unit and run as a business designed to extract the highest possible rents from its subjects, unconstrained by any consideration other than their own power. This differs from the definition of Grossman, who, in a context which sets states in competition with organized criminals as public service providers, defines *all* states as maximizing units and therefore as kleptocracies (Grossman 1995: 143 *et seq.*; see also Baumol 1995: 83–84). This is a provocative thought indeed, but it is not one we develop here.

2 Negative reception is all important. During the 2001 United Kingdom General Election campaign the Deputy Prime Minister punched a demonstrator in view of the TV cameras. A horrified Prime Minister, reportedly about to dismiss him, changed his mind within hours as evidence of public amusement and support began to emerge.

3 This complex conspiracy is reported generously but fairly by Emery (1994).

4 We make the same point in Chapter 2 in relation to Italy's President Berlusconi.

5 Nixon worked covertly to increase support during the primaries for the eventual winner, the unelectable George McGovern, and to damage the more credible contender, Edmund Muskie. In particular Nixon feared as his potential nemesis the undeclared Edward Kennedy, waiting in the wings to answer a call but vulnerable to any revisiting of the Chappaquiddick affair (in which, allegedly

drunk, he had driven his car off a bridge, run away and left a girl passenger to drown). Nixon's strategy was hence to attack Mr Kennedy's character and family at every opportunity (Emery 1994: 106).

6 For examples of how Ferdinand Marcos rewrote aspects of Filipino law during his presidency to suit his own and his family's interests see Carbonell-Catilo (1986); Pedrosa (1987); Coronel (1998).

7 US companies are liable to fines of up to $2 million per violation. For individuals (officers, directors and stockholders) the maximum penalty is a $100,000 fine and five years' imprisonment, as well as civil penalties, suspension or expulsion from the securities business and export licence withdrawal.

8 For a helpful review of developments in transnational policing (in the broadest sense of the word) see Schneider *et al.* (2000).

9 This Index, which measures foreign businesspeople's perceptions of corruption in different countries, has been praised by, among others, Lancaster and Montinola (1997). Though utilizing an ingenious methodology and having considerable political impact, it inevitably excludes many hidden forms of pecuniary corruption such as money laundering and political donations, as well as subtle forms of non-pecuniary corruption, often involving social status enhancement.

10 Approximately £32,000 sterling.

11 Clive's response to the Parliamentary inquiry of 1773 into his conduct as Governor General of the East India Company.

12 For further information see ⟨http://www.jubilee2000uk.org/faq_corr.html⟩.

13 These contributions have been described as a rare example of money dirtying. Clean funds were dirtied by being passed through secret bank accounts and companies in Switzerland, Panama, Gabon, the Bahamas and Lebanon before being passed to the Campaign for the Re-Election of the President (Clarke and Tigue 1976: 17, 124–127, 135).

14 Though even here we should note that many ordinary Filipinos continue to express nostalgia for the days of Ferdinand Marcos.

15 The European Union's corruption and anti-corruption strategies (and the relations between them), which justify a full-length study in their own right, do not receive detailed consideration here, though we return briefly to them in Chapter 7.

16 Happily the Foreign Corrupt Practices Act 1977 applies only to individuals and corporations, not to the state itself.

2 The idea of political corruption (II): the contribution of political economy

> there is one human motivator that is both universal and central to explaining the divergent experiences of different countries. That motivator is self-interest. . . . Endemic corruption suggests a pervasive failure to tap self-interest for productive purposes.
>
> (Rose-Ackerman 1999: 2)

In this chapter we consider, *first*, the contribution of political economists to the study of political corruption. We show in particular the utility of Olson's classic theory of collective action for addressing corruption, and advise anti-corruption strategists to place less emphasis on ethical imperatives than on striving to create a consonance between public and private interests: in a fallen world it is generally more effective to address people's worst than their best natures. Even this, however, is almost impossible to achieve in high-corruption countries, because if the organs of government are so thoroughly corrupted that corrupt behaviour is normal behaviour, what internal leverage can be brought to bear on them?

Second, we address the issue of rent-seeking, described by one of its leading theorists (Tullock 1989, 1993) as politicians' pursuit of private interests when such interests conflict with public duty. We accept this definition but argue that rent-seeking, even of this extreme kind, is but an extension, albeit quite possibly a grotesque and deplorable one, of normal political behaviour.

Third, we introduce the subject of economic liberalization, a policy considered by many to be conducive to lowering levels of corruption. Liberalization, according to this line of argument, drives out corruption by forcing the rigours of the market into economic transactions previously subject to distortion as a result of monopoly state activity. This occurs by squeezing out the non-productive capital involved in bribe payments, contracting corruption and so on, ensuring, in a process of economic Darwinism, the survival of the fittest and most efficient providers. Conversely, where state economic intervention is extensive, corruption thrives as a natural, inevitable and arguably desirable market response to the market imperfections such interventions create. These imperfections occur either because the intervention is designed to hand rent-seeking opportunities to politicians, bureaucrats or other suppliers of goods or services, or, in social policy in particular, because it is intended as a corrective to the negative impact of economic downturns or inequalities in wealth or income distribution. The good intentions behind such policies, however, are, to economic liberals, inevitably submerged by such undesirable concomitants of any form of monopoly provision as inefficiency, the elevation of provider over consumer interests, a lack of accountability and transparency, and opportunities for a range of what in Britain are sometimes called 'Spanish practices' at all levels.

In the abstract this position seems to us to have considerable force, but we shall argue that it is, for all its theoretical elegance, insufficient to meet the 'real time' challenges posed by political corruption. Though successful 'hits' can be made against low-level corruption (see for example Klitgaard 1988; Klitgaard *et al.* 2000), because entrenched corruption cancerously infects previously healthy organs of the polity it denudes the body politic of the only internal means by which corruption can be brought under control. So whereas in low-corruption countries an independent judiciary, generally honest police force and a free press, for example, remain healthy, when these organs are themselves corrupted or suppressed the process of liberalization can itself only be corrupt. Hence, for the most part, states acquire the quality of liberalization that their leaders deserve and high corruption can only be addressed, to the extent that it can be addressed at all, by the external intervention of international donors or trading partners, or by international governmental or non-governmental organizations.

Finally, closely associated with this problem is the longstanding (and now generally unfashionable) view that corruption can have beneficial effects. We consider the work of a number of proponents of this thesis and offer a qualified repudiation. In some cases the argument seems simply to be wrong; in others, though the argument is not logically faulty it has nonetheless been overtaken by events, failing to ring true on the anvil of experience. In other situations again the line is that though corruption is in many respects damaging, the side-effects of the cure are greater than the costs of leaving it alone. In our view this latter claim is, however, best reframed as a tactical challenge of how, when and at what pace to tackle the problem. To take it as a recipe for inaction underestimates corruption's infectious character and corrosive effects.

The political economy of corruption

> Things fall apart; the centre cannot hold;
> Mere anarchy is loosed upon the world,
> The blood-dimmed tide is loosed, and everywhere

The ceremony of innocence is drowned;
The best lack all conviction, while the worst
Are full of passionate intensity.
(W.B. Yeats, *The Second Coming*)

The insights of political economists are especially relevant to the analysis of political corruption. Underpinning much of the literature of political economy is the assumption that human action, whether that of politicians, voters, bureaucrats, the judiciary, pressure groups or multinational corporations, is rational, purposive and self-seeking, designed to achieve what such theorists refer to as utility maximization. This insight permits the development of reasonably precise policy prescriptions in relation to corruption in high- and, particularly, low-corruption countries.

With only modest adaptation Mancur Olson's classic theory of collective action has considerable explanatory power in relation to political corruption (Olson 1965, 1982). In his earlier, seminal, book Olson takes as his focus goods collectively produced which no one can be excluded from consuming, and asks why a common interest in producing a public good does not automatically lead to collective action in pursuit of it. The fact that it does not creates what Olson calls a 'free rider' problem. In a large group, because the contribution of each individual to the production of the collective good is negligible, everyone knows that whether or not the good is produced is independent of his or her own particular contribution to it. As will be obvious, this theory owes much to Jeremy Bentham's felicific calculus (Bentham [1789] 1970), according to which humans have, like other animals, two sovereign masters, pleasure and pain, and no choice other than to pursue the former and avoid the latter.

Two examples unrelated to political corruption help clarify the point. Suppose, *first*, that an individual strongly supports the work of a large charity but knows that the impact on that work of any donation he or she can afford to make will in practice be non-existent. Economic logic leads us to conclude that, the act of giving away money being painful, without the intervention of other variables no donation will be made. It is, after all, part of utilitarian logic that it is perfectly possible for individuals to maintain a genuine *commitment* to decency, integrity, civic pride and any number of other values but not to *act* in accordance with them.

Second, the British Museum, anxious to maintain free entry while facing grave financial difficulties, invites visitors to donate £2 to help it do so. This is a small sum, about the price of a sandwich in London, whereas, taking major charging attractions like the Tower of London as comparators, a compulsory charge would be around £12. Visitors accordingly encounter collecting boxes at different points as they proceed from the top of the steps into the Great Court. In this case Olson's motivational logic suggests

that, *ceteris paribus*, the *worst outcome* for any individual would be the introduction of charges. The *next worst outcome* would be the retention of 'free'
admission to which that individual contributed £2. The *best outcome* – the
free rider solution – would be for everybody else to pay the £2 to enable
admission to remain free, but for the individual not to do so him or herself.
This solution would, after all, make no practical difference to the museum
but would enable the free rider not only to enjoy its many delights for nothing but also to spend the £2 on a sandwich lunch afterwards. So £2 offers an
identifiable benefit to an individual in the way that it does not to a multi-
million pound organization such as the museum.

Of course if this were all there was to it everyone would be a free rider and
the whole structure of voluntarism would fall apart: our role models would
be Scrooge and Shylock, not the selfless heroes and secular saints whom,
typically, we admire rather more. That this is not so is as obvious to economists as it is to anyone else. For example, in relation to political corruption
Pizzorno asks how political economists would explain its *absence* where the
benefits are high and the risk of discovery and punishment very low (cited in
LaPalombara 1994), while Cartier-Bresson (1997), in a Rousseauesque state
of nature argument, points out that social networks frequently exist prior to
the onset of political corruption.

It is because human beings are complex organisms that determining what
causes pleasure and pain is not straightforward. It is also clear from experimental psychology as well as common experience that human behaviour is
eminently manipulable. Hence it becomes a desirable aim of public policy
to create a consonance between individual happiness and prosocial actions.
In the case of our first example one's pain at writing a £20 cheque to
Oxfam might be mitigated by pleasure deriving from the belief that one's
contribution would have a discernible impact on Oxfam's work. If this
were so for appreciable numbers of people, such a charity would be wise
to do whatever it could to foster such a belief. Indeed many charities have
done just this. For example, some international children's charities have
developed the tactic of personalizing donations through sponsorship schemes
whereby recipient children report periodically to their benefactors on the
uses to which their donations have been put. This transforms the otherwise
impersonal unilateral act of charitable giving into a bilateral one based on
reciprocity: the pain of paying the direct debit is offset by the pleasure
which derives from receiving periodic letters in return, and knowing that
one has actively contributed to a measurable good. In another context the
linking of charitable giving to multi-million-pound lotteries is a more
obviously self-interested variation on this theme – a lottery ticket both
benefits charities and gives the purchaser inexpensive fun and an outside
chance of becoming rich – a perfect harmonization of altruism and self-interest.

In our second example, among the British Museum's visitors will be
many who will anyway derive greater pleasure from paying than from not
paying. This may be for a host of reasons – habit, conscience, embarrass-

ment, commitment to a Rousseauesque general will, because they are rich (personal wealth potentially, though certainly not inevitably, neutralizes the disincentive) or to impress their girlfriends. Clearly, encouraging the rejection of free riding is or should be a strategic priority for the museum. Nonetheless, the technical problems involved in eliminating the negative effects of utility maximization should not be underestimated. For example the fact that visitors pass several collection boxes at different points is designed as a negative incentive, basically encouraging potential free riders to crack under pressure. But for three main reasons this may constitute a perverse incentive not to donate. *First*, the existence of so many boxes encourages the hope that one's fellow visitors will assume one has put one's £2 into an earlier box or intends to put it into a later box: this naturally diminishes the likelihood of shame. *Second*, it is not clear whether one is expected to donate on entering or leaving. Accordingly there is always the possibility that one intends to make one's donation on the way out, having gauged the 'value' of the visit before deciding how much to give. The free rider leaving the museum will, of course, 'pass' as having donated on entry. *Third*, the existence of several dispersed collection boxes increases the proportion of visitors seen by others not to be donating. This invites the thought that one might even, by donating, be subsidizing the visits of other free riders. Accordingly the siting of the boxes potentially creates behavioural contagion[1] by offering an easy technique of neutralization ('everyone is at it'). Hence not donating appears statistically normal.

Switching back to corruption, those who justify it as a victimless crime, as a crime whose victims are simply a grand abstraction – the state, the people, the tax or customs authorities – from which no one really suffers, or as a harmless and universal activity are espousing a free-riding philosophy. According to this argument the minute proportion of total revenue extracted by the individual corrupt person, though too small to be missed by the victims, may transform the life of the free rider. Hence corruption becomes a game with a winner but no losers. As a result the sum of human happiness is increased, and the entire affair is perfectly in tune with Bentham's felicific calculus and the attainment of the greatest happiness for the greatest number. Just as children's charities and the British Museum have to develop policies to change the behaviour resulting from this belief, so is it imperative for the public policy of countries wishing to control corruption to do the same. It is not a matter of moralizing, which, if one accepts the logic of Olson's utilitarianism that it is perfectly normal for people in a position to do so to exploit opportunities to their own advantage, will have minimal and brief effect. The necessity, rather, is to create a consonance between public and private interest.

Susan Rose-Ackerman (1978, 1999) has been especially adept at designing penalty systems to reduce the attractiveness of free riding precisely by bringing prosocial behaviour into line with individual self-interest. Similarly relevant is the work of Francis Lui (see in particular Lui 1986), whose China studies postulate a distinction between high- and low-corruption equilibria broadly in line with our own concepts of high and low corruption. In high-corruption situations auditing an official is costly because other corrupt officials have an incentive to protect the suspect, whereas in low-corruption ones corrupt officials receive less protection because a higher proportion of their colleagues can be encouraged to report misconduct: an honest majority almost always resents, or can be brought to resent, a dishonest minority. Low compensation and weak monitoring systems are associated with high corruption, and in such situations bribing politicians and bureaucrats becomes a rational as well as a normal act. Not only is it reasonable for both bribers and bribed to anticipate, at worst, lenient punishment, but the act of reporting is liable to be damaging to the whistle-blower and to be at best futile and at worst counterproductive.

Rescuing a fundamentally sound organization from a temporary fall from grace, therefore, is a qualitatively different act from tackling a corrupt status quo. Where the scales are so heavily tipped in favour of continued corruption Lui argues persuasively that harsh penalties are required to rebalance them (Lui 1986: 231). Nonetheless the usefulness of this formulation is somewhat diminished by the fact that it is predicated on the improbable assumption that in such a situation the criminal justice system has remained unsullied. It is, however, more characteristic of high-corruption countries, including China, for the executive to dominate the judicial system as convincingly as it does the legislature and the military.

In addition, since the threat of punishment without the possibility of reward is an ineffective motivator, this is anyway only half the story. In a classic paper Banfield proposes a 'carrot and stick' approach, inducing loyalty through salary policies, using the threat of sanctions to make the consequences of exposure more serious and monitoring agents' activities by systematic audit to increase the likelihood of detection (Banfield 1975). Generally the greater the stake individuals perceive themselves as having in their own society, the less likely they are to offend against it, since the effectiveness of sanctions is increased by the amount that miscreants stand to lose as a result of them. Hence, increasing the perceived likelihood of detection is also likely to have reductionist effects.

Political economists offer the crucial insight that, in politics as elsewhere, ethical rhetoric for the most part is just words, while corruption is a subset of normal behaviour involving the pursuit of pleasure. It follows that the problem of political corruption is not that it is abnormal but that it is perfectly normal. And it emerges not from individual acts of villainy (these certainly exist, but they are more properly regarded as symptoms than as causes) but from the political structures which permit it to go unpunished. Unchecked power permits corrupt leaders to abandon the felicific calculus's aim of achieving the greatest happiness of the greatest number, and to replace it with their own aim of achieving their own greatest happiness at whatever pain to others. This cost may initially be negligible, but corruption has an inexorable logic of expansion, and as corruption expands honesty contracts, with the result that, unless halted at an early stage, the corrupt momentum becomes virtually unstoppable.

In low-corruption countries the way forward is, in principle if not in practice, relatively clear. Positive incentives can be based on transforming an individual act into a transaction by creating a structure that consistently rewards some forms of behaviour and punishes others. The achievement of a bilateral modality creates an exchange-value for any action: a good (or non-corrupt) act is rewarded, a corrupt one punished. Such incentives change the weighting of the felicific calculus by increasing the likelihood that failure to behave in a non-corrupt way will cause more pain than pleasure. The technical challenge then becomes twofold. *First* there is a need to recalibrate the calculus so that pleasure and pain attach to the targeted actions at a level which redirects behaviour with optimal efficiency and effectiveness (something to which Bentham paid meticulous attention). *Second* comes the necessity of achieving effective, consistent and impartial enforcement.

But criminal and employment policy are only part of an economics-derived anti-corruption strategy which also includes trade, fiscal, financial, social and macro-economic policies of daunting scope and integration:

> lowering tariffs and other trade barriers; unifying market exchange and interest rates; eliminating enterprise subsidies; minimizing enterprise regulation, licensing requirements, and other barriers to market entry; privatizing while demonopolizing government assets; enhancing transparency in the enforcement of banking, auditing, and accounting standards; and improving tax and budget administration . . . civil service reform, legal and judicial reforms, and the strengthening and expansion of civil and political liberties . . . improving administrative procedures to avoid discretionary decision making and the duplication of functions, while introducing performance standards for all employees (related to time and production); determining salaries on the basis of performance standards; reducing the degree of organizational power of each individual in an organization; reducing procedural complexity; and making norms, internal rules, and laws well known among officials and users.
> (Buscaglia n.d.)

To political economists, politicians pursue the public good primarily to obtain private benefits, and 'formulate policies in order to win elections, rather than win elections in order to formulate policies' (Downs 1957: 28). In analysing the pressures to political corruption in weak democracies Heymans and Lipietz identify as most significant:

> the high costs of mounting election campaigns, the power of economic elite groups in political parties, the politicisation of the state apparatus by elected officials, and the desire of the latter to compensate for political uncertainty by building up a capital stake through corruption.
>
> (Heymans and Lipietz 1999: 30)

In larger and more sophisticated societies, particularly those with strong party discipline and high levels of inter- and intra-party competition, the situation has already been reached where, on the felicific calculus, bribery involves far greater risks than benefits, and hence more pain than pleasure. In addition, as honest government is a part of the stakes in party competition, and securing election or re-election is the prime aim, it is in no one's interests to engage in it. In Great Britain, vote buying, endemic until the mid-nineteenth century, virtually disappeared with the extension of the franchise, the creation of a model non-corrupt bureaucracy, increased party competition, judicial supervision of the electoral process and increased levels of punishment under the Corrupt and Illegal Practices Act 1883. With very rare exceptions direct electoral manipulation of this kind is unknown because the conditions in which it flourishes – aristocratic patronage, weak enforcement procedures, low literacy and incomes, and poor ballot administration – no longer exist. In addition, such corruption would be unrealistically expensive and almost certainly detected and punished.

In such societies, however, brokerage does not disappear but operates in a more sophisticated way. Today it is more likely to involve trading policy commitments, networking opportunities, high-profile meetings with senior members of the executive or the exchange of honours for party donations; while newspaper owners and editors may be offered a wide range of privileges, sometimes of a non-pecuniary kind. Such approaches, because they normally stay within the letter of the law, give the political entrepreneurs undertaking them reason to claim they are not corrupt, simply the beneficiaries of democracy in action. And, precisely because political corruption is indeed an extension of normal human political behaviour involving crossing a faint and mutable line into unacceptable forms of politics, this is precisely correct.

To Jeremy Bentham democracy perfectly matches the felicific calculus because the voters get policies that benefit them (and which therefore make them happy), the politicians get re-elected (which makes *them* happy), and, the latter being consequential upon the former, the perfect virtuous circle is created. Democracy is not, however, quite so simple. In pursuing the support of sectional interest groups, parties inevitably allow their policies to be influenced, not as part of a socially desirable process of meeting the wishes of, and securing legitimacy among, a heterogeneous electorate, but for more subterranean purposes. The one-nation rhetoric of a party governing 'in the interests of all' gives way to an approach involving the covert paying off of political debts, if necessary in a manner that sacrifices the public good to private interest. The trade-off between paying such debts (and securing the funding) and achieving electoral popularity by enacting either sound government or populist policies is itself part of the woof and warp of democratic politics. It is this that makes political corruption so hard to distinguish from daily politics, and that leads us to turn now to a fuller discussion of the concept *rent-seeking*.

Rent-seeking

> But what is a government itself but the greatest of all reflections on human nature? If men were angels, no government would be necessary. If angels were to govern men, neither external nor internal controls on government would be necessary. In framing a government which is to be administered by men over men, the great difficulty lies in this: you must first enable the government to control the governed, and in the next place oblige it to govern itself.
>
> (James Madison, *Federalist*, 51)

Clearly the rise of multi-national corporations, some of them richer and more powerful than nations, increases opportunities for clandestine interstitial activities. In the United Kingdom the Labour Government of 1997–2001, elected in part on an 'anti-sleaze' ticket, nonetheless legislated a temporary exemption from a proposed ban on cigarette advertising for Formula 1 motor racing, following a £1 million party donation from its Chief Executive (hastily returned when the transaction, which the government claimed was coincidental, attracted negative publicity). Almost inevitably, the high cost and abrasively competitive nature of elections in developed countries mean that election costs exceed donations, while the decline in party loyalty and membership which has characterized political behaviour in much of the developed world has caused the number of small donations from committed individuals to collapse. Hence parties in power almost always attempt to blur the boundary between government information and party propaganda to achieve free beneficial coverage, while opposition parties engage in such strategies as are open to them in order to compete effectively:

> it is difficult to see how such a party can raise money, unless it engages in the kinds of morally dubious fund-raising methods suggested earlier: taking a 'cut' of taxes raised for the production of public goods, or taking bribes from individuals with a private interest in decisions affecting the public sphere . . . parties need to draw some material benefit out of political power, if only to pay for the costs of organisation.
>
> (Hopkin 1997: 263)

Situations such as these, entailing the pursuit of private interest at the cost of the public good, or 'the use of resources in actually lowering total product although benefiting some minority' (Tullock 1989: vii) constitute *rent-seeking*. A 'rent' is a resource available to politicians to dispense as a quid pro quo for activities that might include individual bribe-giving, party donations or delivering votes in return for policy commitments. Rent-seeking is an especially strong feature of politics in the United States, where weak party discipline combined with Congressmen's urgent need to raise campaign funds makes them especially vulnerable to interest groups.

Rent-seeking is one of the major themes to emerge from the political economy of corruption. Its definition is controversial. Tullock offers the following formulation, more restrictive than some:

> The use of resources to obtain through the political process special privileges in which the injury to other people arguably is greater than the gain to the people who obtain rents.
>
> (Tullock 1993: 22)

Rent-seeking in this definition, though it may well entail lobbying, fundraising and exerting democratic pressure, is not synonymous with such activities. All pressure groups and political lobbyists engage in pressurizing politicians – that is their job. So Jewish voters may have had a greater influence on US foreign policy in the Middle East than the Muslim League, and the National Rifle Association may well have influenced domestic policy more successfully than the anti-gun lobby, but that is simply how politics works. The causes may be right or wrong, but those who lobby for them are playing straightforward pressure politics of a kind central to the democratic process. This is presumably so even if the result, to quote Tullock, is that 'the injury to other people arguably is greater than the gain to the people who obtain rents'. Lobbying fuels the American political process in particular, and, according to Tullock, only tips into rent-seeking when it is knowingly and (normally though not invariably) clandestinely pursued so as to set private against public interest. Rent is paid when the party or politician self-interestedly takes what is offered although doing so conflicts with his or her public duty. A rent is, in short, very close to a bribe.

The distinctions involved are, however, subtle, for actions deemed rent-seeking by an unfriendly commentator might equally be considered normal politics by an observer of sunnier disposition. Opposition parties will claim one thing, governments the opposite; the press and other opinion formers will have their say, and so, ultimately and critically, will voters. So Tullock's definition is no simpler to apply than other similar ones which seek to bifurcate the corrupt and the non-corrupt. While extremes of corruption and habitual corruption are usually easy to spot, it is seldom possible to draw and hold an absolute line between the pure and the corrupt. For the most part, small-scale political corruption is better regarded not as a breach of ethics (a concept deriving more from the rhetoric than the reality of politics) but as an error of political judgement or a piece of bad luck.

Democracy in action can never be entirely clean, and both corruption and its subset rent-seeking have electoral costs as well as political, economic and personal benefits. Hence wise politicians weigh these before they embark on activities, including perfectly innocent ones, that may, justifiably or not, leave them vulnerable to media or popular opprobrium. Situations where they fail to do this can be as replete with irony as they are devoid of political judgement. So the Premier of New South Wales, Nick Greiner, so concerned about corruption that he instituted an Independent Commission Against Corruption, became one of its earliest victims when he was judged to have 'overstepped a line which to him and many of his counterparts in Australia and his predecessors in New South Wales was blurred if not invisible' (Williams 2000b: 146).

Perhaps the classic demonstration of this point is in the Keating Five case in the USA, which stemmed from the neo-liberal deregulatory policies of the Reagan administration. During the 1980s, savings and loan companies (thrifts) faced problems stemming from the fact that they were no longer prohibited from involvement in the high-risk commercial real estate sector. This led to a number of thrifts running into financial difficulties. The regulatory body, the Federal Home Loan Bank Board, responded by unsuccessfully seeking a new regulatory framework through legislation. Matters came to a head in 1989 with the spectacular and widely publicized collapse of the Lincoln Savings and Loan Association. The Chairman of Lincoln's parent company, Charles Keating, responded by complaining to the House Banking Committee that the Board had a vendetta against him. The Board, meanwhile, claimed to have been pressed to discontinue its investigations by five senators, subsequently known as the Keating Five, who had received campaign contributions totalling over $1.3 million from or through Keating in return for representing his interests in the course of the investigation. The senator most implicated, Alan Cranston (Democrat, California), insisted plausibly that:

> he had done nothing which the vast majority of other senators had not done on previous occasions, and that his activity was nothing more than the normal process of politics in which campaign support is traded for a willingness to help contributors with their problems.
>
> (Philp 2002: 43)

Keating himself, meanwhile, cheerfully confessed: 'One question . . . had to do with whether my financial support in any way influenced several political figures to take up my cause. I want to say in the most forceful way I can: I certainly hope so.' Investigations by the State of California, the US Department of Justice and the Senate Ethics Committee followed, to determine whether these senators had acted improperly. The investigations as a whole concluded that all the five had indeed acted improperly, albeit that they were differentially culpable. It proposed, largely unsuccessfully, legislating to impose restrictions on campaign funding practices.

Such a line is very fine indeed and it must be possible that a differently constituted Ethics Committee in a different political climate would have arrived at a different conclusion. If in marginal cases the existence or otherwise of political corruption requires *post hoc* forensic determination where the main facts are not in dispute it is hard to claim that a clear line exists between corrupt and clean politics. It does, however, seem reasonable to conclude that a political system which resists transparent legislation is not averse to its own politicians and bureaucrats engaging in rent-seeking, and that such rent-seeking is indeed an integral part of normal political activity.

This is not to suggest, of course, that no judgements can or should be made, or to deny that it is simple to spot and deplore extremes of corruption and rent-seeking. For this reason Whitehead, summing up his findings on presidential corruption in Latin America, is surely correct to be scathing about some scholars' excessive ambiguity or cultural sensitivity, for even in the absence of a clear and agreed point of delineation one should not entirely abandon common sense and common observation:

> some writers shuddered at the thought that they might be imposing values derived from Western industrial society on conduct which was perceived quite differently in a 'non-Western' context. However, in the case of flagrant personal enrichment by Latin American rulers . . . those not enjoying the spoils are just as likely to resent the illicit privileges of their top rulers in Latin America as people in the United States. . . . Of course at the margin there are still problems of definition about what constitutes abuse of office, but I am little troubled by this objection since so few of the individuals discussed in this chapter operated anywhere near the margin.
>
> (Whitehead 1983: 146–147)

Even such extreme behaviour as that of Whitehead's presidents, however, constitutes a set of recognizably *political* manoeuvres occurring as a product of political structures which at least permit and frequently facilitate them. Other examples abound. In Italy for example, the two premierships thus far of the entrepreneur Silvio Berlusconi reflect the consequences of ineffective campaign funding restrictions even more decisively than does the Keating Five case. Berlusconi formed a populist right-wing party Forza Italia (FI) immediately before the 1994 election, in good part with the predatory aim of protecting his business interests against the possibility of a left-wing government supported by an 'upstart' judiciary nationalizing his media empire. In addition to owning all three of Italy's main commercial television stations, Berlusconi owned numerous other media outlets including books, magazines and newspapers. He was a populist chairman of AC Milan Soccer Club and owned a vast range of insurance and other commercial interests. FI's remarkable victory was secured by its astute exploitation of the vacuum that followed the demise of the Christian Democrats (which had ruled Italy virtually uninterruptedly since the end of the Second World War) and their Socialist coalition partners following the corruption scandals of the early 1990s (Nelken 1996; della Porta and Vannucci 1999). Though the FI Government fell ten months later Berlusconi returned to power in 2001, aided by a campaign designed by his own marketing and public relations experts, including repeated Forza Italia propaganda transmitted by his media empire, frequently in the guise of news designed to raise public concern about threats to Italy's integrity from communists and immigrants.

Berlusconi's political success stemmed from the failure of Italy's competition legislation in the 1980s to prevent him securing a media monopoly. It also reflected his achievement in securing delays to court hearings to beyond the period permitted by Italy's statutes of limitation, ensuring that his criminal record (bribery, perjury, illegally funding political parties and corporate fraud) involved conviction but not sentence.[2] This may appear to be rent-seeking on the grand scale but it also entails Berlusconi adroitly exploiting legal avenues to secure election through the democratic process. So it would be wrong to dismiss Berlusconi, as many have, as an individual villain exploiting public position for private benefit. All societies contain characters like Berlusconi but not all states elect them to power. Hence, since his election was not the result of fraud, it is to the nature of the Italian legal and electoral systems that one must turn if one wishes to understand the reasons for his rise to power.

Rent-seeking interests economists *first* because on the felicific calculus it normally achieves the opposite of the greatest happiness of the greatest number, breeding a cynicism which may itself spawn further pain through generating additional costs. These include an uncertain business climate, a loss of tourist revenue, high levels of individual and organized crime (often involving high levels of violence) and declining inward investment. Inward investment is especially vulnerable because, in environments full of restrictions, procurement of goods or services can necessitate securing separate approval from each bureaucratic layer, all of which function as monopolies concerned with their own rent-seeking and not at all with expediting consumers' passage through the maze.

The market response to this chaos is the emergence of 'fixers' as middlemen. The mechanism, however, is restricted by three factors: the fixers are themselves in competition with the bureaucrats; they lack recourse to arbitration in the event of breaches by any party; and, unavoidably, secrecy prevents them from advertising and competing for custom in the open market. Hence:

At one tier, private agents compete for the rent or revenue which has been contrived by intervention. At a second tier, agents employed in government seek that share of the same rent or revenue which accrues to them in their roles as creators of the rent or revenue seeking opportunities, or which they are able to obtain in their capacity as enforcing or monitoring agents. Further tiers are added to the hierarchy of contests if the latter officials and bureaucrats are organized in a hierarchical structure . . . and if transfers are made between different levels of the bureaucratic structure.

(Hillman and Katz 1987: 138)

Second, corrupt business arrangements, where disputes clearly cannot be resolved by recourse to law, present serious enforcement problems often soluble only by the employment of local enforcers in the form of gangsters. Hence in Russia:

there is a steady flow of individuals trained in the use of arms and without other employment, such as disbanded army soldiers, and former police and KGB officers . . . non-state enforcers of rules (such as rackets and mafias) have to a considerable extent displaced the state in the process of post-communist transformation because they have been doing a better job than the state in reducing the transaction costs of exchange and production.

(Humphrey 1999: 200)

Such costs offset any benefits from the low price of labour and are liable to cause inward investors to relocate to countries where procedures are more cheaply manoeuvred. Not surprisingly, therefore, corruption and economic growth rate are negatively related (Mauro 1995).

Rent-seeking entails investing in unproductive political capital rather than in economically or socially productive public goods. High levels of defence expenditure in less-developed countries seldom reflect a dispassionate view of national need, but rather that the secrecy associated with the arms trade offers more scope for kickbacks than does health and social expenditure. This ensures that the public pays several times over for its own victimization. *First*, policy is diverted from the public to the private good. *Second*, the 'dead' costs of rent-seeking demand that rent-seekers impose higher prices to cover their costs. *Third*, because rent-seeking aims to restrict competition, officials who believe, say, that a free market system would reduce their corrupt opportunities will resist necessary economic reforms irrespective of the public good. *Fourth*, a mass of unnecessary regulations is likely to be created, designed ostensibly to restrict future rent-seeking activity but in fact to facilitate it. *Fifth*, rent-seeking typically entails politicians or bureaucrats exercising their power to set prices at below market value in return for bribes. *Sixth*, and crucially, rent-seeking impedes the free trade of democratic politics itself by creating market imperfections stemming from secrecy and conspiracy, so depriving voters of the opportunity to exercise rational and informed choice through the ballot box.

Because the logic of such rent-seeking is expansionist, once high corruption has been reached, the system, by that time itself corrupted, loses the capacity to self-correct. This breeds yet further conflict and political instability in a downward spiral whose end, in the absence of intervening variables, is entropy. For example, when corruption in Cambodian universities is such that only by bribery can one obtain a degree, the degree itself becomes worthless except in Cambodia. Hence a whole generation of Cambodians is unemployable on the international job market and Cambodia's regional as well as international isolation is perpetuated.[3] In Kenya under President Moi rent-seeking was estimated to have accounted for 38 per cent of GDP in the 1980s (Tullock 1993: 76); while in 1992 a third of banking assets were virtually worthless as a result of political interference (Rose-Ackerman 1999: 10). In Fiji, where the heads of the National Bank were political appointees (one new Chief Officer even arriving with a bodyguard of soldiers), the management systems were compared by the World Bank to 'driving at high speed on a highway in a car without a dashboard and a steering wheel'. Loans were made both under political pressure and to employees and associates. One branch, in Rotuma, had $5 million outstanding loans, including a $2 million loan to a company whose CEO was a director of the Bank, but only $150,000 in deposits (Findlay 1999: 81–82).

In the last chapter we adopted a 'signpost definition' of political corruption as involving 'the use of public position for private advantage or exceptional party profit, *and* the subversion of the political process for personal ends' (Summers 1987: 14; italics added). It will be clear that, however fundamental rent-seeking may be to the democratic political process, in its extreme form rent-seeking meets the criteria for both limbs of this definition.

Political corruption and economic liberalization

> We may observe in Africa today that, contrary to the teachings of the neo-liberal rubric, measures of privatization and financial liberalization can lead to a plundering of the economy as widespread as did the processes of nationalization, and perhaps in an even less orderly manner.
>
> (Hibou 1999: 71)

The post-1970s global trend towards free trade internationally and economic liberalization at home is by no means new. The question of whether free trade is the most assured pathway to economic growth and political freedom has been longstanding in British political history at least since the eighteenth century and arguably since the sixteenth. The United States, though like most countries averse neither to single-issue mercantilism around election time nor to regarding free trade as more a one- than a two-way street,[4] has formally regarded international free trade as a major foreign policy goal for much of the post-independence period. US regional policy in particular, both in Central America (for example building the Panama Canal) and the Pacific Ocean (where Japan and Hawaii were initially the prime targets), has long been geared to opening the world economy to US markets.

Domestically, for most countries economic liberalization means selling off national corporations and utilities into private ownership. This may lead to the creation of a genuine market, or, more often, to a quasi-market wherein the aim is to simulate market conditions by tactics such as contract competition, league tables, target-setting, incentivization and central regulation. At the same time quasi-markets present politically convenient ambiguities, particularly concerning residual governmental involvement, as a result of which direct government intervention often remains an option at propitious political moments (Harris 2003). Selling off is often accompanied by fiscal changes to benefit risk-taking entrepreneurs and a tightening of anti-monopoly legislation; and populist gestures in the form of underpriced share offers or high-profile and popular items of public expenditure typically follow.

While debtor countries may approach liberalization reluctantly and under pressure from the World Bank or IMF, stronger countries may proceed by joining powerful regional free trade zones which then act in a mercantilist manner towards non-member states by creating tariff barriers and restricting the movement of labour. OECD and WTO policies, intended, inter alia, to achieve a common basis for international trade among members, reflect global pressure to manage and regulate nation state and regional mercantilism. Where it has been achieved, this (theoretical) level playing field, while controversial in other respects, has affected political corruption by removing such interstices as the sweetheart deals and punitive tariffs within which it formerly operated. Nonetheless, because economic liberalization emerges from the polity, it displaces but does not eliminate pre-existing corrupt propensities. Partly for this reason, introducing liberalization in weak states has been well described as changing the steering wheel while driving the car (Cusimano 2000b: 14). As we argued in the last chapter, though successful economic liberalism is a predictor of low corruption, liberalization itself is not a cure for corruption. In the absence of a strong democratic state and a strong civil society, imposing it can be a high-risk strategy; although it is also true to say that the performance of predatory governments may be such as to lead international organizations and others seeking to do so to believe there is little to lose. As long ago as 1972, for example, Scott observed:

> We can nevertheless identify certain conditions under which the extent
> of market corruption . . . is likely to increase . . . the growth of a large
> commercial elite with little formal access to influence . . . the greater

the scale of government activity . . . the more widespread market corruption will become . . . because large-scale government entails many transactions where no personal ties exist . . . the use of cash and other material incentives becomes more likely.

(Scott 1972: 89)

Prior to liberalization, in weak, particularly pre-industrial, states corruption typically operates through a network of vertical patron–client relationships within which access to resources is dependent upon brokers whose power is in turn determined by their ability to control resources. The corrupt transaction entails exchanging the client's loyalty for the patron's protection and support. Liberalization inevitably attenuates such relationships by removing their monopoly status and subjecting them to competition from the numerous new corrupt opportunities emerging. *Ceteris paribus*, such opportunities, by enhancing the power of the client, transform not just corruption but the political, economic and social relations from which it emerges and which strongly influence its character and degree. So liberalization, far from being a panacea for corruption control in high-corruption countries, characteristically contributes, at least in the short term, to the bad becoming worse. It is for this reason that for the most part states get the liberalism their leaders deserve.

It is important to distinguish the process of economic *liberalization* from the attainment of an economy based on economic *liberalism*. Where liberalism is achieved and the doors are thrown open to competition and free trade, the structures supporting political corruption should in theory, if other necessary conditions prevail, be undermined. Nonetheless considerable challenges are involved in achieving this. The introduction of liberalization does not cause corrupt politicians and bureaucrats simply to go away, but rather to engage in *defensive* manoeuvres to maintain their rent-seeking channels and *offensive* ones to exploit the hitherto unimaginable opportunities presented by liberalization. Official attempts to control demand, whether by fiscal policy or by Chinese-style restrictions on internal mobility and occupational change, themselves create new rent-seeking opportunities for bureaucrats in particular unless the basic structures of state, economy and society are sound – where, that is to say, low corruption already exists. In the absence of such structures the system is always liable to spin out of control, potentially falling, wholly or partly, into the hands of organized criminals with access to international supply sources. The areas of economic activity most vulnerable to such predation include commodities designed to meet such illicit consumption preferences as drugs, gambling, nuclear, chemical, biological and conventional weaponry, fake designer goods, pornography and prostitution. In addition, criminal networks frequently colonize the market in highly taxed imported goods and those with a high mark-up, including alcohol, tobacco, compact discs, perfumes and cosmetics. The remarkable yields deriving from such activities enable the networks not simply to become rich but also, if they wish, to invest their wealth in embedding themselves in the political system by tactics such as threats, bribery, blackmail, buying popularity and demonstrating genuine usefulness to the ruling group. Hence:

> In Somalia, we have seen criminal warlords or drug gangs take over the streets and shantytowns. In Rio de Janeiro, Brazil, drug gangs have taken over the provision of some governmental functions and services. In Peru, drug traffickers, such as Chachique Rivera's group, paid teachers and other local civil servants 100 dollars a month to maintain public services in jungle drug towns and supplement their meager government salaries. Throughout the Andean drug production areas Colombian drug traffickers fund satellite dishes, electric generators, water purification systems, soccer equipment, widen and improve roads for landing strips, and pay salaries to buy local cooperation and support.
>
> (Lupsha 1996: 27)

Further examples of this are to be found in those Eastern European countries where criminals operate by corrupting local politicians and bureaucrats, including the police, whose co-option leads to increased arms availability and, therefore, to more street crime. This in turn creates pressure for more efficient crime control which an impoverished as well as corrupted police force cannot satisfy. Accordingly, a vacuum appears, to be filled by criminals and paramilitaries (including dispossessed members of the security, military and police forces as well as current members of such forces engaging in 'moonlighting'). Criminal gangs are recruited, or recruit themselves, to maintain order in countries where the official forces lack skilled personnel, adequate arms, resources, loyalty or political legitimacy. Once in a position of power, they perpetuate that position by terror, or, more subtly, by shoring up a corrupt regime while at the same time maintaining or enhancing their own legitimacy by achieving peace and security for the people.

In such a situation not only is political corruption maintained in new guises, but the relationship between order and disorder is turned on its head. When the state itself is privatized by criminal elements, as has occurred not only in weak sub-Saharan African states but also in several former Soviet republics, order is imposed by the street-level functionaries of criminal gangs. The state itself, meanwhile, is gradually transformed into a vast criminal enterprise in which the binary opposition of order and disorder ceases to have meaning.

In much of the less-developed as well as the developed world, economic liberalization has shifted responsibility for public service provision from the public to the private sector in a manner bound to impact on both political and bureaucratic corruption. Prior to liberalization, high levels of competition for government appointments typically existed in many less-developed countries. Most such countries also lacked any cultural commitment to the notion of public service, key posts often being auctioned, with successful bidders naturally seeking to maximize the utility they had purchased (Scott 1972: 12; Williams 1987; Wade 1989):

> A corrupt civil servant regards his public office as a business, the income of which he will ... seek to maximize. The office then becomes a 'maximizing unit'. The size of his income depends ... upon the market situation and his talents for finding the point of maximal gain on the public's demand curve.
>
> (van Klaveren 1989)

In the longer term, economic *liberalism* undoubtedly offers the hope of reducing corruption benefits through introducing competition in areas currently under monopoly state control (Rose-Ackerman 1978; Hillman and Schnytzer 1986). Nonetheless, the process of *liberalization* offers new opportunities for corruption. Nor should we assume that existing corrupt dynamics will not persist in a privatized system; indeed they can be exacerbated, as has occurred in Russia, the Ukraine and other former Soviet republics as well as many African countries and those in south and southeast Europe, including Turkey (Baran 2000: 134). Where effective regulatory structures are not created, non-accountable monopolistic corporations simply replicate the functions and ethos of government. Creating non-corrupt regulatory structures then becomes more than challenging: as is clear in much of sub-Saharan Africa, corrupt structures are not easily prevented from self-perpetuation, and few corrupt politicians and officials acquiesce in surrendering the source of their wealth to private corporations.

The evidence that privatization creates short-term opportunities for corruption is persuasive, confirming suspicions widespread in many countries undergoing economic liberalization (Baran 2000: 143). Such opportunities can result from former state-owned enterprises being driven into the hands of those sufficiently enriched by prior corruption to become viable purchasers. In many LDCs the internal political economy is such that the only viable purchasers are members of the corrupt ruling elite or their families, and their main purpose in bidding is to retain monopoly power and, in consequence, their rent-seeking capacity. In fact, in a challenge to western models of privatization based on the prior existence of a form of communal ownership, Hibou claims that entire states have themselves been privatized by such predatory elites:

> the privatization of the economy can be defined more widely than simply the cession of public enterprises to private actors. It can include the acquisition, the creation or the conquest of markets by various

means by persons linked to those in power but operating in a private capacity. In this sense, the privatization of the economy today is truly massive and in effect is the main form taken by the economy of plunder.

(Hibou 1999: 72)

A state may be privatized by the capitulation of government to criminals, by its being so infiltrated by criminals as to be effectively under criminal control, or by a parallel government being instituted. Any successful challenge to legitimate government involves the surrender of the state monopoly over internal and external security services, border control, taxation, customs and excise, and other trappings of statehood. Hence the choice facing aid donors, creditor nations, potential inward investors and ordinary people in privatized states is not between the legitimate and the corrupt, simply between different types of corruption.

Several former Soviet republics are in effect run by gangsters, their street-level enforcers frequently former members of the military, police and security services. So in Russia, 'Nothing is easier than to slip over from the bodyguard to the bandit role in relation to a business you work for each day' (Humphrey 1999: 221). Nonetheless, even within the more traditionally restricted, neo-liberal, definition of privatization, major problems have to be overcome if it is to assist in reducing political corruption. As has been rightly said, 'the fundamental structures of power within a given state will almost certainly be replicated within its civil society' (Theobald 2000: 154). It follows that while mature democratic states can, by tradition and regulation, keep corruption's ubiquitous potential in check, the problem in the less-developed world and among societies in transition is overwhelming. Market competition is very unlikely to be free of major imperfections, the rigours of competition will not quickly or easily squeeze out corrupt and other counter-competitive practices, and liberalization will be driven by the same corrupt forces which previously monopolized governmental rent-seeking.

Turbulence is especially likely in countries where Weberian principles of bureaucratic impartiality are absent, and which lack any culturally ingrained conception of public service or any system for maintaining a distinction between individual and collective interests. For example, in the banking and financial sectors of much of sub-Saharan Africa granting non-reimbursable loans has long been an important aspect of clientelism, and there is no reason to believe liberalization will change this. On the contrary, financial liberalization has created a free-for-all, with vast new opportunities for corporate fraud emerging, while, in countries non-compliant with international banking regulations, money laundering has been simplified as a result of the easing of such controls on the origins of funds as previously existed.

In much of Africa, for several reasons the liberalization of financial markets has had disruptive consequences, not least because many African countries combine high levels of administrative centralization, incompetence and corruption with judicial weakness. *First* is the fact that in countries where the stabilizing effect of a public service ethos is lacking, turbulence surrounding economic liberalization simply creates new opportunities for illegitimate competition for resources, and such competition merely provides those already enriched by corruption with the opportunity to consolidate power, wealth and influence. So, aided by the fact that independent auditing of private companies is rare in sub-Saharan Africa, and loss-making companies in particular offer a useful cover for illicit transfers, liberalization has transformed entrenched political corruption into an anarchic rent-seeking opportunity for corporate fraud. *Second*, liberalization has shored up the power bases of corrupt regimes by creating new sources of patronage by which corrupt rulers can buttress existing client networks and create new ones, and weaken both unpopular ethnic groups (Uganda, Tanzania and Zimbabwe) and potential competitors (Cameroon and Nigeria) (Hibou 1999: 73). Once these corrupt elements are in control of privatized industries, in addition to any financial return from the industries themselves they offer new opportunities for laundering a whole range of criminal activities. These include smuggling and customs evasion, central to Africa's formal as well as informal economy, the distinction between the two having little meaning in a context where the state's active involvement in the informal economy is itself often an element of political corruption. This is particularly but not exclusively the case in such entrepôt states as Benin, Gambia and Togo, where the illicit export of diamonds, ivory and rhinoceros horn, for example, far from being the province of small-time crooks, is largely controlled by the power elites (Hibou 1999: 80, 89).

Third, some forms of pseudo-liberalism provide especially rich pickings. Notable are those which create hybrid organizations by selling off only part of a state's holding in a company, so creating arm's-length state or private sector bodies to manage monopoly services (Heymans and Lipietz 1999; Agbese 1998; White 1996; Rose-Ackerman 1999; Beare 2000a). Even developed countries often find monitoring the behaviour of such agencies difficult, and it appears that in sub-Saharan Africa, where for all the numbers of enterprises earmarked for privatization very few 'pure' sell-offs have actually taken place (Hibou 1999: 72), pseudo-liberalization simply makes a bad situation worse. *Fourth*, in many countries liberalization has been associated with rolling back the state's responsibility for internal security. This has been manifested in a weakening of border controls, normally introduced under pressure from international trading corporations[5] or as a policy of regional organizations. Weak border controls facilitate new opportunities for international organized crime by removing the costs and uncertainties associated with bribing border guards and customs officials, and by creating large and diverse internal markets with greater economic potential and many more hiding places. We return later to the relationship between such organized criminality and political corruption. *Fifth*, not only in China but also in many Latin American and sub-Saharan African countries, economic liberalization has not been matched by such characteristics of political liberalization as democracy, transparency, accountability and press freedom. Transparency in particular has little meaning in a society lacking civil liberties and a strong civil society, for there is little point in being open to scrutiny if the scrutineer is liable to be corrupt. Hence, in the absence of independent investigative or reporting machinery, only politically inspired attacks on political corruption will normally emerge. *Sixth*, in newly privatized sectors where the regulatory agencies on which the probity of privatized concerns depends are immature, corrupt incentives are regularly made available to members of the regulatory staff themselves. In some cases the regulators are even drawn from the ranks of the organizations being regulated, and in such situations it would stretch credulity to suggest that the main purpose of their presence is to root out corruption. Following Mexico's privatization of shrimping in the Bay of California, for example, inspectors were introduced, more as a sop to the United States, with which the North American Free Trade Agreement was at the time being negotiated, than as a serious attempt to address the problem of environmental degradation. For these inspectors, their term of office offered a unique opportunity for personal enrichment which they would have been implausibly saintly or humanly foolish to ignore (Vásquez-León 1999).

Seventh, the management of privatization itself offers scope for corruption. In Turkey under the Özal regime in the early 1980s, economic liberalization was accompanied by political pressure to award contracts to sympathetic businessmen in return for kickbacks to politicians and bureaucrats (Baran 2000: 134). Valuing industries is an imprecise art, and at the shortlisting stage, not only corrupt decision-making but also the power to supply favoured bidders with access to 'inside track' information about unpublished considerations offer scope for bribery (Rose-Ackerman 1999: Chapter 3). *Finally*, any belief among corrupt politicians and officials that in the longer term economic liberalism will succeed in squeezing corruption out of the system is liable to increase the incentive to maximize illicit opportunities before they disappear.

Nonetheless it is reasonable to ask: if not liberalization, then what? Entrenched corruption is, as we have seen, logically insoluble by internal structures which have themselves been corrupted; nor is covert support for revolutionary forces a feasible way of challenging corruption. On the contrary, few strategies could be better designed to increase it, as the experience of US foreign policy in Central America and the Middle and Far East in particular amply demonstrates. While the short-term effects of liberalization may be negative, however, it is at least possible that in the longer term order will emerge from chaos, and that the shifting of traditional patriarchal social and political relations will create the opportunity for more open international trading relations. Clearly the leverage of strong over weak nations is a potentially vital tool, but the deployment of such leverage in the past, notably to force liberalization on debtor countries in the wake of the oil price rise of 1979, had overwhelmingly negative consequences. In fact it was this more than anything else that contributed to the spiralling debt crisis of the 1980s which has led both to widespread impoverishment and to numerous opportunities for corrupt private enrichment, and from which the global economic system is only now extricating itself. The problem, therefore, is acute. If no action is taken to encourage liberalization, existing corruption continues unabated in political and economic circumstances likely to exacerbate it. But if liberalization is forced on weak and corrupt states corruption will also be exacerbated, and quite probably be accompanied by economic chaos and severe political instability.

Clearly the aim must be to achieve a situation in which corrupt vested interests are more motivated to enforce reduced levels of corruption than to engage in endemic rent-seeking. But how to achieve it is a great problem in international relations:

> in the desire to contain the transsovereign threats of international crime, nuclear smuggling, etc., that come from the weakened states of the former Soviet Union, the United States pushes for rapid economic privatization, trade liberalization, and democratization. However, rapidly opening societies and economies can further destabilize states, further exacerbating the very transsovereign problems the United States wishes to contain. The post-Cold War security dilemma is how to open economies, societies, and technologies (in order to increase security) without making transsovereign problems worse (and thereby decrease security).
>
> (Cusimano 2000b: 32)

The final years of the last century and the early years of the present one have seen both the World Bank and the International Monetary Fund admitting to past mistakes and speaking in terms more of partnership than coercion. This is likely to lead to the need to distinguish ever more clearly those LDCs with which partnership is possible from those with which it is not. Here there are, as we shall see later, possible early glimmerings of recipient countries in Africa in particular acknowledging the need for aid and loans to be reciprocated by moves towards improved governance. To western governments such signs may appear too little too late, but to political leaders in a continent where political instinct supports an 'all for one and one for all' approach, and which repudiates reciprocity by claiming publicly that financial assistance is a minimal recompense for slavery and colonialism, they are a major step. If the formation in 2001 of the New Partnership for Africa's Development (NEPAD) does indeed mark a greater willingness among reform-minded African nations to bid for support on their own merits there may be scope for progress. It would be premature to be overly optimistic, however, and the refusal of NEPAD's fifteen members to condemn publicly the corrupt Zimbabwe election of 2002 sent entirely the wrong signal to the west. Nonetheless, it appears clear that only by a consensual approach of this kind is progress likely to be made; and, this being so, the partialization of Africa for the purposes of aid, loans, debt relief and trade would be a significant step forward for all parties.

The costs and benefits of corruption

> the irony to be noted is that government strategies that may be commonly regarded as good and sensible often create demands for, and facilitate the supply of, illegal goods and services. In this sense much of the harm inflicted by criminal enterprises is an unintended consequence and the hidden cost of otherwise desirable or legitimate policies.
>
> (Passas 1993: 303)

Most of the writers who have argued that in the right time and place corruption can be beneficial were writing in the context of the different international context of the 1960s–1970s. Nonetheless they are sometimes cited as though their views were applicable today, when the weight of argument has swung away from this belief. *First*, Myrdal argued that political corruption could enable enterprising companies to cut through the maze of bureaucratic regulation (Myrdal 1968). This line of argument, while doubtless attractive to the western businessman or woman approached by a prospective broker, appears innocent to the near inevitability of a corruption-friendly environment perversely incentivizing the creation of more red tape to extend the scope for bribery. For example, in numerous countries including India (Das 2001), China (Cheung 1996; Smart 1999), Mexico (Vásquez-León 1999) and the Philippines (Hutchcroft 1998; McCoy 1999; Kang 2002), oppressive and unenforceable regulations have been created to facilitate corruption. Normally this is done either by encouraging officials to subsidize low salaries by bribery or by creating opportunities for entrepreneurs to create a web of illicit relationships with state officials and consumers. In China this activity was until recently aided by the existence of a dual pricing structure virtually guaranteeing major market imperfections by permitting commodity purchasing at state rather than market prices. For example, in Nanjing the same 1,000 tons of steel was purchased and resold 223 times among eighty-three companies and *danwei* (workplaces) over several months without leaving the warehouse, the price rising from 1,663 to 4,650 yuan per ton (Johnston and Hao 1995) as speculation increased. So like many arguments in favour of corruption, Myrdal's sacrifices long-term economic and political stability on the altar of short-term solutions.

Second, in an argument which in essence rehearses the advantages of economic liberalization but applies them to corruption, Tilman claims that corruption can equilibrate an unbalanced market (Tilman 1968). By this he means that intrusions into the market by state-run or other not-for-profit services, often in the form of counter-cyclical corrective interventions in areas such as health and welfare, create imperfections leading to inefficiency and restrictive practices. Corruption, by injecting the rigours of competition, can, according to this argument, help restore the political economy to Pareto optimality. A variation on this theme is Huntington's view that corruption, because it attacks traditional and therefore counter-competitive practices, is, at least in smallish doses, a desirable concomitant of modernization (Huntington 1968; see also Padhy 1986: 16–18). So corruption injects the rigours of the market into economies previously driven by state decision-making designed to buck the supply–demand nexus. In a related argument speed payments have gained support from economists who believe they reduce the cost to the state of employing bureaucrats by transferring salary costs to consumers, and constitute an effective rationing system by permitting those to whom time is most important to jump the queue.

There can be little doubt that the greater the market distortions imposed by government and the greater the relative size of the government sector, the greater are the incentives to cut corners. An experiment conducted in Peru, a high-corruption country, in which an attempt was made to set up a legal government company without bribery, demonstrated that an activity which took 3.5 hours in Florida took 301 days there (Walter 1985: 16–17). Certainly many state-run enterprises, whether deriving from Maoist principles in China, loosely Marxist-Leninist ones in the former Soviet Union, liberal democratic ones in the United Kingdom and France, or presidential predations in the Congo, Nicaragua, Indonesia and the Philippines, bear characteristics of this kind. Such enterprises are prone to both high- and low-level corruption, gross inefficiencies and the elevation of provider over consumer interests by restrictive practices and industrial relations disputes in which consumers lack an effective voice. This latter problem is especially likely in the skill-based, high-wage economies of the west, particularly at times of economic boom when labour is at a premium. Nonetheless, to cite corruption as a solution to such problems seems rather odd to anyone to whom corruption, which itself distorts market systems by rendering social and economic interactions uncertain and unpredictable, is part of the problem. The near inevitable involvement of organized criminals, attracted by corrupt possibilities as flies to a honey pot, means that major enforcement problems unavoidably arise. In particular, once the state has surrendered its monopoly over force the door is opened to violence and disorder and to the criminals taking charge of the state itself, a position they are unlikely to surrender without a prolonged and bloody battle.

Third, Nye, in a classic paper best remembered now for its definition of political corruption as 'the use of reward to pervert the judgement of a person in a position of trust', develops a cost–benefit matrix to identify the circumstances in which corruption respectively helps and hinders development (Nye 1967). He argues that corruption can solve a number of problems, including economic development, national integration and governmental capacity, though his support for this view is heavily conditional and he concludes that only in specified situations do the benefits of corruption outweigh its costs. A key dimension of this is that political corruption enables politicians to invest their capital in a manner more economically beneficial than would be the case if the money were spread thinly among the populace. Certainly corruption leads to capital formation: a whole range of corrupt politicians from Mobutu to Somoza and from Trujillo to Duvalier stand testimony to that. But, as Nye concedes, the supposed benefits of corruption entirely depend on the decision of these politicians to invest their rents internally and not overseas. With this proviso it is perfectly plausible to argue that an injection of corrupt capital would stimulate the economy more than the same sum being spent on basic foodstuffs by ten million poor people. Nonetheless, research subsequent to Nye's paper indicates all too clearly the extent of the predilection among corrupt leaders for Swiss bank accounts and western investments, to say nothing of western pleasures. In addition, corruption has a strongly negative impact on inward investment, while the instability of indigenous banking systems, itself a product of corruption and a partial illustration of the power of money-launderers over the host banks, normally leads to massive capital flight. This in turn creates a vacuum in the country's political, economic and financial structure, always liable to be infiltrated by organized criminals in the manner described earlier.

In spite of the seeming weakness of arguments in favour of corruption it is true that specific forms of corruption, being comprehensible and inevitable, may demand a pragmatic response. As Williams wryly observes, 'To the moralist, corruption is always an evil, but political leaders recognise that it is sometimes preferable to the likely alternatives' (Williams 1987: 6–7). Similarly, in a stimulating and robustly expressed study based on research in New York City, Anechiarico and Jacobs (1996) argue that anti-corruption attempts are to corruption what Prohibition was to drinking: all too often they simply make things worse.[6] New levels of bureaucracy and control follow, their logical outcome being the all-seeing Panopticon, conceived in the eighteenth century by Jeremy Bentham and revisited in the twentieth by George Orwell in the form of Big Brother. Expressed otherwise:

> If the market mechanism is suspect, the inevitable temptation is to resort to greater and greater intervention, thereby increasing the amount of economic activity devoted to rent seeking. As such, a political 'vicious circle' may develop. People perceive that the market mechanism does not function in a way compatible with socially approved goals because of competitive rent seeking. A political consensus therefore emerges to intervene further in the market, rent seeking increases, and further intervention results.
>
> (Krueger 1974: 302)

It does not, however, follow that the presence of political corruption per se is preferable to its absence, rather that a calculation of the costs of eliminating it needs to be made. In the short term at least and in certain situations anti-corruption efforts may indeed produce a cure more dire than the disease (Gong 1994). There is also a powerful argument that concentrating law enforcement on money laundering simply diverts criminal money into illegal rather than legal expenditure (see Fiorentini and Peltzman 1995: 24) with little or no benefit and, possibly, some harm. Nonetheless, given the contagious character of political corruption and its near immunity in countries of high-threshold corruption, it seems desirable to discourage activities which lead to the influence of criminal gangs insinuating themselves more than can be avoided into national political elites. The costs of permitting institutionalized corruption to continue, and in the process inevitably further to entrench itself, should not be underestimated. The tactical decision, by donor governments and international financial organizations in particular, of when and how to press for change is one thing; but any decision to regard the permanent existence of institutionalized corruption as preferable to its eradication would be entirely different.

In an exemplification of the short-term costs of corruption control Smart shows that in China 'eradicating certain kinds of low-level corrupt activities could potentially increase the overall costs to the society of corruption from the top down' (Smart 1999: 114). Localized corruption, conducted through the relationship system of *guanxi*, can restrict the privileged status of inefficient state enterprises to the overall benefit of efficiency and competitiveness, bringing, but only in the short term, productive outcomes (Smart 1999: 118). Similarly, in kleptocracies, where, corruption being the norm, the appearance of rival criminals should, by introducing competition, drive down the cost of rents, there is a strong argument that competition, at least in the short term, expands the market (Grossman 1995). Certainly in many parts of sub-Saharan Africa so chronic are the impediments to business dealing and so embedded the political power structures in the informal economy that businesspeople prefer to deal informally rather than formally. But a commercial preference for dealing through an informal system, far from being a prescription for corruption, is simply indicative of the unsurprising fact that where no non-corrupt option exists businesses act pragmatically.

Numerous studies across academic disciplines demonstrate the long-term deleterious effects of corruption. Economists point to the market imperfections created by corruption: in particular, in a Gresham's Law of corruption, contracts go to high bidders who factor in generous graft payments while efficient suppliers are squeezed out (George 1988; see also Mauro 1995; Rose-Ackerman 1999). Corruption therefore becomes a source of institutional inertia in public sector organizations as well as being detrimental to market reforms in LDCs. Similarly, when senior posts go to well-connected individuals or those prepared to pay for them rather than to the best qualified, there is a double economic loss. *First*, key tasks are being performed less than optimally, and *second* the more able rejected candidates will either seek to leave the country or be co-opted into crime rings better able to recognize and reward the market value of their skills (Murphy *et al.* 1991).

The negative impact of corruption on foreign aid and inward investment is also considerable (Bhargava 1999). This view is reflected not only among economists, who point to the disincentives stemming from the bureaucratic hurdles facing overseas investors, but among public administrators (for example Caiden and Caiden 1977), and criminologists (such as Klitgaard 1991; Leiken 1996). Criminologists in particular show that institutionalized high-level political corruption is a fountainhead for white-collar and organized crime, administrative inefficiency and judicial corruption. After all, if criminals can buy their way out of trouble, legal deterrence is minimal and the political economy of justice stands on its head: if the criminals employ and corrupt the professionals, they are effectively running the system.

Institutionalized corruption is hard to root out because the existence of corrupt networks means honest auditors can seldom be sure that they are not reporting to, as well as on, corrupt officials (Lui 1986). Naturally many auditors and regulators are themselves corrupt or compliant with corruption. For the honest individual in a corrupt system, therefore, the risk of reporting corruption to the surreptitiously corrupt is ubiquitous; the consequences of doing so are potentially fatal. Hence corruption breeds corruption, and a corruption trap (Rose-Ackerman 1999: 3) is set.

Where corruption is the norm the collective pressures to conform facing honest deviants are overwhelming and potentially life-threatening. *First*, in Turkey the Motherland Party of Turgut Özal, a former World Bank employee, came to power in 1983 on an anti-corruption free market platform; but Özal quickly succumbed to the lure of bribery by contractors. On his death in 1993 an anti-fundamentalist coalition came to power, again professing opposition to corruption. Again, however, corruption re-emerged. Tansu Çiller, the young reformist leader of the True Path Party, quickly formed a coalition with her political enemy, the Islamist Party of Necmettin Eberkan, which had secured less than 20 per cent of the popular vote, in return for Eberkan's opposition to corruption investigations against her (Baran 2000: 136).

Second, in the Philippines following the replacement of the iron-willed Ferdinand Marcos by a popular but politically weak successor Corazon Aquino, democratization decentralized rather than reduced corruption. So powerful local elites used their new power bases to engage an increasingly diverse range of national politicians and bureaucrats in corrupt practices, and the situation became at best unpredictable and at worst chaotic (Hutchcroft 1998: 13; Heymans and Lipietz 1999: 29–30). In 2001 the circumstances surrounding the fall of the erratic and dissolute former film actor President Joseph 'Erap' Estrada, popular with the people but dubbed by *Asiaweek* the 'Best Reason to Doubt Democracy', demonstrated that corruption continued to oil the political machine in Manila as well as in the regions.

Third, in Spain, a weak political system characterized by low party member-ship and high levels of patronage and personalism contributed significantly to the problems involved in replacing Franco's forty-year dictatorship, inhibiting 'the assumption of individual responsibility, the taking of organi-sational initiatives, and collective action' (Heywood 1994: 7). *Fourth*, similar problems in Italy resulted from failures in nation-building going back to unification (Donovan 1994), the decentralized regional government system introduced in the early 1980s creating opportunities for corrupt practices at regional level which were left largely untouched by central government. *Fifth*, in Uganda, despite genuine advances by President Museveni and the National Resistance Army to root out both political and bureaucratic corruption since 1986 (Kpundeh 2002), a World Bank mission in 1998 still identified:

> systemic problems in the government's revenue and expenditure management, public procurement systems, the civil service reform pro-gramme, the deregulation of the economy and the privatisation and reform of state enterprises. Its findings included the estimate of Uganda's Auditor General that between ten and 20 per cent of public funds are being misused or diverted.
>
> (Watt *et al.* 2000: 37)

And *sixth*, Riley, in his study of the Stevens regime in Sierra Leone, notes:

> In order to maintain political control with a weak economy in decline, those in key political positions have to divert and corruptly use public funds. This diversion of funds affects the presumed development strat-egies of the regime. Success at maintaining political control has meant failures in administrative efficiency and development planning and the growth of a large parasitic 'state class'.
>
> (Riley 1983: 204)

Conclusion

> Again, the many are more incorruptible than the few; they are like the greater quantity of water which is less easily corrupted than a little. The individual is liable to be overcome by anger or by some other passion, and then his judge-ment is necessarily perverted; but it is hardly to be supposed that a great number of persons would all get into a passion and go wrong at the same moment.
>
> (Aristotle, *The Politics*, 1286a)

In this chapter we have considered, *first*, a small part of the extensive politi-cal economy literature, in particular that drawing on the felicific calculus.

In Bentham's simple model, in a democracy being re-elected is what makes politicians happy; this in turn results from their pursuing policies that make the people happy; ergo, everyone is happy. But in real-world politics things do not work like that. Lobbyists, party managers, the media, constituents and large donors mount different forms of pressure, with politicians and parties pulled in different directions by competing interest groups. And, as election costs exceed funds, donations from large corporations are necessary. But large corporations are accountable to their shareholders and are not in the business of altruism, so if they pay the piper – often covering their bets by donating to all main parties – they will try to call the tune. For this and other reasons all politicians have, as part of the day-to-day business of politics, to manage the dissonance between public rhetoric and private ambition just as corrupt ones have to manage that between public probity and private corruption. The difference is not so great as one might imagine.

Second, we addressed the complex issue of rent-seeking, that central characteristic of political corruption in which politicians exploit public position to further private ends at the expense of the public. Here we considered in particular Tullock's interesting and forceful distinction between 'normal' politics and rent-seeking. We found, however, that while it was analytically persuasive its utility was restricted to fairly extreme cases. Most politicians, like most professionals, are concerned with their private interest: they want to be re-elected, they want to be promoted, they want to have a secure, pleasant and affluent lifestyle and they will take action, sometimes of a covert kind, to further those ends. These may be very normal political activities, but at a certain point they may become detrimental to others, and at a further point they may be deemed corrupt, by law if a law exists or by powerful determiners such as the World Bank if not. In saying this, our aim is by no means to minimize or normalize corrupt behaviour. Rather it is to stress that the route from normal to corrupt politics is often short, and the frontier post unmarked. But once the frontier has been crossed the momentum increases, and, even though one may not know when one has reached it, the point of no return is seldom far down the track.

Third, we considered some of the experiences of countries that have undergone economic liberalization, and how those experiences affected corruption. Liberalization, like political corruption, emerges from and remains part of the polity, so the character of pre-liberalization politics shapes the nature and character of the liberalization process. Where the state is corrupt so will liberalization be; indeed liberalization may well, as occurred dramatically in China, multiply existing opportunities for corruption by disturbing the previous equilibrium and offering unrestrained possibilities of wealth accumulation. Where, on the other hand, the bureaucracy is honest, the judiciary free and the political system mature, in spite of inevitable mishaps liberalization will broadly reflect these characteristics. In particular, safeguards built into mature political systems will manage the inevitable new tensions between public service and private profit with the minimum possible conflict.

Nonetheless, it is hard to see any long-term solution to the entrenched corruption of many less-developed countries that does not include economic liberalization. The creation of even an imperfect market causes a disturbance to a corrupt status quo which, after an initial period of chaos, has the potential to open a country to world trade in a manner likely ultimately to be beneficial. In fact for a country where the nature and extent of corruption are such that internal means of eliminating it are weak or non-existent, a loosening of the reins of traditional authority supported by enhanced international trading opportunities appears the only feasible means of salvation. The leverage of strong over weak nations is immense, and a hard-nosed approach by such nations to inward investment, food aid and debt relief offers at least some scope for reform by so pressurizing corrupt vested interests that enforcing reduced levels of corruption becomes preferable to endemic rent-seeking. This is no panacea, but such leverage as may shake the more negative aspects of the sovereignty of weak and corrupt nation states appears at present to be the only approach to bringing them into the international trading community in such a way as to increase their growth rates and per capita GDP. We return to this point in later chapters.

Fourth, we reviewed briefly some of the literature that balanced the costs and benefits of political corruption. While it is true that there are situations in which, if political corruption were magically removed, new problems would arise, this fact is, we believe, best seen not as an argument for corruption's beneficial effects but as a demonstration of the need for system reform to be carefully judged. To suggest that high levels of political corruption can be, as it were, amputated from the political system ignores the fact that corruption and politics are interlinked. So just as a predominantly non-corrupt system will self-correct to deal with corrupt individuals and the legislative or political flaws that facilitated their corruption, so will a predominantly corrupt system self-correct to maintain its corruption following a purge. Corruption cannot solve a problem of politics because it is one of the symptoms of that problem, and a disease cannot cure itself.

The next two chapters offer contrasting one-country analyses of corruption. China has been and remains a high-corruption country; the United Kingdom, a former high-corruption country, is now low corruption. By tracing the contrasting patterns of corruption in these two states it is hoped that we can learn something about the challenges faced by China, and those who interact with it, if corruption is to be brought under control; and about the historical processes by which the United Kingdom successfully achieved an acceptably low level of political corruption.

Notes

1 A psychological theory based on the premiss that more people will follow others in committing a bad act than will initiate the act themselves. It is a common observation that when one person crosses a road when the 'red man' is showing, many more follow immediately.

2 During his second premiership Berlusconi came under further investigation following allegations, unresolved at the time of writing, about the deployment of offshore slush funds, as well as unproven personal links to Mafia killings (Ginsborg 2001).

3 The level of university salaries in Cambodia assumes corruption will provide a supplement to basic income.

4 In fact historically the United States has been quick to impose punitive tariffs on countries it believes to be hindering US exports. Most notably Super 301, a provision of the Trade Act 1974, requires the US Trade Representative to report annually on the foreign country practices which impact the most negatively on US exports for purposes of retaliation.

5 For succinct but insightful commentaries on the reduced activities in this area of the US Customs Service and the additional demands placed on the Service not only by the sheer weight of traffic (430 million people entering the US annually) but also by developments which include containerization, the exponential increases in the numbers of private aircraft, international couriers and international express mail, see Flynn (2000).

6 A similar point is made by Naylor about the active pursuit of money laundering, which he considers an 'artificial crime' (Naylor 1999: 61). Naylor notes: 'Few would disagree with the fundamental moral principle that society should strive to strip criminals of illegal gains. However, on the subsidiary issue of how much collateral damage society should be willing to sustain to implement that principle using current tools, the amount of disagreement could be considerable' (Naylor 1999: 42). For further discussion of this issue see Chapter 5 below.

3 National political corruption (I): the People's Republic of China

In 1994, in the province of Hubei, 20 percent of the cotton harvest was lost because the district government had issued a decree that required everyone to buy a certain brand of substandard pesticide, which was produced by a company owned by the local party secretary . . . A peasant sent a letter of thanks to the party secretary because his wife, after a violent quarrel, had tried to commit suicide by drinking the stuff, but had survived because it was a harmless imitation.

(van Kemenade 1997: 12)

The experience of corruption in what is now the People's Republic of China (PRC) has deep historical roots (Lau and Lee 1978), though there are differences among scholars as to the relationship among corruption, culture and (particularly Qing Dynasty) political administration (Yang 1994; Leonard 2001). China's success over the centuries in resisting western cultural influence means that its institutions of government developed quite differently from those exported to the colonies by the European powers. Checks and balances, the separation of powers, the concept of natural law, accountable democratic government and the ethos of public service had no place in the Chinese imperial tradition. Political accountability through independent audit was therefore inconceivable, and to this day, in spite of advances made since the mid-1990s, neither culturally nor organizationally is the idea of a national leader's decisions being subject to judicial review at all plausible.

Following the 1949 Revolution, in the absence of any civil sphere the National People's Congress (NPC), and not the judiciary, is at least formally the ultimate judicial as well as constitutional arbiter. The status of judges remains low: fewer than 10 per cent of them have a university degree, and graduates are disproportionately located in urban areas. There is widespread nepotism in appointments, and, in spite of some reform attempts, judicial misconduct remains common both through personal predation, made possible by the variable control of self-interested judicial discretion (Woo 2000), and through the continued subordination of judicial decree to the will and interests of the state. According to the *China Discipline Inspection and Supervision Daily*, in 1993 136 prosecutors, judges and senior policemen in Jiamusi city, near the Russian border, were purged, reprimanded or transferred because of their connections with organized crime. In a city in southern Hunan, Mao Zedong's home province, 270 out of 515 hotels, restaurants and dance halls (some of them effectively brothels) were owned and run by Party and government officials, including judges, prosecutors and senior officials of the People's Armed Police (van Kemenade 1997: 19).

Nationally, in 1998, action was taken against 2,512 judges and other court personnel and 1,557 procuratorate[1] personnel who had acted illegally (Hao and Johnston 2002: 593). Judges remain functionaries, not members of the powerful independent profession familiar in the west; their duty is not only, indeed not primarily, to interpret statute law but to reflect 'morality' as expressed in Party documents and leadership speeches (Ocko 2000: 80). For example Judge Wang Airu was appointed in Shaanxi Province despite having been barely educated to primary school level simply because he was a 'dance patron' of a senior local official (Fong 2002). In Shanxi Province a 2001 investigation revealed that eighty-nine judges in rural areas had been unlawfully appointed. On Hainan Island, a spectacularly corrupt province whose economy has been largely fuelled by organized smuggling and other forms of criminality, 1,718 cases of judicial malpractice were uncovered between 1997 and 2001.

Only in 2002 did the Supreme People's Court introduce an official examination, a requirement for new judges to be graduates, a disciplinary procedure and an obligation on judges to make an 'independent' decision regardless of pressure from government or powerful individuals. Since, however, the judiciary remains an arm of government, with the cases it is permitted to adjudicate being politically determined and the status of its employees low, how this will operate in practice, particularly at times of unrest, remains to be seen (Fong 2002); but there is room for scepticism.

Until recently no discourse of individual rights existed; indeed the notion of individuals having 'rights' against the state simply made no sense. Even such discourse as exists today is largely the product of an increasing awareness among the Chinese leadership of the expectations of the western powers and international organizations with which China is increasingly enmeshed. While there has undoubtedly been a greater willingness among the leadership to pay lip-service to the concept in return for such tangible benefits as admittance to the WTO in 2001 and the award to Beijing of the 2008 Olympic Games, this lip-service has not been translated into fundamental constitutional change.[2] The intellectual bureaucracy governing China for two millennia of imperial rule denied the validity and prohibited the expression of opinion contrary to official knowledge, and this culture, though modulated by the new generation of leaders, has by no means disappeared.

The role of experts was traditionally convergent, not divergent, contributing to the scientific improvement of the official discourse on terms laid down by the ruling elite rather than questioning authority. In Platonic style, Chinese orthodoxy rejected the errors of opinion in favour of the objective truth of knowledge. Non-compliant scholars were dismissed from court or punished severely for their objective errors.

In this chapter we shall show that the power structures of contemporary China, as they evolved through the republican, classical communist and socialist market eras of the twentieth century, have retained strong elements of these cultural traits. This is so although their concrete expression has been subject to two major transformations and countless lesser modifications. They have also, overlaid as they are by a hierarchical and authoritarian political and economic structure supported by strong information control, helped shape Chinese political corruption in ways quite different from those of the west. Kwong, for example, believes this affects Chinese corruption in five ways:

> First, the dependence on the higher authority for resources encouraged managers to inflate their needs to obtain more supplies. Second, the strong pressure to conform encouraged them and their subordinates to fabricate reports on their achievements to please those above. Third, the ability of supervisors to dispense resources offered opportunities for bribes – subordinates would give anything to get what they needed. Fourth, the control of resources also offered administrators opportunities to use them for their own benefit. And fifth, the people's dependence on these officials discouraged them from reporting illegal activities, thus increasing the anonymity of corrupt officials . . . every level of every ministry tried to minimize its responsibilities and maximize its resources.
>
> (Kwong 1997: 54)

This chapter is divided into the periods between the 1949 Revolution and the death of Mao Zedong in 1976, and the socialist market period from 1976 to the present. Within this framework for the most part it proceeds chronologically. This is for two reasons. First, most readers will not be China specialists and will require basic information as well as analysis. Second, it is impossible in China to separate political corruption from political structure and activity. Though Chinese ideology consistently claims that corruption must be viewed individualistically, this argument does not stand up to serious analysis: on the contrary, political corruption emerges precisely from the Chinese polity. Hence, though this book is about political corruption, this chapter addresses also the politics *of* corruption in China as the only means of grasping its Hydra-headed character.

Corruption in the classical communist period (1949–1976)

> to kill only mosquitoes and flies, but not fight tigers.
> (Contemporary comment on *San-fan* and *Wu-fan*, Mao's anti-corruption
> campaigns of 1951–1952)

Prior to 1949 corruption was endemic, and public cynicism about the predatory character of the Kuomintang (KMT) government contributed significantly to Mao Zedong's success in mobilizing mass support. For example, in the latter stages of the Republican period (1911–1949) offices were openly bought and sold as business propositions; families of the purchasers were placed in lucrative jobs; and additional levies were exacted from those wishing to receive a public service. Instances exist of taxes being demanded twenty years ahead of the due date, and of junior staff being forced either to work unpaid in their manager's private interest or to pay a fee to be permitted not to do so. Complaints were rare but, when made, further bribes were normally able to buy the silence of senior officials (Kwong 1997: 79–81).

In the classical communist period it was virtually impossible to distinguish either between political and administrative corruption or between political corruption and the political process. The parallel horizontal structures between Party and state and the vertical power structures which determined the character of local control right down to the village unit left neither space for, nor concept of, civil society. In a situation where not only economic crime but also simple profit-making were deemed acts of theft from the people, western distinctions between legitimate commercial activities, torts and crimes were meaningless. All forms of enterprise were self-evidently counter-revolutionary political acts demanding a political response. Any suggestion that their legality or otherwise was determinable by independent investigation and adjudication would have been judged not only absurd but itself counter-revolutionary. In such a political context every act is judged through the filter of orthodoxy, every departure from it deemed an error demanding expiation and correction.

Corruption under Mao, therefore, had to address this reality. The dangers involved in displaying sudden wealth gravitated against pecuniary corruption. The character of the commune system encouraged collective corruption from which all members of a work unit benefited. The associational aspects of the traditional concept of *guanxi*[3] invited, with a strength that defies translation, nepotistic or reciprocal corruption such as banqueting, drinking and gambling. Inevitably this breeds corruption:

> to run even a legal business or obtain basic services, networks have to be
> 'gratified'. . . . In order to ensure supplies, promote sales, and maintain
> long-term contractual relationships, some work units give gifts and

favorable terms of trade to others . . . managers give 'gifts' and banquets to officials whose help might be needed in future. . . . One work unit spent 365,000 yuan to organize 219 banquets in one year. Although these practices are a form of embezzlement, they are directly linked to the imperatives of *guanxi*.

(Hao and Johnston 2002: 594)

In an era lacking any concept of privacy, corruption naturally lost much of its clandestinity, assuming rather the character of a conspiracy, either among corrupt partners or between the players of roles which in the west would be designated 'perpetrator' and 'victim'. 'Victims' were also in all probability perpetrators further down the line, but even if they were not their response would be more likely to be a resigned shrug or a torrent of private oaths than an official complaint. Partly this was because, for all the Beijing-inspired campaigns designed to undermine the culture of deference and to report the depredations of one's superiors, there was seldom anyone sufficiently trustworthy to complain to. But primarily it was because the situation was one of privation not deprivation: that was simply the way things were and always had been.

Feudal restrictions on individual liberty for the most part slid effortlessly into Mao's proletarian dictatorship. In other respects, however, Mao sought to rid the country of its imperial and Confucian heritage. A land in which Confucian ideas – respect for one's superiors, the idealization of the family, the near God-like status of teachers and intellectuals – were dominant was not exactly fertile ground for his central ideas of permanent revolution and unremitting class struggle. Equally, *guanxi* was bound to lead to partiality in employment and procurement as well as to nepotism, maintaining the blurred boundaries between public duty and private interest such that the distinction between what was legal and what was not was seldom clear.

Such cultural traits, boosted by the inevitable periodic hits of *tang-yi pao-dan*, the sugar-coated bullets of contemporary capitalism, would challenge the creation of the kind of state to which Mao, to the end as much a dangerous romantic as an authoritarian moralist, aspired for China. Achieving scientific socialism by means of permanent revolution constituted the prime political objective of the classical communist period and the consideration underlying Mao's seemingly incessant political campaigns.

Corruption attracted strong condemnation, but primarily because Mao regarded it both as part of the 'filth and poison' of the past and as a symptom of the contemporary dangers of *tang-yi pao-dan*. It followed that the corrupt required both punishment, often administered in public for the dual purpose of shaming the miscreant and confirming the class consciousness of the punishers, and re-education by ideological instruction. Accordingly anti-corruption campaigns were designed only incidentally to deal with individual corrupt acts. Mainly they served broader political ends by striking at the root cause, capitalist contamination, thereby contributing to the attainment of the perfect, objectively correct, scientific socialist state.

It is this intermeshing of corruption and politics in Mao's China that helped give political corruption its particular inflexion. China lacked not only a clear cultural distinction between public and private but also the political and organizational distinctions embedded in the separation-of-powers doctrine. The particular nature of Chinese corruption is highlighted in Mao's subjugation of both economic and judicial considerations to the class struggle. The dreadful consequences of the subordination of economics to politics are not central concerns for this book, but the relation between law and politics is, since the nature of the legal system was fundamental to Mao's enterprise.

One of Mao's early ambitions was to purge from office as many former KMT officials as possible. Many KMT adherents were continuing their former corrupt practices while also infecting communist officials, so damaging the Revolution's moral purity and hence continued success. The 1951 Statute on the Suppression of Counter-Revolutionary Crimes was accordingly intended to remove unrepentant KMT dissidents and to suppress, by execution or by re-education in 'reform through labour' institutions, hundreds of thousands of supposed enemies of the state. These included not only political dissidents but intellectuals[4] as defined by the Ideological Reform Campaign, and members of both the bourgeoisie and religious organizations. The Campaign heightened previous practice rather than introducing something new, however: in 1950 for example there had been some 30,000 mass trials in Beijing alone, probably attended by some 3.4 million people (Brugger and Reglar 1994: 185).

Meanwhile in rural areas Mao had launched his Agrarian Reform Law in 1950. This entailed the confiscation of land and its redistribution among poor peasants, the denunciation of corrupt or criminal landlords in *pidou* or 'speak bitterness' meetings, mass trials, the execution of 1 to 2 million landlords[5] and the murder of many more by the peasants. This activity was condoned by Mao in his 'not correcting excesses prematurely' policy. The programme succeeded in redistributing 43 per cent of cultivated land to 60 per cent of the rural population (Teiwes 1997: 36).[6]

In 1952 Mao introduced a Statute of Penalties for Corruption (*tanwu*). This statute was concerned with the seizure, theft, fraud or appropriation of state property, using extortion to obtain another's property, accepting bribes and any other activities that involved using one's position to benefit oneself. In short, officials who crossed the boundaries separating the public from the private were guilty of corruption (Kwong 1997: 12).

The counter-revolutionary and anti-corruption statutes remained the only public legal documents on criminal justice for more than two decades (Kwong 1997: 7), becoming the springboard for Mao's first two anti-corruption campaigns. The Three Antis (*San-fan*), which began in December

1951, was launched to fight the three evils of corruption, waste and bureaucracy. The Five Antis (*Wu-fan*) of 1952 was designed to attack the five evils of bribery, tax evasion, theft of state property, cheating on government contracts and stealing state economic information. Mao later also said that these campaigns could not have been started without the agrarian reform policy, which had increased proletarian solidarity and destroyed much of the political status, psychological security and economic base of counter-revolutionary elements.

Meanwhile, popular feeling about political and administrative corruption was being carefully fanned through the media. *Renmin Ribao* (*The People's Daily*, still today the official organ of the Party's Central Committee) had just reported 1,670 cases of corruption in different departments of state. Soon afterwards 15,000 cases in Sichuan Province were exposed. High-profile criminals included district Party secretaries in Tianjin, and the Mayor of Wuhan and his deputies (Kwong 1997: 82). *San-fan* was directed at Party members and particularly cadres[7] as well as state officials (not all of whom were Party members, though the proportions that were increased steadily throughout the 1950s).[8] *Wu-fan* was directed at private businessmen.

Neither of these campaigns was targeted only or even mainly at specific provable acts of corruption. More importantly, they were designed to remoralize the populace, to weaken powerful elements which might in future pose a threat to state security, and to strengthen the class unity and hence political allegiance of the people. *San-fan*'s main targets included urban cadres in contact with bourgeois and overseas influences (and therefore most susceptible to *tang-yi pao-dan*) and intellectuals.

The thought reform policy, *sixiang gaizao*, later to be taken to its logical conclusion by the Cultural Revolution, entailed newspaper-reading teams being sent to workplaces to inform workers about the campaign and to lead compulsory 'speak bitterness' meetings. In these meetings passivity was not permitted, and repeated confessions of previous errors of thought were demanded with increasing degrees of vitriol. Family members who denounced family members and workers who denounced employers were praised; those who failed to do so (and their families) were punished both formally and, by public stigmatization, informally. Consistent with the principle of mass justice, the proletariat was also involved in interrogations, trials and punishment, an involvement designed to achieve the further political purpose of weakening Chinese cultural traits such as unquestioning respect for superiors (Teiwes 1997: 39). *San-fan*

> acted as a status-degrading ceremony. Those regarded as 'corrupt' by the CCP [Chinese Communist Party] were condemned at mass meetings. Even their family members and relatives were urged to denounce them. The CCP stressed that wives had the obligation to denounce the wrong-doings of their husbands, and children of their parents. . . . Those attending the broadcast trials were instigated to condemn the culprits

before they were sentenced to death or long-term imprisonment. . . . The proceedings were intended to undermine the status of the class enemy and to mobilize the masses in the accusation process. As a consequence of this 'mass line' supervision, the proletariat became educated in the essential elements of class struggle.

(Lo 1993: 25)

Wu-fan was boosted by official visits to homes and workplaces designed to mobilize the workers. Street corner loudspeakers were set up to communicate directly with the illiterate masses, both to arouse the people's consciousness of class struggle and to increase the pressure on capitalists and other counter-revolutionaries. All businesses were ranked on a five-point scale, from 'law-abiding' to 'completely law-breaking', on the basis of decisions made in mass meetings, committee meetings and private interrogations by *Wu-fan* committees and proletarian teams under their control:

The 'most serious cases' were turned over to special revolutionary People's Tribunals . . . empowered to make arrests and to pass sentences, which could include specification of sums of money to be repaid to the government, fines, confiscation of property, 'surveillance', 'reform through labor', prison terms, and death. Any death sentence, or prison sentences over ten years, required higher approval, however.

(Barnett 1964: 142)[9]

Enhancing the power of the Party by eliminating dissident elements was considered crucial in the immediate post-revolutionary period. Corruption trials helped create a climate stressing workers' duty to report corrupt officials to the authorities. The campaigns had three main political purposes and consequences. *First*, they achieved a dramatic increase in proletarian solidarity and Party loyalty, moving the still-to-be-won class struggle to the centre of popular consciousness. This enabled the campaigns to produce a crop of young leaders to be harvested by the Party later in the decade. The strengthening of trades unions in the workplace and the creation of CCP branches there also provided the state with permanent sources of intelligence about the crimes of capitalists (Teiwes 1997: 40). *Second*, the fines and confiscations imposed on businessmen under *Wu-fan* were substantial: they have been estimated (very roughly indeed) as providing up to 10 per cent of the state's total budget for fiscal year 1952–1953 (Barnett 1964: 159). This income was vital during the economic chaos of the post-revolutionary period, particularly given that the national economy had been further weakened by the cost of military involvement in the Korean War, a conflict into which Mao had unenthusiastically stumbled. *Third*, while the financial penalties weakened the capitalists' economic base, violent attacks and unremitting propaganda weakened their physical and psychological security.

This is said to have led to some 200,000 suicides in addition to the 500,000 apparently resulting from the Statute on the Suppression of Counter-Revolutionary Crimes (Teiwes 1997: 37).

The softening of the bourgeoisie's economic base and morale enabled the Party to introduce a policy of 'state economy helping private economy'. This policy, whose precondition was the collapse of capitalist enterprise, involved the state recycling the capitalists' fines to purchase bargain basement share stock from, make loans to, and place orders with, private enterprises in difficulty, so securing sufficient leverage to ensure compliance with its philosophy and policies. Taming capitalism was a necessary step on the road to its destruction, so the public–private partnerships resulting from *Wu-fan* constituted a significant contribution towards achieving Mao's revolutionary ends.

In 1956 the Hundred Flowers Campaign was introduced. This was optimistically envisaged as an educative process which, by inviting new ideas (the hundred flowers being allowed to bloom) and intellectual critique, would demonstrate rationally the objective superiority of Mao's brand of Marxism-Leninism.[10] The agitation resulting from this Campaign, however, taught Mao that dissidents and potential counter-revolutionaries permeated all population strata.[11] Understandably, therefore, the Hundred Flowers gave way to the Anti-Rightist (or Rectification) Campaign of 1957. In the cities the Rectification Campaign entailed up to 500,000 suspected rightist elements, including many intellectuals (whom, contrary to the Confucian tradition, Mao had always regarded with suspicion), being sent to the countryside for hard labour (*xiafang*) or required to perform ostentatiously humiliating and 'face-losing' jobs. Hence many reports exist of, for example, professors being demoted to lavatory cleaners at their own universities.[12] In rural areas the Campaign concentrated on those who had questioned the wisdom of agricultural collectivization.

These activities led on to the Great Leap Forward of 1958, designed to maximize peasant and worker productivity. This was to be achieved by distinctively Chinese means rather than by the former Soviet approach of the Five Year Plan which, to First Secretary Khrushchev's chagrin, was peremptorily discarded. The Leap saw over 120 million households belonging to 740,000 agricultural collectives reorganized into 26,000 people's communes, which were to remain the basic political unit in rural China until 1984 (Kwong 1997: 39).

The economic logic of this was that by combining households into communes, economies of scale in agricultural production would maximize the efficiency of human labour and facilitate the use of scarce machinery. The political logic was to create a single unit of human existence by combining the political, administrative, military and economic apparatuses, so weakening rival organizations such as private enterprise and the family (Schram 1966: 294). However, unrealistic targets were set, figures were concocted to claim success in meeting them, and lack of expertise among

the peasants charged with tasks such as iron smelting or agricultural production led to tragi-comic chaos. For example, a campaign to kill birds (because
they ate the grain) was so successful that a plethora of insects survived to eat
it instead. Additionally, the poverty of China's transport and communications infrastructure meant that grain frequently failed to arrive at its
intended place of consumption (Wright 1989: 44). In fact it is now known
that agricultural output in 1960 was only 75.5 per cent of that of 1958 and
that light and heavy industrial output similarly declined steeply year on
year up to 1962. The result was 'the most devastating famine of the twentieth
century in China (and probably in the world)' (Lieberthal 1997: 110).
Estimates as to the number of deaths vary enormously, but the total is
unlikely to have been fewer than 20 million and may have been as high as
50 million.

Intellectuals were pressured to become propagandists, while creative
artists, many of whom had learned to write in deniable historical metaphor,
were either a cog and screw in the revolutionary machine or poisonous
weeds in need of uprooting (Brugger and Reglar 1994: 233). Senior cadres
(*lingdao ganbu*) had all-embracing political, economic and social functions,
providing their members with employment, housing, eating facilities, health
care and education, as well as being responsible for dealing with infractions
such as minor criminality and breaches of Party discipline. So ordinary
members became totally dependent on the commune and, in particular, on
the *lingdao ganbu* whose authority over them was all encompassing:

> authorization from the work unit was required to travel, to buy a train
> ticket, to check into a hotel, to get married, to transfer to another
> work unit, to locate to another area, and, depending on the population
> policy of the time, to have a child . . . because these authorizations,
> opportunities, and amenities were granted by one's immediate super-
> visor, there was a strong inducement for the staff to follow his/her
> directives.
>
> (Kwong 1997: 53)

Following the economic and political chaos of the Leap Mao's political
stock fell sharply and a period of doubt and questioning set in, with intellectuals increasingly able to exercise critical freedom. Mao, however, began to
reaffirm his authority at a crucial month-long Party conference in Lushan
in 1959, where he purged his openly critical Defence Minister, Peng Dehuai,
for 'right opportunism' and conspiring with his Soviet foe Khrushchev
(Saich 1981: 39–44).

Mao had largely re-established his former supremacy by 1962, however,
and the following year he boldly reasserted the centrality of the class struggle
when he launched his third anti-corruption campaign, the 'Four Cleans'
(*Siqing*, or the Socialist Education Movement). This was targeted initially
at how cadres determined work points, kept accounts, distributed supplies

and handled warehouses and granaries. This campaign, generally regarded as a direct antecedent of the Cultural Revolution, again stressed Mao's belief that corruption was attributable to bourgeois tendencies among inadequately supervised landlords and rich peasants. It led to an open power struggle with State President Liu Shaoqi and other revisionists, ostensibly over the question of whether corruption was itself a proper and necessary target for intervention or, as Mao continued to believe, a mere epiphenomenon of subversive or counter-revolutionary tendencies.

Liu (to be insultingly dubbed 'China's Khrushchev' at the time of his purge during the Cultural Revolution) and his wife Wang Guangmei had spent time studying conditions in the countryside. Liu had been in Henan Province, while Wang had for five months stayed incognito in a commune near her native city of Tianjin:

> They ascertained that corruption was widespread and that many basic-level cadres opposed the Party (as did a large percentage of the peasants) . . . they felt that counterrevolution had a grip on a large portion of rural China and that draconian measures would be necessary to rescue the situation. Mao may well have agreed with this diagnosis – but he subsequently disagreed strongly with the measures taken to effect a cure.
>
> (Lieberthal 1997: 138)

Liu boldly, not to say recklessly, followed up this research with the publication of his 'Revised Later Ten Points' in September 1964. This concentrated on bureaucratic corruption among the ordinary cadres, *yiban ganbu*, heavily protected by the patronage system and supported by Mao himself, whom he accused of personal extravagance (normally categorized as *bu zheng zhi feng*, or inappropriate bourgeois behaviour), mammonism, bribery, extortion, misappropriation of funds and nepotism. Mao responded furiously by attacking Liu's 'apparently leftist, but in fact rightist' line. *First*, he objected to Liu's concentration on corruption at the expense of the need for broader rectification. *Second*, he objected to the harsh penalties to be imposed on the *yiban ganbu*, whose exposed corruption, since overseas capitalists could scarcely be blamed for it, clearly threatened the edifice of his scientific socialism. *Third*, he objected to work teams being parachuted in to supervise cadres contrary to the Mao Zedong Thought doctrine that rectification should emerge from the masses. In his 'Twenty-Three Articles' of January 1965, ignoring Liu's and Wang's evidence he reaffirmed the centrality of class struggle and extended the focus of *Siqing* to politics, economics, ideology and organization. This explicitly transformed an anti-corruption campaign into a full-blown political and ideological movement; and, in a particularly bold tactic, he extended the class struggle by identifying even upper-middle peasants as enemies of the people.

In 1966 Mao began the process of creating the structures by which *Siqing* could be intensified and incorporated into the Great Proletarian Cultural Revolution.[13] This saw Party and state administrations dismantled and replaced by revolutionary committees made up of representatives of the proletariat in an attempt 'to purify the country of inequality, corruption, and elitism through mass mobilization' (Harding 1997: 247). Tens of thousands of cadres and their family members were executed or re-educated under a renewed and vigorous *xiafang* policy; many senior politicians, including Liu Shaoqi and Deng Xiaoping, were purged. In the midst of the ensuing chaos, though after the brutal excesses of the Red Guard phase which ended in 1969, the Tenth National Congress of 1973 was reminded that:

> In 1966 . . . Chairman Mao already pointed out, 'Great disorder across the land leads to great order. And so once again every seven or eight years. Monsters and demons will jump out themselves. Determined by their own class nature, they are bound to jump out.' The living reality of class struggle has confirmed and will continue to confirm this objective law . . . to constantly consolidate the dictatorship of the proletariat and seize new victories for the socialist cause, it is necessary to deepen the socialist revolution in the ideological, political and economic spheres, to transform all those parts of the superstructure that do not conform to the socialist economic base and carry out many political revolutions such as the Great Proletarian Cultural Revolution.
>
> (Wang 1973: 45–46)

The years between the Leap and the associated rift with the Soviet Union in 1958, on the one hand, and on the other the death of Mao and the arrest of the Gang of Four in 1976, are the apotheosis of Mao's experiment in classical communism with a Chinese flavour.[14] At this time petty corruption, from senior officials to village cadres, was virtually ubiquitous, and, though certainly not popular, a fact of life played out by local unwritten rules and generally accepted fatalistically if not uncomplainingly. Corruption continued throughout to be officially promulgated as individual criminality stemming from lack of ideological purity (such as the pursuit of private wealth), not as an institutional or systemic problem. Mao's 1965 response to Liu's 'Revised Later Ten Points' indicates clearly his view that concentrating on corruption as criminality was a revisionist ploy designed to direct attention away from the task of rectifying the ideological error of which corruption was but a concrete manifestation.

The path towards this conclusion had begun to be cut during the immediate post-revolutionary period. The abolition of lawyers and the creation of a legal system appropriate to a one-party state[15] in the 1950s had led to an approach to corruption largely unconcerned with such minutiae as the burden of proof. Mao's early attempts to construct a legal system based on the Soviet model quickly gave way to informal and ad hoc measures driven by unpublished and frequently ignored laws and regulations. The process which ultimately led to the effective abolition of the legal profession had begun with an anti-lawyer campaign in 1952 closely associated with *Wu-fan*, and culminated in 1957 when the Rectification Campaign imposed criminal sanctions on uncooperative judges and defence lawyers guilty of taking their clients' side against the state.[16] The abolition of the Ministry of Justice had followed in 1959, when legal personnel were sent to conduct speedy and summary trials jointly with local cadres, and local mediation committees were instituted to deal with petty criminality. Following the Leap, communes and adjudication committees in the work units (*danwei*) had assumed law's everyday discursive functions of moralizing and educating. The power of *lingdao ganbu* (senior cadres) as sole providers of life's necessities meant they were well placed to undertake broad-based surveillance and corrective duties and to impose sanctions ranging from small fines or reparative penalties to expulsion from the Party or demotion at work. More serious political crimes were dealt with either in secret or, conversely, in mass educative trials.

Law as an activity lacked status, esteem and hence connections; law as a system was concerned less with proof of infraction than with the correction of a lifestyle potentially damaging to the harmony of Party and state. In communist Chinese jurisprudence the idea that the law functioned to protect civil society against the state simply and literally made no sense. As no separate civil society existed, law's function was to further the interests of the state by representing the proletariat in the class struggle waged against capitalists and their running dogs, as well as against errant comrades hit by *tang-yi pao-dan*. The idea of law as protecting individual rights was redolent of the contract-based commercial exchange necessitated by capitalism's unique contradictions and alienation, and was by definition inapplicable in a one-class and therefore legitimately one-party state.

The main function of the legal system hence became the political one of strengthening the unity of Party, state and people. Administrative codes warned against dereliction of duty, false accusations, shifting blame, living lavishly and other bourgeois activities. The 1957 Regulations on Reward and Punishment of State Administrative Personnel, for example, had inveighed against behaviour such as gluttony, drunkenness, gambling, deceit and sexual impropriety on or off duty. As private ownership was prohibited and displays of ostentatious wealth dangerous, corruption frequently assumed a non-pecuniary character, with officials spending state resources on lavish banquets, luxurious offices and spacious official residences. The 'iron rice bowl' policy of a job for life precluded both competition and effective reward and sanction. This, combined with Mao's regrettable failure to create such political conditions as would have remoulded human nature into a state of prelapsarian innocence, effectively guaranteed the proliferation of the very sins his policies were intended to eradicate: endemic underperformance, laziness, absenteeism, deceit, uncompetitiveness and waste.

Many corrupt acts committed by officials were designed to secure benefits for their work units rather than (or as well as) themselves. The offence of *benweizhuyi*, or departmentalism, involved putting the interests of one's own department ahead of those of the larger collective. This normally entailed exaggerating performance, so enabling one's department (and hence oneself) to bask in the glory of being the first to meet one's quotas, so cheating honest comrades of their just recognition. Alternatively it led to quantities of raw materials or commodities (steel and concrete were especially attractive) being 'lost' in the accounts and stockpiled for private sale for the benefit of the commune or individuals within it. Fines for underperformance could often be similarly lost by bribing state inspectors.

The line between unacceptable nepotism and the cultural importance of reciprocity in Chinese culture was impossible to draw definitively, particularly in the absence of the forensic skills and independence characteristic of western judicial systems. This was particularly so since, for all Mao's efforts to mobilize the peasantry and workers against landlords and employers, in traditional Chinese society senior people remained entitled to many privileges and were subject to minimal levels of scrutiny (Kwong 1997: 17–18). Accordingly the Chinese political economy under classical communism lent itself to a mode of corruption both pervasive and elusive, and to particularistic and politically motivated modes of scrutiny reflecting, if not the macro-politics of Beijing, then the micro-politics of village gossip and malice.

Corruption became the norm, but the line between corruption and non-corruption remained unclear. Corruption was popularly repudiated, but reciprocity and subservience continued to be applauded. There were no independent legal or audit system and no free media. The People's Armed Police was underpaid and institutionally corrupt. All-powerful and effectively unaccountable leaders were regarded with fear and respect. In the absence of a private sector, or even of any concept of personal economics, all corruption was officially defined as theft from the people, and pursuing profit became a politically subversive act. In such a context corruption itself and all responses to it could only be political. The corrupt were perceived to be such not because of system failure but because they had been hit by *tang-yi pao-dan*, capitalism's sugar-coated bullets.

Corruption, therefore, was above all a symptom of wrong thinking. While of itself it deserved condign retributive punishment, where the offence was non-capital the attack on the cause also demanded political re-education, both for individual reformation and general deterrence. So by this logic a western response based on a given burden of proof and individualistic sentencing principles of, say, proportionality and equity or gravity and intent would have been nonsensical. The only function of punishment in this context was to strike at those forms of corruption presented by the leadership as objectively the most damaging to the Chinese polity. Hence when, on a utilitarian calculus, punishing individuals was deemed detrimental to the interests of the state, offenders would remain unpunished;

and these offenders were almost invariably the most powerful or well connected. In Mao Zedong Thought the larger unit is always more important than the smaller units of which it is composed, and this can entail sacrificing the individual for the greater good. To think otherwise is to make the objective error of bourgeois individualism.

Corruption under the socialist market (1976 to the present)

> It does not matter whether a cat is black or white, so long as it catches mice.
> (Deng Xiaoping)

> It doesn't matter whether the cat is black or white, it doesn't even matter whether the cat can catch mice. What matters is that the cat does not get caught.
> (Hinton 1990)

Politically, the years immediately following Mao's death were primarily taken up with the establishment of the succession. The Gang of Four, including Mao's controversial third wife Jiang Qing, were arrested and tried. A stopgap leader, Hua Guofeng, supposedly Mao's chosen heir,[17] became Party Chairman and Premier. In his Two Whatevers policy (whatever Mao said had to be obeyed and whatever Mao decided had to be upheld), Hua embarked on an attempt to reconcile Mao's theories with the modernizing ambitions of Zhou Enlai. Deng Xiaoping, meanwhile, destined to be the dominant figure in Chinese politics for the next decade, was rehabilitating himself after his dismissal by the Gang of Four in 1976. His main concerns were to consolidate his power base with the People's Liberation Army, secure the election of his associates to the Politburo and its Standing Committee, and undermine Hua. So Deng explicitly repudiated the Whateverists, advancing instead the ostensibly pragmatic but in fact Mao-hostile slogan, 'Practice is the sole criterion for testing truth'.[18]

Hua was forced to resign first as Premier in 1980 (his replacement was another liberal, Zhao Ziyang) then, in 1981, as Chairman of the Central Committee and the Military Affairs Commission. Here he was replaced by, respectively, Hu Yaobang, after Deng Xiaoping the decade's most significant figure, and Deng himself, whose seniority Hu explicitly, and certainly not spontaneously, acknowledged in his acceptance speech. From now until the 1989 disturbances Deng's political dominance went largely unquestioned.

It would be wrong to regard Deng's political and economic approach as simply a repudiation of Maoist dogma. In fact Deng, though possessing in abundance the survivor's ability to be the first to test the wind and then blow with it, was rather a conservative figure, no more an enthusiast for the capitalist road than he was the political visionary some have implied. His era was characterized by equivocation and inconsistency, as well as by the ruthless discarding of both allies and loyal but less politically nimble subordinates. Many of his utterances presented economic liberalization as a necessary evil to enable China to compete internationally; and as late as 1985 he was ruling out the possibility of wholesale departures from socialism (Baum 1997: 372). One scholar characterizes this, perhaps a little imaginatively, as a traditionally Chinese *fang-shou* (relax and control) cycle:

> As early as the spring of 1979 . . . this ambivalent pattern of relaxation and control, *fang* and *shou*, began to display recurrent, periodic fluctuations and phase changes . . . characterized by an initial increase in the scope of economic or political reform (in the form, e.g., of price deregulation or intellectual liberalization), followed by a rapid release of pent-up social demand (e.g., panic buying or student demonstrations); the resulting 'disorder' would set off a backlash among party traditionalists, who would then move to reassert control.
>
> (Baum 1997: 341)

Hu Yaobang was an able, but irascible and unpredictable man, prone to errors of judgement at home and abroad. He had longstanding enemies, and his unfortunate tendency to collect more, including powerful ones, was exemplified in his refusal to intervene to prevent the execution for corruption of a young relative of President Li Xiannian in 1986 – a grave breach of *guanxi*. This only increased the hostility towards him of the Party gerontocracy, most significantly Deng, who was anyway becoming increasingly concerned about Hu's growing westernization. When in 1987 Deng made a speech widely read as a veiled attack on Hu, his enemies exerted mounting pressure for his dismissal for six 'crimes' including political rightism and economic irresponsibility. A few months later the Politburo replaced Hu as General Secretary with Zhao Ziyang (Baum 1997: 399–401).

We return to Hu later, when we describe events leading to the Tiananmen Square incident. It is now time, however, to explain the economic changes affecting China up to 1987, and the nature of their impact on corruption in an era when, in Hu's own phrase, formerly applied only to revolutionary martyrs and their families, 'to get rich is glorious'.

Deng's policy of economic liberalization at home and an 'open door' to international trade and commerce, initially via the four original Special Economic Zones, involved a dramatic departure from the previous control economy. This policy had been approved at a historic meeting of the Party's Central Committee in December 1978, when the main task was identified as economic development, not political struggle. Beginning with experimental worker bonus systems instituted by Zhao Ziyang, initially in Deng's home province of Sichuan (Saich 1981: 168–169), the new processes of decentralization, increasing reliance upon market forces and acceptance of the private economy profoundly affected the political system. The policy, which combined a less regulated economy with a largely unchanged totalitarian political system, the 'socialist market', was to initiate unparalleled economic growth and political turmoil. Naturally it also created previously unimaginable opportunities for economic exploitation, particularly by cadres, including, through decentralization, lower-level ones than hitherto. Because cadres retained key decision-making powers in procurement, for example, it has even been suggested that they were among the main beneficiaries of Deng's reforms (Hao 1999: 407).

Though Party and state were intertwined from central government through neighbourhoods, villages and individual work units down to individual families, the theory of state control was daily confronted by the reality of chaos and deviance. Even Mao's centralism had seldom offered an effective mode of government, and often in the provinces during the classical communist period it had been said with a shrug that '*shan gao huangdi yuan*', or 'the mountains are high and the Emperor is far away'. Deng's policy of simultaneously maintaining a one-party state, decentralizing political power and encouraging selective economic liberalization was clearly challenging, both to explain and to follow. This is particularly so since 'whenever the central government fears even a temporary loss of control over some aspect of China's economy or society, its first impulse is to recentralize' (Feinerman 2000: 313).

In 1982 the Twenty-second Plenary Session of the Standing Committee of the Fifth National People's Congress passed the 'Decision on Severe Punishment of Serious Economic Crimes'. In his Party Rectification Campaign (*Zhengdang*) of 1983–1986 Deng aimed to purge the Party of corrupt and decadent elements.[19] Emergency measures were introduced to ensure swift and severe punishment, with responsibility for cases involving murder, robbery, rape, bombing, arson and sabotage devolved to provincial Higher People's Courts (Woo 2000: 183). The main political goal, however, was to censure

> factionalism and leftism together with corruption. As the latter crime was so rampant in the bureaucracy, the censure of corruption could be used selectively to denounce those factionalists and leftists whose errors could not be established due to difficulties in obtaining past evidence on their relationships with the Gang of Four.
>
> (Lo 1993: 50)

The campaign began with a significant attack on crime of all kinds by Premier Zhao Ziyang, certainly at Deng's behest. In his speech to the Sixth NPC in 1983 Zhao broadened his attack on increased street crime to embrace corruption by cadres, and called for strong measures to deal with all criminals, naturally including counter-revolutionaries. Leading cadres in particular had lost much of their traditional status and perquisites under liberalization, and had increasingly adopted western styles of corruption, including bribery and embezzlement. The ensuing campaign involved the attenuation of the rights of defendants, mass trials, truncated appeals and summary executions (Baum 1997: 354); but at its heart was a reworking of Mao's *tang-yi pao-dan* theory that corruption stemmed from incorrect thinking as a result of bourgeois influence.

Maintaining an authoritarian power structure, albeit of an unprecedentedly decentralized kind, while encouraging economic liberalization created two parallel but symbiotic economies. State-owned enterprises (SOEs) maintained responsibility for major products such as power, natural resources and commodities such as steel and cement, while the burgeoning private sector manufactured other goods but was necessarily dependent on the power sources and raw materials which remained the province of the SOEs. SOEs, however, were slow, inefficient, subject to poor quality audit and increasingly large budgetary deficits. Their workers were underpaid in relation to private sector staff and hence resentful, fearful for their jobs (a new experience following the abandonment of Mao's iron rice bowl policy) and of low morale. Accordingly they were more than willing participants in bribery, embezzlement and extortion.

Deng's decision to manage these parallel economies by a dual pricing system led, particularly during the high inflation and economic growth of the early 1980s, to many opportunities for corruption, with raw materials being traded repeatedly at escalating prices without ever leaving the warehouse. Buying at low state prices (through bribery) and selling high on the commercial market (with generous discounts), with the spoils divided among senior employees, became commonplace. This had strongly negative economic consequences. In 1983 the state collected 890,000 tons less steel than stipulated in the central plan, yet 330,000 tons were available in the market (Kwong 1997: 97).

Deng's attempts, from the mid-1980s, to reverse these problems by phasing out dual pricing had catastrophic consequences, including mass withdrawals of savings, panic buying, a run on consumer durables and the denuding of currency reserves by the importation of luxury goods. The government's response, printing money, led inevitably to yet higher price inflation not only of luxury goods but also of staples such as food and rent. From 1985 protests by workers, intellectuals and students against inflation, corruption, economic inequity, human rights abuses and the absence of intellectual freedom led to unrest of a kind not seen in Chinese cities since the late 1970s. Crime of all kinds again escalated and in 1985 alone a million new security personnel were recruited. This was followed by a further crackdown in 1986, using the familiar techniques of 'mass trials, heavy sentences, perfunctory appeals, and, in the most severe cases, immediate executions' (Baum 1997: 386). Very unusually, given that relatives of high-ranking officials (*gaogan zidi*) were normally exempted from severe punishment, a relative of President Li Xiannian was among those executed in the face of the President's unsuccessful plea to General Secretary Hu Yaobang to intervene. Hu, as we have seen (on p. 80), was to pay a high price for this decision.

Corruption was further stoked by the decentralization to the provinces of key elements of administration, including policing and tax levying. In the case of taxation the provinces entrusted collection of sometimes complex and discretionary taxes to low-ranking personnel, so that paying taxes often became in practice optional. Quite apart from the economic consequences for the state, this extended corruption from leading cadres, traditionally unaccountable on the Confucian ground of seniority, to administrative or even ordinary ones. Corruption networks became common, and fines levied by cadres (few crimes were processed judicially) for economic crimes were usually discountable by bribery. Hence the conjunction of increasingly westernized modes of corruption and traditional Chinese social relations created an inexorable expansionist logic, reciprocal favours both increasing the numbers of people involved and tying them into a *guanxi* network (Kwong 1997: 99).

Inevitably, economic liberalization introduced such 'evils of capitalism' as smuggling, speculation, fraud and rampant corruption as well as further political destabilization. The effects on the newly affluent eastern seaboard Special Economic Zones such as Guangdong,[20] Hainan and Xiamen, where a Klondike mentality was readily visible, were predictable and obvious, though increasingly they permeated the country. By the same token permitting cadres greater economic freedom engineered not only numerous corrupt opportunities but a boom in the import of luxury goods, fuelling inflation yet further, diminishing China's foreign currency reserves and contributing to increasing budgetary deficits (van Kemenade 1997: 10). Yet a further problem was the punitive but complex and variable taxation levied by the state on private enterprises, liable for a profit tax of up to 55 per cent. This situation had been worsened by the decentralization of tax collection to local areas at the beginning of the reform era, a policy designed both to energize and create an income stream for provinces and sub-provincial units. In fact it denuded central government of revenue (Fewsmith 1997: 515–517),[21] leading to endemic underreporting of profits, tax evasion and bribery of (and in some cases violence against) tax collectors (Kwong 1997: 126). Decentralization also invited heightened low-level corruption:

> Low-ranking officials demand money for routine services such as stamping forms, which used to be free of charge. Maintenance and repairs of water pipes or telephones are no longer carried out without the payment of a bribe in addition to the service fee. In some of the smaller cities, the Public Utilities Company turns off the gas and electricity if 'special levies' are not paid on time.
>
> (van Kemenade 1997: 15)

The continued inadequacies of the legal system, meanwhile, continued to sustain high levels of corruption, ensuring that it was dealt with privately and by methods themselves frequently corrupt:

> Transgressions of administrative rules and sometimes even laws were handled internally by the work organization; administrators would refer legal cases to the courts only if they believed that the accused were guilty of serious offenses. . . . When rules were broken, the party secretary qua administrator was prosecutor, investigator, judge, and executor of justice all rolled into one. . . . This combination of the judicial roles and the administrator's discretionary power in meting out rewards and punishments made their authority unassailable.
>
> (Kwong 1997: 128)

By 1988 the economy was officially recognized as having spiralled virtually out of control. Many employers were paying unauthorized wage increases and bonuses. Policy proposals for the decontrol of urban rents were known to exist. In the rich south-eastern Guangdong Province, household purchasing power in the first quarter was 55 per cent higher than in the same quarter in 1987 (Baum 1997: 416). In consequence consumer demand for luxury goods fuelled inflation while the poor faced a significant decline in purchasing power. Vegetable prices rose by almost 50 per cent over the previous year, and whereas in 1985 food had accounted for 42 per cent of the average worker's spending, by 1988 this had risen to 60 per cent. Meanwhile there was growing panic among investors stemming from corruption and instability in the banking sector. These phenomena combined with a further surge in popular protest against political corruption and street crime to provoke yet further violent demonstrations. *Inside China Mainland* spoke of the inestimable damage to the CCP done by:

> The decay of party discipline, bribery and corruption, covering up for friends and relatives, deceiving and taking advantage of good cadres and party members, open violations of the law . . . being covered up through 'good connections' of various kinds.
>
> (cited by Baum 1997: 422)

In a foreshadowing of the events of 1989 there was increasing unrest among students protesting in favour of democratization and human rights, beginning in Anhui Province but followed by demonstrations in Shanghai, Beijing and elsewhere. It was Hu Yaobang's lenient approach to these disturbances which led to his replacement, with Deng's support, by Zhao Ziyang (Lo 1993: 57–58). In Beijing power struggles arose between conservatives, led by Li Peng, and liberals, including Zhao Ziyang and the Shanghainese future Premier Zhu Rongji. Deng, for the moment aligned with the liberal cause, secured agreement to widespread price liberalization of meat, sugar, eggs and vegetables, followed a few weeks later by cigarettes and alcohol. At the annual summer summit (1988) in the resort town of Beidaihe, however, conflicts increased, and, unusually, were reported in the official media. The ensuing articles were followed by rumours of further deregulation. These, combined with the fact that inflation, now running at over 20 per cent, was more than twice the level of interest rates, led to mass withdrawals of savings and panic buying. In the face of a scale of unrest which was to Party leaders disturbingly reminiscent of the rise of Solidarity in Gdansk, Deng now abandoned his *fides Achates* Zhao, supporting Li Peng and Vice-Premier Yao Yilin's demands for a price freeze and a slowdown in economic liberalization to 'rectify the economy'. Accordingly, in December price controls were reintroduced on thirty-six categories of goods.

Hu Yaobang, meanwhile, continued to enjoy strong popular support, including that of numerous students who attributed to him, not Deng, responsibility for rehabilitating several of the new generation of Chinese leaders, including Zhu Rongji (Becker 1998), and for promoting economic opportunity and human rights. Hu's sudden death of a heart attack on 15 April 1989 in the midst of the political unrest triggered an outpouring of popular venom against Deng, now widely reviled as a conservative influence.[22] On 24 April, students from twenty-one Beijing universities formed the Beijing Provisional Federation of Autonomous Students Associations as a vehicle for expressing their discontent. Later that day, during Zhao's absence in North Korea, Li Peng convened a Politburo Standing Committee meeting which approved a forthcoming hard-line editorial in *Renmin Ribao*, committed itself to a firm response to disorder and contemptuously dismissed the students as pawns of counter-revolutionaries.

Meanwhile signs of civil unrest were beginning to surface in a number of major provincial cities. Opinion polls showed majority support for the protesters' attacks on political corruption, and there were rumours of the formation of workers' protest movements to parallel and support the Provisional Federation. Within days, between 50,000 and 150,000 students were boycotting lectures and mounting anti-government protests. On 25 April the government refused to recognize the Federation, agreeing only to meet individual students from the prestigious Qinghua University, an offer peremptorily rejected by the demonstrators. On 4 May[23] a mass march took place, joined by several hundred journalists, whose influence was to increase in the ensuing weeks.

In the face of mounting protests, including a 3,000-student hunger strike commencing on 13 May, Zhao proposed publishing the incomes and emoluments of political leaders, and independently investigating allegations of *guandao* (profiteering by officials). The Politburo Standing Committee, however, aware that Zhao had lost Deng's support, voted him down. Zhao, now a desperate man, responded by obliquely attacking Deng for criticisms of the students made (partly as a face-saving measure) to Soviet First Secretary Gorbachev following a meeting in Beijing. On 18 May, Zhao and Li Peng went to meet the protesting students. Li left quickly, but, to his subsequent fury, Zhao stayed to talk to them sympathetically and apologetically, implying they were 'right'. Zhao resigned later that day; the next day Li Peng declared martial law.

On 4 June, when the troops, which had for some time been hovering in Beijing, moved into Tiananmen Square, the protests were focusing primarily on political and administrative corruption; but as events unfolded a much broader-based civil protest emerged. The deaths of an unknown number of student protesters,[24] combined with mass arrests as the protest movements were declared illegal, provide an exemplary case study of the consequences of lacking a democratic political forum and independent legal system within which to engage disorderly protest. In such a situation a zero-sum game was probably unavoidable.

In the short term the incident heralded the 'not hamstrung by details' policy, leading to the detention and punishment of numerous suspected counter-revolutionaries. In the longer term the resultant political trauma contributed to the emergence of a new generation of politicians, though not to a new political system. The emergent politicians included future President Jiang Zemin, a Shanghai anti-corruption activist who had replaced Zhao Ziyang, and his Shanghainese protégé Zhu Rongji.

An early consequence of the Tiananmen Square incident was the promotion of a new round of anti-crime, including corruption, campaigns. Badly shaken, as was the entire leadership, Deng made a conciliatory speech highlighting the need to catch and punish corrupt high-level officials. Meanwhile the Supreme People's Procuratorate claimed that three times as many corruption cases had been uncovered in 1989 as in 1988 (as well as a 30 per cent increase in common criminal cases). In the wake of this, and within days of the incident, Li Peng ordered a crackdown on corruption in specified provinces.

Meanwhile, Deng initiated a further anti-corruption campaign, led by Qiao Shi, a senior member of the Politburo's Standing Committee, this time targeting the 'ulcer' of official profiteering (*guandao*). Liberalization had led to the creation of around 360,000 new companies by 1987, of which 250,000 were believed to be acting to some degree corruptly. The opportunities offered by these companies led many cadres, with official encouragement, to plunge into the business sea (*xiahai*) with predictable results. Both *lingdao ganbu* and *gaogan zidi* (relatives of senior officials) manipulated their official and private roles, using their influence to favour companies with which they or their families were associated. Once again, however, virtually all the 330,000 prosecutions stemming from this campaign appear to have been, and certainly were popularly perceived as being, of 'small potatoes' only.

The campaign advanced quickly. In July the expulsion of hundreds of corrupt Party members (whether for corruption itself or simply in a political purge is unknown) was announced in *Renmin Ribao*. In the same month the Politburo decreed that *gaogan zidi* should be barred from engaging in private business and that Party officials should no longer have access to such traditional perquisites as imported cars and private food supplies. Heavy fines were imposed on five of China's largest semi-private corporations, and the Governor of Hainan Province was dismissed (Baum 1997: 467–468). Between 1988 and 1993 the Central Commission for Discipline Inspection disciplined 730,000 members and expelled 150,000 (Johnston and Hao 1995).

Still, however, corruption remained endemic to the system. Major corruption surrounded the Three Gorges Dam project on the Yangzi River, where some 5 billion yuan, over 12 per cent of the first-year budget, were said to have been embezzled. Other construction contracts suffered similarly, to the extent that the phrase 'bean curd projects' came to be used to describe those unsafe buildings and bridges where inferior manufacture and poor design meant that their life span was short and their threat to health and safety great.

Launching his own anti-corruption campaign in 1993, Jiang Zemin described corruption as a virus threatening the survival of Party and state, albeit that he qualified this with the traditional warning that, nevertheless, anti-corruption campaigns should not undermine 'reform enthusiasm'. An early, and probably token, victim of the campaign was the wife of the Governor of Guizhou Province, executed in January 1995. Safely installed as Vice-Chairman of the provincial Discipline Inspection Commission, she had instituted the corrupt Guizhou International Trust and Investment Corporation, diverting the money of Hong Kong investors to her son, who in turn had used it for financial and property speculation in Shanghai and Shenzhen (van Kemenade 1997: 20). Naturally she had few connections in Beijing.

In 1995 Jiang extended the campaign to include Party leaders and their families. Again in the best tradition of such campaigns he did so in good part for reasons of realpolitik. He quickly authorized an investigation into the interlocking affairs of two of China's largest corporations, Shougang Steel and Xingxing Industrial Corporation. Zhou Beifang, son of a friend of Deng Xiaoping and a business associate of Deng's son Deng Zhifang, was implicated by the inquiry and resigned from his post. The scandal also brought down members of the Beijing city government, who had been embezzling public money to invest in Shougang. As many as sixty cadres were interrogated, and a vice-mayor, Wang Baosen, apparently committed suicide.[25] Most significantly Beijing's First Secretary, Chen Xitong, an ally of Deng, was successively removed from office, from membership of the Party Politburo and from the Party. In addition, very unusually for a man of his seniority, he was then turned over to the judicial system, where he became one of the first people to be dealt with under the 1997 Penal Code, and therefore a test case for the promised independence of the system. Under Article 383 of the new Code bribery in excess of 100,000 yuan was a capital offence where aggravating circumstances existed. In the case of Chen the sum involved was well over half a million yuan (the true figure is unknown, but believed to be much higher than the quoted figures), and this, combined with his seniority, prima facie constituted aggravating circumstances. Accordingly, liberals demanded Chen's execution to rectify the fact that the death penalty had almost never been imposed on senior officials. In the event, Chen, having been sentenced to the relatively modest term of sixteen years' imprisonment, was subsequently released on medical parole. While liberal protests continued, Jiang's deft and ruthless political handling of the case impressed many Beijing watchers:

> In a single stroke Jiang Zemin moved against one of the most entrenched local leaders in the country, made a bid for popular support in the campaign against corruption, and acted against powerful people who might oppose him in the future, including the Deng family.
>
> (Fewsmith 1997: 521)

There have been other signs of an approach to high-level corruption that at least acknowledges in principle the existence of the rule of law.[26] In particular Zhu Rongji took responsibility for the Three Stresses Campaign, launched by Jiang in 1998, to uphold state ideology and the one-party system, to ensure obedience to central government and to combat corruption. At this time Zhu was under domestic and international pressure to emphasize China's attack on corruption and its increasing adherence to the rule of law. This led to a great intensification of activity, with all senior officials required to attend day-long 'criticism' sessions reminiscent of Mao's 'speak bitterness' meetings, in which lower functionaries were pressed to denounce their superiors' conduct (Conachy 2000). A number of reasonably senior executions followed: in March 2000, for example, Hu Changqing, a Deputy Governor of Jiangsu Province, was executed for taking bribes of 5.45 million yuan after no more than a cursory trial and appeal. The summary nature of Hu's trial and his immediate execution, however, simply indicated his lack of political influence.

A much more significant execution was that of Cheng Kejie, from Guangxi in the Zhuang Autonomous Region. Cheng was Vice-Chairman of the 9th National People's Congress Standing Committee (1998), a protégé of Li Peng, now NPC Chairman, and the most senior official executed by the People's Republic. Cheng's execution quickly followed that of one of his associates, Li Chenglong, vice-mayor of Guiyang city, also in Guangxi. Cheng was executed in September 2000 for accepting bribes totalling 40 million yuan in connection with land sales and business contracts. The money was said to have been gambled away in Macau during holidays with his mistress, Li Ping (who was sentenced to life imprisonment), though this seems unlikely to be a complete explanation. The tone and content of the condemnation by the Central Commission for Discipline Inspection were clear and familiar: 'Cheng's degeneration happened because he abandoned his ideals and belief in communism, fell victim to the temptations of women and money and took advantage of the power endowed by the Party and the people to make personal gains'.

Nonetheless, the bulk of corruption cases were still dealt with extra-judicially by the Party's Discipline Inspection Commissions, which continued to operate at all levels of the system. Corruption remained endemic. In 1998 the Commissions punished 158,000 officials, 5,357 at county or department level, 410 at prefecture level and twelve at provincial or ministerial level (Hao and Johnston 2002: 584). The following year, according to the Commission's Chairman Wei Jianxing, though the total fell to 132,447 the number at ministerial level rose to seventeen, with nearly 20,000 companies run by the People's Liberation Army, the police and legal departments also being closed down. Systematic frauds hitherto unparalleled in size and scope were increasingly uncovered. In 2000 in Guangdong Province, bordering Hong Kong, officials issued fake export certificates permitting companies to claim up to 50 billion yuan in tax rebates. The police there routinely supplemented their incomes by corruption: many were involved in the entertainment and sex industries, some conspired with prostitutes to blackmail the latter's clients by misuse of their powers of arrest and sanction:[27]

> Bribery of local tax officials is seen by many entrepreneurs as just another way to keep expenses down. . . . Some judicial and law enforcement officials resort to blackmail, ask for and accept bribes, practice graft, and bend the law for the benefit of their relatives and friends. Police bureaus in some areas have reportedly charged 'fees' for providing protection. Some police officers in prisons or educate-through-labor schools (*laodong jiaoyang*) extort money from prisoners or their families. Others take advantage of criminals who want to shorten their sentences or be released on parole, to see non-prison doctors or to request time off, often obtaining private services in exchange.
>
> (Hao and Johnston 2002: 592)

The Yuanhua case in the south-eastern port of Xiamen involved at least ninety-one government officials said to have taken bribes (in cash and kind) from the corrupt businessman Lai Changxing, head of the Yuanhua (Fairwell) Group,[28] and over 200 other defendants, almost all under Lai's control. Lai bribed city officials to permit him, probably from the early 1990s, to smuggle goods including telecommunications equipment, crude oil, rubber, cars and cigarettes, evading taxes to a probable value of around 50 billion yuan. The extent of the operation was such that Lai's clients, and therefore Lai himself, controlled virtually every arm of city government. For example, the Head of Customs Administration and at least three other senior customs officials were heavily bribed, as were the Deputy Director of the Fujian provincial police and a vice-mayor of Xiamen (Lawrence 2000). Following the belated investigation (seemingly instigated on the instructions of Zhu himself), leading officials including the Vice-Minister of Public Security and Head of the Anti-Smuggling Leadership Group and the Deputy Party Secretary in Fujian Province were dismissed and expelled from the Party. Criminal trials ensued over the following two-year period.

It is inconceivable that the corruption of so many senior officials was not common knowledge among the power elite in Beijing. In particular it is widely believed that Lin Youfang, wife of Jia Qinglin, formerly Party Secretary in Fujian Province, who moved to Beijing in 1997 as Beijing Party Secretary and Politburo member, was heavily implicated. Jia was a protégé of Jiang Zemin, and his wife appears to have escaped prosecution only because the family was under Jiang's *baohu san* – the collective umbrella of *guanxi*. By early 2001 167 cases involving 273 defendants had been accepted by local courts, and 213 defendants in 119 cases convicted and sentenced.

In response to the continuing corruption crisis, as part of the Three Stresses Campaign the Central Commission for Discipline Inspection introduced new rules on the use of public funds and official privileges in 2000. These barred senior officials from accepting gifts or money and members of their families from running businesses or taking positions within their areas of responsibility. At the same time *Renmin Ribao* published an authorized four-part article on corruption.

Politically the government increasingly sought, doubtless with the experiences of the Soviet Union and Yugoslavia also in mind, to reverse Deng's policy of decentralization, blame lax local cadres for the problem of corruption and put Beijing placemen in key positions in provincial administration. In spite of significant reforms since the classical communist period, however, the legal system remains substantially deficient and, in practice, organizationally subservient to the executive. It is true that the official *China Today* website claims that the Supreme People's Court 'exercises the highest judicial right independently by law, without any interruption by administrative organs, social organizations or individuals', and the courts now have greater influence than hitherto in respect of non-sensitive criminal matters. Nonetheless the power and status of the SPC are in no way analogous to those of its western counterparts. It remains inconceivable, for example, that the SPC would be permitted to create a constitutional crisis by acting against the wishes or interests of the General Secretary or the Politburo.

In addition, though the number of lawyers in China more than doubled between 1995 and 1997, less than one-quarter of them have law degrees. While the 'lawyers' law' enacted in 1997 changed the definition of 'lawyer' from 'State legal worker' to 'legal personnel who provide legal service to society', and lawyers' status from salaried cadre to self-employed (Hao and Johnston 2002: 600) the legal system as a whole remains under state control. In the medium term it seems unlikely that international pressure to end this will be more than politely encouraging.

In Xiamen, and wherever else the 'black economy became mainstream, and virtually all the city's most senior officials were working against the interests of Party, Province and Beijing' (Lawrence 2000), corruption and smuggling, though ultimately destructive, in the short term fuel the local economy. It remains the case therefore that, in the words of a senior government researcher:

> if you take measures that are too stringent, you run the risk that the party will collapse. And if it comes to implicating senior leaders, the priority is to protect the party, not the economy.
>
> (cited in Rosenthal 2000)

Successful corrective action always faces the risk of creating recession. While owners of expensive restaurants, sellers of luxury goods and others who benefit from economic growth are the first victims of recession, the trickle-down effect is all pervasive. Hence extrication becomes extremely delicate, as even the most well-intentioned reforming regime has to tread delicately between further embedding corruption in the national political economy and proceeding with such zeal as to create a cure worse than the disease.

Conclusion

Scholars advance different and sometimes contradictory explanations of Chinese corruption, depending on their disciplinary origins and political sympathies. In an intriguing analysis Fan and Grossman argue that corruption serves the economic function of a compensation and incentive scheme, with efficient cadres permitted to engage in corruption and inefficient ones controlled through censure of their criminality (Fan and Grossman 2001). Hao and Johnston articulate five mutually reinforcing causes: systemic and structural problems, increased incentive and opportunity, a crisis of values, deficient legal and supervisory mechanisms and cultural factors (Hao and Johnston 2002: 585). Certainly from the Revolution to the present, from *San-fan* to the Three Stresses, both corruption itself and anti-corruption campaigns have retained their strong political flavour and purpose. The campaigns' overt purpose of dealing with corrupt individuals has been consistently subverted by two imperatives: *first*, the macro-political imperative of strengthening the interests of both Party and state (and, therefore, those of the people, declared synonymous with them); *second*, the micro-political determination of successive Beijing Leviathans to strengthen their own positions by removing dangerous rivals, and the utility of such campaigns for aiding them to do so.

Corruption in China has its roots in the political process, including the way in which economic changes have been implemented. The political structure vests power in a small oligarchy of effectively unaccountable politicians, military leaders and officials. Secrecy is maintained through media control, fear and punishment. Civil liberties are respected only when they are harmless or at propitious political moments; otherwise they are repressed. Centralization of power presents insurmountable obstacles in a country so vast, complex and variable that even undertaking an accurate population census has recently proved impossible. Conversely, decentralization of administration *to* the provinces has led to more corruption, while organizational decentralization *by* the provinces extends corruption downwards, with lower-level cadres obliged to form corruption networks with their superiors. Such corruption has permeated the People's Liberation Army, with as many as 10 per cent of new recruits emerging as '*guanxi* soldiers', sent money by their parents for 'relationship-building' purposes as a means of corrupting the promotion system, with deleterious consequences for both efficiency and morale (*Daily Sun* 2002). These alliances of convenience are held together by a combination of self-interest and the knowledge that anyone in the network can both bring down and be brought down by anyone else. High corruption combined with *guanxi* and its protective umbrella means the risks involved in reporting it far outweigh any possible benefits. If criminals can bribe their way out of trouble, legal deterrence is minimal and the economy of justice stands on its head: the accuser is exposed to the risk of prosecution or persecution while the offender walks free. In a situation where anyone and everyone might be corrupt and in the absence of independent investigative or reporting machinery, whistleblowing is dangerous if not impossible, as well as entirely pointless. Covering for those under investigation becomes a necessary self-protective device.

Punishments for convicted officials, though severe, are erratic. The probability of detection is slight, the gains from corruption immense. In a (still) low-wage economy the proceeds of even an act of minor corruption are likely to be the equivalent of many years', even a lifetime's, wages for *yiban ganbu*, ordinary cadres. Corruption is therefore a rational act. In a culture in which corruption by institutions is perceived as a victimless crime with many beneficiaries, and corruption by individuals as a semi-legitimate perquisite, it is hard to see how it could be effectively detected or extinguished other than at the behest of political leaders. And to the age group fond of characterizing itself as the 'Five Noes Generation' – no education (because of the Cultural Revolution), no work (the abolition of the iron rice bowl), no family to look after one in old age (the one-child policy), no universal health care and no pension – corruption may appear the only escape route. This generation is caught between systems, tumbling into the very interstices between communism and capitalism that the corrupt are able to exploit. And in a world in which 'everybody else is doing it', doubtless one would be a fool not to join them.

If political reform comes it seems more likely that it will originate outside China than within. In China itself it is inconceivable that the General Secretary and the Politburo will voluntarily surrender power, and the strength of the PLA is such that it is unlikely to be wrested from them by civil disturbance. Nor is the dispute with Taiwan at all likely to lead to any concessions of this kind. On the other hand, with WTO membership a reality since November 2001, China will eventually be forced to make adjustments to some of the more criminogenic or otherwise dysfunctional aspects of its public administration.[29] WTO membership appears initially to be more widely regarded in China as providing trade and tariff benefits than as imposing reciprocal obligations; and the liberalization timetabling is at present incomplete. But to implement the Normal Trading Relations Policy throughout the country, Beijing will have to surmount many of the same obstacles that have beset its anti-corruption campaigns. The shelter provided for local companies by provincial administrations, frequently both corrupt and protectionist in character, is contrary to the WTO's National Consistency Policy. Transparency, also demanded by the WTO, will pose structural problems, since in China law is normally subordinate either to local custom and practice or to internal and unpublished memoranda or regulations. China will also be forced to accept the jurisdiction of the WTO's Dispute Settlement Body when other member states lodge complaints about its trading practices. For a country that has so long and vigorously argued for a traditional interpretation of national sovereignty in relation to human rights, the legal system, territorial disputes and capital punishment, this will be a bitter pill indeed, and China will certainly contest pressure to change with great vigour.

Such pressure seems very unlikely to be brought, at least in the near future, since any such requirements will almost certainly not be enforced aggressively by the WTO over the initial phase of Chinese membership. Even assuming the Organization treads delicately, however, while China may hope its low-wage economy will lead to unsullied economic improvements overall, a new external trading environment will inevitably do short-term damage to some local economies. The extent and duration of this damage and its internal social, political and economic consequences will be crucial to China's long-term adaptation.

As China integrates increasingly into the world trading community, however, and as the time of the 2008 Olympic Games approaches, Beijing may find its practices of coercion and military suppression attracting increasingly telling international pressure. At this time any continuation of the rise of human rights on the international agenda will quite possibly mean that, on the safe assumption that China remains in the WTO, it will be forced to concede that its present policies can no longer be convincingly defended by reference to a Westphalian concept of sovereignty. The suppression of Falun Gong, the treatment of secessionists in areas such as Xizang Zizhiqu (Tibet) and Sinkiang Province, the widespread deployment of forced confessions (Conner 2000), compulsory internal mass movements of population, capital punishment without a transparent and independent legal system[30] and the management of intellectual dissent may come to have increasingly unavoidable international consequences. Following the failure of the Seattle Round in particular, the WTO is increasingly sensitive to the international politics of mass protest, and may well move to create a broader forum for debate. In such a context Beijing will find it increasingly difficult to maintain a domestic politics that operates in so starkly different a way from that of the developed world.

The likelihood, therefore, is that these external processes will eventually force changes in China that are currently undeliverable, and that shifts in the character and extent of corruption will follow. Since there is currently no internal reason for political reform (on the contrary, Beijing has taken the lessons of Eastern and South-Eastern Europe as warnings of the perils of democratization), any impetus for reform will, however presented, probably be external. If future circumstances create either irresistible pressure to reform or a conjunction between political liberalization and the interests of Beijing's power brokers, the political structures necessary for exposing and dealing with corruption will, doubtless, materialize. Otherwise, probably, they will not.

Notes

1 The Supreme People's Procuratorate (SPP), abolished in the Cultural Revolution but revived in the new Constitution of 1978, 'operated between the public security forces and the people's courts, rather like the District Attorney's office does in the United States' (Saich 1981: 125). The SPP reports to the NPC and its Standing Committee. Its reinstatement, alongside certain free speech guarantees, was intended to signify the growing strength of the rule of law. We shall argue, however, that where law remains subservient to politics any such guarantees are conditional, and rescindable in circumstances falling well short of the constitutional safeguards existing in most western countries.

2 For a stimulating theoretical consideration of this and related points, see Hall and Ames (1999, particularly Part 3: 'The cultures of democracy').

3 This cultural phenomenon means that corrupt relationships are protected by formal as well as informal networks (*baohu san* refers to the 'collective umbrella' of *guanxi*). In addition the distinction between what is legal and what is not is seldom clear: 'what is acceptable reciprocity one year may be redefined as corruption the next . . . [depending] on transactional or political relationships' (Smart 1999: 112; see also White 1996; Zhu 1999).

4 For a striking eye-witness account of the campaign in Yenching University Beijing, a private, US-aided institution taken over by the state in April 1951, involving the denunciation of the President and leading professors, see Barnett (1964: 126–130).

5 Like all figures in this chapter this one must be treated with circumspection. In Mao's China in particular, facts were of use only to the extent that they contributed to his revolutionary ambitions. No reliable official statistics were kept, though many were manufactured by proponents and opponents alike. Such figures as are quoted here are best estimates only.

6 Society at this time was divided into the Proletariat, comprising the Five Red Categories (poor and lower-middle peasants, workers, revolutionary soldiers, revolutionary cadres and dependants of Revolutionary Martyrs), and class enemies, comprising the Seven Black Categories (landlords, rich peasants, reactionaries, bad elements, rightists, traitors, spies) (Lawrance 1998: 14). Prior to the Great Proletarian Cultural Revolution Mao was to reclassify upper-middle peasants as Black, but even under the original categorization Mao's own father, a rich peasant, would have been deemed a class enemy.

7 Cadres are holders of leadership positions within state organizations, though not necessarily the Party. There are three main levels of cadre: *lingdao ganbu* are leading cadres with power and prestige, *xingzheng ganbu* are administrative cadres, *yiban ganbu* are lower-status ordinary cadres. They are central to the day-to-day governing of China.

8 It is a common misconception that Party membership is widespread. At the time of writing the Party officially claims some 60 million members, a little over 5 per cent of the population, disproportionately older men, in its 3.5 million branches.

9 For a detailed account of the campaign in Shanghai see Barnett (1964: 144–152).

10 This is not, however, a universal interpretation. To others the HFC was from the first a ploy to 'smoke out' dissidents prior to purging them in the Anti-Rightist Campaign (Lo Tit Wing, personal communication).

11 For a concise account of the failure of the Campaign see Teiwes (1997: 77–81).

12 Wright (1989), in a very readable book written to accompany a radio series, includes graphic accounts of these and other experiences.

13 The events of the Great Proletarian Cultural Revolution are not germane to this book, though readers seeking a concise and accessible account are referred to Saich (1981: Chapter 3).

14 The undesirability of importing Soviet communism to China had been a consistent feature of Mao Zedong Thought, as well as of Mao's realpolitik. The policy, which obviously brought tensions with the Soviet Union, was influenced by the arrogance with which, from the first, the CCP had been treated by Stalin (whom Mao nonetheless admired), his representatives Borodin and Zinoviev, and, latterly and starkly, by Khrushchev. During and after the Leap, First Secretary Khrushchev had made no secret of his contempt for the commune system, to which he had responded by cancelling aid, including support for China's nuclear programme, and withdrawing Soviet advisers.

15 Though it is not strictly correct to describe China thus, there being several competing parties, the fact that only parties operating within the communist paradigm are permitted to exist probably justifies this common shorthand.

16 The activity of law (it would be wrong to call it a profession) was not officially reinstated until 1980, and then as a state-funded activity of largely unqualified practitioners which had to reconstruct itself from nothing at a time of rapid economic growth, high crime rates and social dislocation. Lawyers became self-employed only in 1996.

17 Though Hua, plucked from an obscure post in Mao's own province, Hunan, was indeed his protégé, his nomination as heir mainly reflected Mao's anxiety to limit Deng's power, and was based on his supposed deathbed utterance to Hua that 'with you in charge I can be at peace'. Hua's opponents had always been sceptical as to his legitimacy, but his position was secured temporarily by his mobilization of public hostility against Jiang Qing and other members of the Gang of Four (See Hua 1977 for his denunciation of the Gang). This did not endure, however, and Hua, regularly humiliated by the Politburo, was destined to be no more than a temporary leader. For an excellent account of the manoeuvrings that precipitated Hua's downfall see MacFarquhar (1997b).

18 This was rightly read at the time as a direct assault on the theoretical communism of Mao Zedong Thought, under which scientific socialism was the sole criterion for testing truth.

19 This was coded language for dealing with the unpunished leaders of the Cultural Revolution. This combination of political self-protection and personal revenge serves as a reminder that under Deng anti-corruption campaigns and political imperatives still remained yoked together.

20 For a thorough account of the endemic corruption and organized criminality on Hainan Island in particular, see van Kemenade (1997: Chapter 7). This gives a flavour of activities in this most corrupt of SEZs: in 1985 '89,000 cars, 2.9 million color televisions and over 250,000 videotape recorders were imported under a duty-free policy for goods to be used locally, and then resold on the mainland for large profits' (Hao and Johnston 2002: 586).

21 The policy was accordingly rescinded by the Third Plenum of the Fourteenth Central Committee in 1993.

22 Within hours of Hu's death posters appeared proclaiming that 'The wrong man has died' and 'It is difficult for one man to illuminate the country, but one man is enough to make the country perish'.

23 This is a significant date. On 4 May 1919 violent student demonstrations had taken place in Beijing, initially against the decision of the Paris Peace Conference to hand former German concessions in Shandong to Japan rather than returning them to China. The protests had quickly broadened, however, provoking widespread revolutionary fervour, and the May 4 Movement, which established an intellectual and political base for the CCP, is conventionally regarded as marking the Party's birth. A student demonstration in Beijing on the seventieth anniversary of this date was hence as meaningful to the demonstrators as it was provocative to the government.

24 The figures were certainly in the hundreds, possibly more. Amnesty International estimated 1,000 and estimates from the democracy movement, naturally, were even higher. The deaths were accompanied by up to 10,000 arrests and almost thirty executions.

25 Unsubstantiated rumours exist that Wang was, with Jiang's support and possibly at his instigation, murdered for political reasons connected with his knowledge of Jiang's behaviour at the time of the 4 June incident.

26 This concept, however, does not translate easily, *fazhi* meaning both 'rule *of* law' and 'rule *by* law'. In countries with a common law tradition, rule *of* law entails the systematic and universal dispensation of justice on the basis of statutes interpreted by an impartial judiciary independent of the state. Rule *by* law, however, has the softer sense of governing by the use of laws, without the implication that the government is subject to law. This distinction, crucial to the understanding of Chinese jurisprudence, and its practical import are well explained in Woo (2000).

27 Sanctions included a humiliating 'chop' in the bearer's passport, identifying the holder as a pursuer of prostitutes. This particularly affected relatively affluent Hong Kong men who had crossed the border, normally to Shenzhen, for this very reason. Local men were more likely to be held in custody until 'bought out' by relatives.

28 Yuanhua was a vast real estate and property development company. It owned a football team, Xiamen's leading theme park and an exclusive holiday resort, Red Mansion, where Lai's corrupt clients were provided with luxury breaks, including sexual favours, as part of their pay-offs.

29 An excellent example of such dysfunctionality was a 1994 case in which the City Council awarded a prime Beijing site to the McDonald Corporation only for the Central Government to issue a contradictory contract allocating the same site to the Hong Kong tycoon Li Ka-shing. Li, as we have already seen in the context of the Cheung Tze-keung case, has extremely close connections with the Beijing authorities.

30 According to Amnesty International, China, with 2,468 judicial executions in 2001, was responsible for some three-quarters of the world's total.

4   National political corruption (II): the United Kingdom[1]

> The cost of transparency in politics is that we will all have to learn to distinguish between a genuine scandal and antics which, however diverting, do not affect the way we are governed.
>
> (Baston 2000: 9)

The United Kingdom of Great Britain and Northern Ireland is a low-corruption country. This is not to say either that it has always been thus or that the UK lacks all forms of structural corruption: indeed we shall show that neither of these propositions is correct. In fact the process by which Great Britain transformed itself in the early- to mid-nineteenth century from a high- to a low-corruption country is a central theme of this chapter. We proceed by offering a brief historical analysis of changing patterns of corruption in the polity as a whole up to the mid-nineteenth century; thereafter we consider issues of governance in relation to central government, local government and the Civil Service. From this analysis it should be possible to identify, *first*, the main factors associated with the decline in institutional corruption and, *second*, the areas in which, and the extent to which, the United Kingdom remains most vulnerable to a resurgence of corruption today.

Naturally the contemporary situation in the United Kingdom contrasts sharply with that of high-corruption countries such as China. There corruption permeates the structures of governance, and, because the primary aim of anti-corruption strategies is normally to eliminate targeted individuals in order to enhance the power of the ruling elite, such strategies are themselves usually symptoms of corruption, not potential cures for it. In high-corruption countries the instruments of governance typically lack transparency, accountability, self-corrective mechanisms, constitutional safeguards and judicial independence. There is, as it were, no reliable political, judicial or bureaucratic thermostat to restore the polity to a functioning steady state following the exposure of corruption. Hence in high-corruption countries whistle-blowing is virtually non-existent, corruption symbiotic and, in the case of junior recruits, effectively compulsory.

In all countries the official line is that political corruption is individu-alistic, not systemic. Though in high-corruption countries opposition groups may associate the characteristics and behaviour of the ruling group with corruption and their own with the common good, this ignores the structural factors which predispose the country to high corruption and which will per-petuate it if such groups themselves come to power. While in low-corruption countries an individualistic analysis is intrinsically more plausible, the wide-spread belief in the United Kingdom in particular in the integrity of existing structures and their capacity to remove the odd 'bad apple' is, though not entirely unjustified, certainly oversimplified.

The Westminster parliamentary system, in contrast to the position in Washington, is characterized by strict party discipline enforced by a com-bination of whipping[2] and prime ministerial patronage. Together these are designed to secure the loyalty of members of the legislature, for most of whom promotion to the executive, entirely in the gift of the Prime Minister, is now (though it was not always) their main career ambition. Party discipline means individual Westminster MPs have little influence on policy-making and little scope to defy voting instructions. In such a tightly controlled system corrupt individuals quickly become an electoral liability to their party. Hence once corruption has been exposed and it is clear that conceal-ment is impossible, except in the case of a favoured few where a decision might be taken to ride out the crisis, the parties normally deal robustly with it.

Naturally under this system fewer rent-seeking opportunities are available to Westminster MPs than to members of the US Congress. In the absence of an institutionalized reward structure Congressmen have little alternative to acting as political entrepreneurs, plucking fruit where they find it, albeit, the United States not being a high-corruption country, within the bounds of political prudence. As we shall see, in eighteenth-century Britain, prior to the emergence of the strong party system, a similar mechanism, royal patronage, was necessary to maintain ministerial authority.

In addition to and antedating party discipline, both Houses of Parliament have historically claimed responsibility for dealing with their own miscreant members, pleading parliamentary privilege as a justification for placing the conduct of MPs (though only when acting as MPs) outwith the criminal law.[3] Parliamentary privilege derives both from the statutory provision of Article Nine of the Bill of Rights 1689 and from case law (Oliver 1997: 126–127). It was for centuries powerfully defended by reference to the Hobbesian logic that a sovereign Parliament answerable to others is a contra-diction in terms: a sovereign body cannot be answerable to any other body or it is that body, not Parliament, which is sovereign. In fact until recently the issue was seldom contentious, since it was assumed that Members were people of honour. Successive speakers ruled that backbenchers[4] from busi-ness backgrounds brought strength to the Commons, that disclosure of interests when speaking[5] was a matter for their conscience and that exhortation to declare them was as far as it was proper to go. It was also the case that, again until recently, backbench salaries were modest, and this naturally encouraged members to pursue extra-parliamentary professional activities.[6] Nonetheless since the 1990s these arguments have succumbed to media and pressure group-initiated demands for external accountability in ways described later.

In truth the self-regulatory system, buttressed since 1969 by a Select Committee on Members' Interests, was never a reliable vehicle for investigating, exposing and prosecuting corruption. Equally the party system is inadequate to protect the public interest against, say, bipartisan collusion over party funding, blurring the distinction between party and government, misusing the secrecy laws, suborning the independence of the Civil Service and the predatory deployment of power, particularly in local government and 'next steps' agencies.

In this chapter we consider the nature of political corruption in the United Kingdom, both as evolving over time and in contemporary politics. Generally we avoid discussions of scandals for their own sake. Periodic attempts by some members of ruling groups to manipulate political and sexual opportunities, illegitimately extend their power and exploit its privileges are almost ubiquitous, and in low-corruption countries the main interest of such attempts for us lies in the nature of the political response they provoke. Nonetheless, in relation to the themes of this book scandals invite further reflection on whether politically corrupt acts are better regarded as qualitatively distinct from political activities or an extension of those activities into areas or acts deemed unacceptable in a particular time and place. If, as we have suggested, in low-corruption countries most individualized acts of political corruption are better seen as errors of judgement, pieces of vulgarity even, than as acts of distinctive wickedness, it is appropriate to regard them as political not moral problems. Hence, as their importance lies more in the political fall-out they provoke than in their intrinsic character, parties will not deal in the same way with the same problem on different occasions. Because their primary concern is with political expediency, and not justice, parties will respond to political problems in a consequentialist manner, based on a judgement as to the most prudent course of action at the time.

Of greater interest than the details of individual improprieties, therefore, is the manner in which the political process of a low-corruption country detects, interprets and responds to them. In a high-corruption country such as China we have seen that political corruption, expressed in the pursuit of both money and power, is locked into the political system and is therefore fundamental to the logic and meaning of politics itself. Similarly we have seen that some African states have been effectively privatized by predatory political leaders such as Mobutu and Mugabe, the enthusiasm of whose pursuit of power correlates closely with the nature and extent of the rent-seeking opportunities available to them once they capture it. We have noted a similar phenomenon in parts of Latin America and South-East Asia. In such countries, analysing politics and not political corruption simply makes no sense, because if one purchases office as one purchases a business and with the same end in mind, utility maximization becomes the primary goal. Hence public capital is only expended on vote buying, coercive enforcement or populist gestures such as capital projects in sensitive locations to the extent that it constitutes an investment in the retention, consolidation or expansion of power, and hence in future rent-seeking opportunities. Such investments are, therefore, corrupt politicians' research and development money, with everything left over representing profit. States such as this contrast with low-corruption countries whose politicians for the most part acquire no more pay or perquisites than they would enjoy in any senior position, and quite possibly less. While in all countries, in politics as elsewhere, seniority offers more opportunities for exploitation and greater scope to act self-interestedly while presenting one's actions as disinterested, inevitable, ubiquitous, even altruistic, the questions about political corruption arising in such countries are of an entirely different order.

The use of the criminal law in political corruption cases is minimal, but only partly as a result of parliamentary privilege. The emphasis is more on such non-criminal sanctions as 'did he fall or was he pushed?' resignations, expressions of public stigma and disqualification from practice. In addition, in England in particular the workings of the class system can lead to informal sanctions for letting the side down or behaving in an ungentlemanly manner. To believe that most political corruption in England is financially predatory is to misunderstand both its historical development and its subtler contemporary manifestations. Accordingly we revisit gentlemanliness later. First, however, because the main area where political conditions in the United Kingdom offer potentially fertile breeding grounds for high corruption is secrecy, we begin with a brief explanatory note.

A note on secrecy

> civil servants are in a relationship of accountability to four sources: their ministers, their departmental and agency superiors, Parliament and 'the people' . . . the constitution only affords full recognition to the first two of these.
>
> (Pyper 1995: 147)

In comparison with the situation in other liberal democratic societies, secrecy laws in the United Kingdom are quite strong, and, self-evidently, secrecy facilitates covert activities including corruption. The four main

Official Secrets Acts of 1911, 1920, 1939 and 1989 are supplemented by conventions designed to delay or prevent the publication of official documents; anybody entering even remotely sensitive employment is bound by them.

Several factors contribute to this cultural characteristic. They include the absence of a written constitution or 'right to know' legislation, the convention of collective Cabinet responsibility which necessitates departmental and Cabinet discussions remaining confidential, the strong legacy of a culturally homogeneous and 'gentlemanly' Civil Service, and an adversarial political system encouraging concealment of potentially embarrassing information (Pyper 1995: 145–146).

In the 1980s secrecy created major political problems. Initially these came in the form of fall-out from the (separate) unpopular criminal prosecutions of three Civil Service whistle-blowers, Tisdall, Willmore and Ponting. This led the Head of the Civil Service to prepare a *Note of Guidance on the Duties and Responsibilities of Civil Servants in Relation to Ministers* (the so-called Armstrong Memorandum). This *Note*, which did not entirely capture the mood of the moment, confirmed that civil servants troubled by a *crise de conscience* had no overriding accountability to the people or to Parliament. On the contrary, their overriding duty of confidentiality remained intact even in the unspoken eventuality of ministerial misuse of secrecy. Further difficulties followed. *First*, in 1986 a senior civil servant at the Department of Trade and Industry (DTI), Colette Bowe, was instructed to commit the party political act of leaking a private letter to discredit the Defence Secretary Michael Heseltine's quest for a European solution to the problems of the Westland helicopter company. *Second*, in 1988 the government sought and humiliatingly failed to prohibit the publication in Australia of a book, *Spycatcher*, by a former secret agent, Peter Wright, an attempt which placed the British tradition of economical truth-telling[7] in the global spotlight, and which could not fail to provoke damaging press criticism.

Third, the 'Arms for Iraq' affair highlighted the potential for the self-protective ministerial abuse of secrecy rules. A manufacturing company, Matrix-Churchill, controlled, as the Foreign Office knew, by Iraqi interests,[8] had been legitimately exporting materials for military conversion during the Iran–Iraq war (Leigh 1993). This practice continued with covert government support following an embargo on arms sales to either combatant, leading, to the DTI's horror, to the prospect of a customs raid. A conflict ensued between the DTI and the Foreign Office, which, knowing the situation, expressed a reluctance to sign further export licences. Nicholas Ridley, as Secretary of State for Trade and Industry, raised the stakes by advising the Prime Minister that Britain had provided Iraq with £1 billion in export credit guarantees and that provoking a default would have implications for the public sector borrowing requirement (Leigh 1993: 10). Alan Clark, a former Trade Minister, raised them further by issuing a denial (subsequently shown to be false) of a newspaper report that he had approved illegal arms sales with 'a nod and a wink'; his successor, Tim Sainsbury, similarly misled Parliament about the issue of the licences.[9] With the end of the war the government was, in 1990, set to lift the embargo, ending all difficulties, when, out of the blue, Iraq invaded Kuwait, provoking the Gulf War and a complete embargo on trade with Iraq. At this point prosecution by HM Customs became unavoidable.

When Paul Henderson, Matrix Churchill's Managing Director and other senior staff were tried for illegal arms exporting, five ministers signed Public Interest Immunity Certificates (PIICs), claiming that concealment of documents vital to the defence was in the public interest. The prosecuting counsel untruthfully advised the judge that the documents, which in fact showed that the government, knowing the purpose of the exports, had acted in contravention of its own embargo, were forensically unimportant. In the event the judge rejected the arguments and the case finally collapsed when Mr Clark conceded under cross-examination that the defendants' claim was correct. This admission almost certainly prevented a miscarriage of justice.

This kind of behaviour, akin to a criminal conspiracy,[10] is relatively unusual in the politics of low-corruption countries. When it is exposed, the almost invariable response is an independent public inquiry, in this case conducted in immense detail and with great relish by an assiduous if slightly maverick judge (Scott 1996), and at least some legislation. Of course the inquiry may well be designed to reduce political embarrassment and the response may be minimal, tardy or both: even in low-corruption countries one should not be naive about practical politics. In the Matrix-Churchill case there were three main responses. *First*, the Prime Minister, John Major, anticipating trouble, made modest but high-profile gestures towards open government in 1993, introducing a Code of Practice for Government and revealing information about the security and intelligence services (respectively MI5 and MI6), much of which had, however, previously been an open secret.[11] *Second*, the incoming Labour administration included a commitment to freedom of information in its 1997 manifesto; but the ensuing Bill was heavily diluted prior to its introduction to Parliament, and even after the Freedom of Information Bill 2000 received the Royal Assent full implementation was delayed until 2005. *Third*, Sir Richard Scott himself complained publicly in 2001 that the response to his recommendations on arms sales had been unsatisfactory.

Nonetheless, in most low-corruption countries, certainly including the United Kingdom, the likelihood of repetition of such scandalous behaviour is, if not negligible, then certainly slight. In any state containing a strong society characterized by legal, public and media pressure and specialist interest-group lobbying it is normally safe to assume that the system will self-correct, if only because the price of repeated scandal would be politically intolerable.

Historical developments in political corruption: the pre-Victorian era

> as each representative will be chosen by a greater number of citizens in the large than in the small republic, it will be more difficult for unworthy candidates to practice with success the vicious arts by which elections are often carried, and the suffrages of the people being more free, will be more likely to center on men who possess the most attractive merit and the most effusive and attractive characters.
>
> (James Madison, *Federalist*, 10)

In early and early modern British history, corruption, etymologically associated (through *rumpere*, to break) with rupture, had two distinct statutory meanings. The first was 'perjury', broadly defined as involving suborning juries, witnesses and justices of the peace (magistrates). The second involved the buying and selling of offices, a proscription for many years honoured in the breach: in fact the predatory notion of public office as private property, not public trust, was to remain a feature of British governance until as late as the nineteenth century.

Certainly by the time of the sixteenth-century Tudor monarchs, the buying and selling of offices and office-holders' exploitation of their position for private gain were both regarded as normal (Hurstfield 1973). Indeed the unpaid or lowly paid nature of many such posts invited or necessitated predation. This laxity in turn helped pave the way for the seventeenth-century Stuart Court, which, under James I and Charles I, possessed many of the hallmarks of institutional corruption seen in contemporary China. Extensive patronage, the selling of office, sinecures, lengthy periods of predatory management and corruption, punctuated by intermittent, politically motivated inquiries whose deliberations normally had the effect and often the aim of weakening one faction and strengthening another, were all present. Again typically of high-corruption countries, participation in, or at least tolerance of, such corruption was de rigueur at Court. Exposing it was beyond the power of any courtier, and attempting to do so would simply have cut him adrift from his own faction, depriving him of the support necessary for survival. The only consequences would have been certain isolation, probable expulsion from court and possible death.

Nonetheless, seventeenth-century perceptions of corruption related not only to court factionalism but also to normal predatory conduct taken to excess – in short, greed. Corruption could, therefore, be a political offence (aligning to the wrong faction) or an error of judgement. For example, fraud and corruption were endemic in James I's peacetime navy, the management of which was in the hands of courtiers who operated the Department as a private fiefdom. But by 1608 reports had reached the King that corruption in naval administration was now of such a kind and degree as to threaten his interests. A Commission was instituted, which found evidence of routine corruption. Some paid-for goods had not been delivered and many goods that had been delivered were defective: unseasoned timber, unsuitable planks, the wrong size masts, rotten cordage, ill-conditioned oakum and inferior canvas were all found. Far fewer men went to sea than the number for whom pay had been claimed, and the quality of recruits was unsatisfactory as a result of bribery and poor recruiting methods (Lloyd 1975: 82). But although the evidence against them was overwhelming, the miscreants were pardoned by the King with little damage done to their persons or careers. This decision resulted from a combination of their security as part of the Lord Admiral's faction, the preferences of (and pressures on) the King himself and the suspects' own tactical adroitness (Lloyd 1975: 100).

Following the so-called Glorious Revolution of 1688 and the replacement of the Roman Catholic King James II by William of Orange, political power shifted from Court to Commons. In spite of early attempts by the Commons to exclude Royal office-holders from membership (notably through the Act of Settlement 1701), the Commons increasingly assumed many of the characteristics of corruption and patronage previously associated with the Stuart Court. In fact, in the absence of a strong party system, as the eighteenth century progressed, the compliance secured by such patronage became, together with regular and semi-official bribery of members, a necessary vehicle for managing the relationship between Parliament and Crown:

> the 'King's ministers' had to rely on the 'influence of the crown' embodied in the patronage network to preserve healthy majorities in the House of Commons. The systematic doling out of places tenable with seats in Parliament, and of contracts, sinecures, reversions, pensions, and leases of crown lands, certainly did create 'a climate [that] was unfavourable to the development of an upright and zealous public service', but the structure of the unreformed constitution necessitated it.
>
> (Harling 1996: 15)

Hence by the middle of the eighteenth century the Westminster system was marked by high levels of corrupt patronage. Holders of sinecures assigned any small amount of work required to others, either as an obligation or for a pittance. Reversions (permitting office-holders to nominate their successors) perpetuated the oligarchic character of the parliamentary system. Government contracts and pensions as well as ecclesiastical preferments were dispensed as bribes or rewards. Safe seats were given for similar reasons or to secure support in the House, though seldom in sufficient quantities to ensure success. So by 1780, when the Dunning Motion on the influence of the Crown heralded the attempts of the significant and influential Economical Reform Movement to destroy the patronage system, only about 200 of 558 MPs were placemen (Harling 1996: 15).

Numerous Acts and Resolutions were passed in the name of the Economical Reform Movement. These included a prohibition on government contractors sitting as MPs, disenfranchising revenue officers, abolishing sinecures, restricting pensions and introducing the notion of accountability in respect of government expenditure (Doig 1984: 45). Commissions were instituted which made recommendations as to salaries, accounting, tenure and promotion. Though the proposals were piecemeal and implementation of reform patchy, the process

> heralded both the acceptance of reforms and the expectation of certain personal standards of conduct and thus made the administrative structure amenable to Victorian reformers' enthusiasm for organization, efficiency and value for money.
>
> (Doig 1984: 47)

There were, in addition, many more indications that major changes could not be long delayed. The politically motivated impeachment for corruption of Warren Hastings in 1795 signalled the end of national tolerance of predatory rule of the kind which had earlier been exercised by the East India Company, and demonstrated that corruption was now an increasingly sensitive political issue. The attacks upon the latitudinarian Established Church following the rise of Nonconformism, particularly in the new northern industrial conurbations, signified a repositioning of the Church of England within the social formation and a new emphasis on justification by deed. If Robinson Crusoe, that model of northern Nonconformism, could, almost a century earlier,[12] create a new society based on puritan attitudes subsequently co-opted into the English class system as the distinctively middle-class virtues of rationality, economic prudence and deferred gratification, how could aristocratic profligacy continue to go unquestioned?

In short it had become clear before the end of the eighteenth century that the prevailing system, as inefficient as it was corrupt, was inadequate to govern a rapidly industrializing country whose political stability had been further undermined by the fall-out from the American and French Revolutions. In particular the country was embroiled in the economically ruinous Napoleonic Wars, to which the government was responding in a recklessly profligate way, aiming to protect powerful domestic interests by a strong mercantilist trade policy and printing large quantities of inconvertible paper money (Harling 1996: 10). In fact the high cost of government exposed the ruling group to the charge of lining their pockets at public expense. Parliamentary criticism increased, and in some parts of the country the Methodist Church in particular became a gathering point for popular discontent which, fuelled by radical orators, came to constitute a genuine political threat. Accordingly Britain reached the crucial point, so often necessary for corruption to be controlled, at which reducing it became an unavoidable price to be paid by the ruling elite to secure their position and stave off the danger of armed revolt.

The political impact of the French Revolution on the British consciousness, though considerable, was moderated by a number of factors. In particular the securing of the Protestant succession in 1688 had demolished all remaining vestiges of divine right theory and the political trappings flowing from it. Similar attempts in France had been resisted successfully by Louis XIV and less successfully by his successors. Divine right theory constituted a powerful intellectual justification for court corruption: as God's secular representative, the King stood above human law and beyond political reproach, holding on trust all property within his realm. So although the theory itself is unlikely to have been persuasive, even to most courtiers, after the Restoration, theories of monarchy deriving from it offered exploitable justifications for the King and his faction to resist accountability. The theory also sustained a ruling mindset that translated itself into class solidarity. Hence the transfer of power, from a King claiming absolute and divinely endowed authority and so demanding deference and subordination to his rule, to an elected Parliament (albeit elected by a very limited franchise), was transformational culturally as well as politically. Power was no longer justifiable on the ground of right, but provisional and contingent: what had been given could be taken away.

The rise of party politics and the vitriolic nature of eighteenth-century political life inevitably set the tone for attacks on the probity and competence of the ruling elite. Not only governments but also politicians generally became fair game for public ridicule or contempt, and the strength of the attacks was exacerbated by the exclusion, no longer with either hereditary or theological justification, of the bulk of the people from the political process. Populist orators and radicals at home exploited public feeling on this issue while the same feeling was more violently and transformationally expressed abroad in the American and French Revolutions. Given the political instability that underlay ostensibly urbane Georgian British society, it is scarcely surprising that the question of legitimacy preoccupied so many seventeenth- and eighteenth-century political philosophers.

These considerations, combined with both the political, economic, technological and social transformations beginning around the 1780s and the high cost of (and high levels of corruption associated with) a lengthy and unpopular war, were to transform political corruption in Great Britain in the first half of the nineteenth century. Both the catastrophic consequences of the economic mismanagement of the Napoleonic Wars and, even more, mechanization and the onset of industrialism meant that the traditional mercantilist policies by which favoured producers were, often corruptly, protected against competition inevitably came to be challenged by the new industrial bourgeoisie.

From the Victorian era to the 1960s

> The evolution of 'good government' . . . involved several transitions . . . from a central administration that was deeply influenced by political considerations to a permanent civil service that was relatively well-insulated from politics; from the notion that civil office was a form of private property to the notion that it was a public trust; and from 'irregular' emoluments to strict salaries, formal superannuation arrangements, and transaction of official business by the appointee in person.
>
> (Harling 1996: 14)

> The more the Empire expands, the more the Chamberlains contract.
>
> (Contemporary [1900] pun, cited in Searle 1987: 65)

Introduction

The emergence of the factory system meant that the workers' time became the employer's money; any interruption to the productive labour of mill and mine workers, whether by absenteeism, alcoholism, ill-health or worker combination activity, reduced the workers' surplus value, which translated into the employer's profit. Accordingly pressures towards a new work ethic and sober lifestyle became inexorable (Weber 1904). So did the need for a dispassionate, formal, efficient and dependable administration, for which the colonial Civil Service, substantially reformed following the replacement of the East India Company as governors of India by the British Government, was an excellent model. Equally necessary were an elected (but heavily bureaucratized) local government system and factory inspectorate, and a poor law which, by the excoriation of able-bodied paupers and the abolition of outdoor relief under the Poor Law (Amendment) Act 1834, discouraged indigence. In the early nineteenth century the new prison-based penal system, which confiscated time as the fine confiscates money, joined the mills and railways as an indicator of the emergence of a new political economy of time. Time was now a commodity to be traded for wages rather than (in the case of a subsistence farmer) a private entity or (as in the feudal system) someone else's property.

Hence with a growing emphasis on efficiency, sobriety and reliability, the emergence of a Weberian rational–legal bureaucracy and electoral reform (with the prohibition of vote buying, accentuation of party competition and judicial supervision of the electoral process), political and bureaucratic corruption began to be brought under control. Both government and public administration were transformed, entirely for the better, during the Victorian era. Victorian government was cheap in comparison with the eighteenth-century British and other nineteenth-century European states, and sound in terms of probity and rationality. It was increasingly laissez-faire in its reluctance to interfere with market forces, oriented towards free trade and with a cautious monetary policy, maintaining throughout a currency freely convertible to gold (Harling 1996: 9).

Gentlemanly conduct

Exemplifying many of the political and administrative changes that transformed political corruption in nineteenth-century Britain was the changing concept of gentlemanliness. Though the traditional idea that the status of gentleman was determined primarily by birth had begun to break down following the Hanoverian Succession in 1714, it was in the wake of the changes associated with the Industrial Revolution that gentlemanly conduct came decisively to refer to character rather than class. So in the seventeenth century John Wilmot, Earl of Rochester, a libertine, serial adulterer, drunkard and pornographer, probably a murderer and certainly financially corrupt (see Goldsworthy 2001), could claim to be a gentleman. He would not, however, have been considered such two hundred years later, when, as a scoundrel and a cad, he would have been unwelcome in many London clubs. By this time governmental and administrative rationality, a Protestant work ethic, unprecedented levels of social mobility and the fact that the bourgeoisie far outstripped most members of the nobility in both wealth and adaptability could be taken for granted.

These changes were accelerated by an agricultural depression and the consequent collapse of land values in the late eighteenth and early nineteenth centuries. This depression clearly posed a threat to the aristocratic and landowning classes whose traditional rural status, which in some areas remained recognizably feudal, was increasingly undermined by rich merchants and industrialists buying themselves into positions of influence. British society remained stratified of course, but much less so than before, and increasingly social, professional, personal and financial acceptability went hand in hand. This process was both symbolized and accentuated by the rise, in the eighteenth and early nineteenth centuries, of the public schools and the gentlemen's clubs around St James's, membership of which was typically determined by party, profession or interest. In terms of political life, for the new middle classes party membership offered such opportunities for career advancement, upward social mobility and new social relationships that for many party and life became inextricably intertwined. Such arrangements opened doors for industrialists (and, by marriage, young women) through which even half a century earlier few could have dreamt of passing, and which were indicative of an adaptability which did much to sustain the system itself. Hence by the early twentieth century, retailers and manufacturers such as Lipton and Lever, newspapermen such as Harmsworth and Aitken, South African millionaires such as Wernher, Beit and Robinson (the so-called Randlords), Jewish bankers and US expatriates such as Waldorf Astor were buying themselves into London society (Searle 1987: 12–14). To those who moved in the circle of that most sociable of monarchs,

Edward VII, the fact that the King's enthusiasm for gambling was all too seldom matched by either luck or skill offered an obvious investment opportunity with a guaranteed return in social, though not, alas, monetary, currency.

Upward mobility of this kind, because it was bestowed by deeds, was contingent, and misdeeds could lead to what had been given being taken away. Nonetheless, schools, colleges, clubs, brigades, occupational groups, trade and commerce associations, churches, guilds and Masonic lodges failed to eliminate corruption, as did membership of the Commons or the Lords. The ties stemming from such institutions did, however, help create a very strong society, which in turn led to the development of norms of conduct which contributed to maintaining corruption at levels well below those of most other countries. Because expected standards of gentlemanliness were counsels of unattainable perfection, however, they inevitably led to surreptitious activities of a male, though not necessarily gentlemanly, kind. For as well as these new and respectable sodalities there were music halls, smoking rooms and brothels where gentlemen were able, if they wished, to participate discreetly in more subterranean pleasures. Such activities were, however, generally concealed by the discretion stemming from class, gender and membership loyalty, the belief that reporting ungentlemanly conduct was itself ungentlemanly having been imbued at an early age and subsequently reinforced in school playgrounds and playing fields the length and breadth of the country.

Central government

So in spite of the public face of Victorian England, political corruption existed, as it would in any economically expanding and socially mobile country, albeit at a lower than average level. From the 1830s successive measures were introduced prohibiting MPs from taking money to steer legislation, transacting private business in the House or voting on Bills where a conflict of interest existed. In 1892 Gladstone required all Cabinet members to divest themselves of directorships of public companies on entering office, a prohibition which, though it lapsed under Salisbury, 52 per cent of whose ministers held such directorships in 1900, was reaffirmed in 1906 and continues today (Searle 1987: 3, 44). Such prohibitions were driven by the unprecedented array of opportunities for corruption opened up by transport and construction in particular, in a situation lacking, at least until mid-nineteenth century, any developed system of local government.

Nonetheless there was widespread scepticism that such proscriptions were sufficient to ensure the highest standards of conduct in public life. MPs themselves, not surprisingly, placed greater emphasis on self-regulation and the need for basic integrity, the exercise of which, because it was perceived as lacking in the politics of countries such as the United States and France, became almost a patriotic duty. In fact, integrity as a peculiarly

British sub-category of gentlemanliness related not only, not even especially, to corruption as narrowly defined, but rather to a whole ethos of public service which assumed a duty to serve the whole nation and indeed the Empire, not a sectional interest.

Such abstract aspirations, though more than empty rhetoric or hypocritical posturing, were by no means invariably implemented. For much of the nineteenth century, maintaining a generally non-corrupt executive proved less challenging than reining in members of the legislature, many of whom had no hope of (or, often, desire for) office. Elite corruption continued to be a major theme of popular newspapers well into the latter half of the nineteenth century. Newspaper stories seldom led to popular protest, however, because corruption was generally regarded as an undesirable but unavoidable by-product of a generally legitimate system. Indeed it has been suggested that the extraordinary reduction in corruption between the eighteenth and mid-nineteenth centuries contributed significantly to the acceptance of the political elite by an increasingly wide and better-informed electorate (Harling 1996: 25).

So while political demonstrations occurred, they had different causes, notable among which were the Corn Laws in the 1840s and the demand for electoral reform in the 1860s. The Corn Laws, which imposed heavy duties on imported corn, in practice from France, had originally been justified on patriotic grounds but were in truth mainly designed to protect the interests of the landed gentry by artificially inflating corn prices to the detriment both of the poor and of national trade. Cobden and Bright, leaders of the Anti-Corn Law League, recognized that abolition, eventually achieved in 1846 after an eight-year campaign, had legitimated the political system, dampening any popular appetite for further protest. In fact, in a clear indication of such legitimation Cobden said of the Conservative Prime Minister Peel, a Protectionist persuaded by the Free Trade argument but shortly afterwards defeated in Parliament by a vengeful Disraeli, that 'If Sir Robert has lost office he has gained a country'. As if to confirm the point, on Peel's premature death in 1850 400,000 labourers contributed to a Working Men's Memorial of Gratitude and the *Northern Star* hailed him a working-class hero (Harling 1996: 255).

In the mid- to late-nineteenth century, anti-corruption legislation continued to attract little interest among voters, while facing strong opposition from vested interests in both parties. Nonetheless, the cumulative effect of legislation to investigate such corrupt political acts as collusion over election petitions, bribery and treating, to disenfranchise corrupt constituencies and to extend the franchise led to such increases in the size of the electorate as to render traditional forms of electoral corruption impracticable. In particular, the Corrupt and Illegal Practices Act 1883 placed limits on election expenditure, increased penalties and redesignated some acts hitherto deemed 'corrupt' as 'illegal', thereby obviating the need to prove corrupt motive. As election expenses fell (from £1.7 million in 1880 to £770,000 in 1900), so did contested election results (from 51 in 1868 to 28 in 1880 and seven in 1895) (Doig 1984: 58–60).

By the early twentieth century, political controversy was increasingly focusing on two problems, both stemming from the transformation of the House of Commons following the universal male franchise introduced under the third Reform Act 1884. These were the inevitable conflict of interests arising when *nouveaux riches* businessmen assumed power, and the temptations of 'new money' for those in power who lacked personal wealth or income but not monetary ambition, and who had, naturally, to keep up appearances. Such controversies, however, were largely *ad hominem*, never threatening the existence, or even challenging the legitimacy, of the political system itself.

So far as the *first* of these problems is concerned, during the Boer War (1899–1900) two contracting scandals threatened to submerge the Chamberlain family. The Chamberlains were rich Birmingham businessmen whose members included Joseph, the Colonial Secretary and a close associate of Powell Williams, Financial Secretary to the War Office with responsibility for contracting, and his son Austen, Civil Lord of the Admiralty. *First*, Kynoch's, a company in which members of the family held substantial shares and whose Chairman was the Colonial Secretary's brother Arthur, was awarded a contract for cordite provision.[13] It came to light, not least through Lloyd George, desperate to divert attention away from his own opposition to the war, that during the tendering process Kynoch's had been permitted to revise their tender. They had also been contracted to supply a large proportion of the substance in spite of still not having submitted the lowest bid. The matter was investigated by a Select Committee, which effectively exonerated the Colonial Secretary of every crime except naivety. *Second*, the press reported that the Chamberlains also virtually owned a small firm, Hoskins & Sons, of which Joseph's second son (and Austen's brother) Neville was also managing director. The family had acquired control of the company, which supplied fittings for the Navy, two years after Austen had taken up his Admiralty post and also after Joseph had falsely denied to the Commons that his family had an interest in any company supplying war goods. Further press investigations, meanwhile, showed that the family also had a large stake in other companies with direct or indirect contractual relationships with the government. Nonetheless, both Joseph and Austen successfully resisted calls for their resignation, Joseph in particular arguing forcefully that this kind of situation was inevitable if successful businessmen, whose participation in government was greatly in the national interest, were to accede to positions of power (Searle 1987: 52–54, 61).

The *second* major concern, the temptations facing impecunious politicians, focused on, *first*, the undesirable company (especially cosmopolitan, particularly Jewish, financiers and entrepreneurs) kept by several politicians, notably Lloyd George; *second*, Lloyd George's dubious financial activities; and *third*, his manipulation of the honours system.

In 1909 Lord Northcliffe advised Lloyd George, at the time Asquith's Chancellor, that critics were pointing to the stark (and therefore politically dangerous) disparity between his ferociously egalitarian platform rhetoric and his extravagant lifestyle. In addition, none of his friends was seen within polite society as respectable, but rather as rich vulgarians who aped the worst but never the best aspects of the King's circle; some, indeed, were suspected of criminality. Questions were particularly asked about the financing of Lloyd George's country house in Walton Heath, which was well beyond his means and had in fact been generously provided by a newspaper proprietor, Riddell. Further, another press baron, Harold Harmsworth, loaned Lloyd George and his political cronies Rufus Isaacs and the Master of Elibank (nicknamed 'the Master of Oilybank' for his unctuous manner and political slipperiness) (Searle 1987: 149) a villa at Cap Martin (Searle 1987: 128).

Lloyd George was thought to be threatening the dignity of his office not only through his choice of friends but more particularly by business dealings redolent of insider trading. In short he was generally believed to have exploited public office for private gain, in particular in that, as President of the Board of Trade, he had bought dock shares while handling the Port of London Bill (Searle 1987: 127). In addition, together with Isaacs and Elibank he had bought Marconi shares when the government was inviting tenders for the construction of wireless stations across the Empire. In this case city rumours led to the postponement of the award of the contract, and the government instituted a Select Committee, whose report showed that this unholy trinity had indeed, through Isaacs's brother Godfrey, purchased American (though not English) Marconi shares. In addition Elibank, as Liberal chief whip, had spent Party funds on purchasing 3,000 shares for the Party itself. The three defended themselves by claiming that since the American and English companies were separate entities no conflict of interest was involved. This, however, was untrue. *First*, the English company had a holding in the American company. *Second*, Godfrey Isaacs, who helped them acquire the American shares, unavailable on the Stock Exchange, at prices below market value, was Manager of the English company. *Third*, the companies employed the same patent, so a government preference for the Marconi system over those of Telefunken and Poulsen would inevitably have benefited all Marconi shares (Searle 1987: 172–174).

In the case of both these scandals the fact that patently untenable positions were sustained points to two familiar lessons. *First*, parliamentary self-regulation is inadequate to censure the most powerful politicians; and *second*, press exposure does not necessarily lead to resignation. For resignations to occur those concerned must normally have lost the Prime Minister's support, but in the case of the Chamberlains and Lloyd George there was little danger of this happening. Joseph Chamberlain (in particular) and Lloyd George were both necessary to Asquith, who was not, anyway, of a quick-firing disposition, while none of the miscreants was of a character to insist on resigning as a point of honour, none of them being that kind of gentleman.

The interrelated issues of party funding, political corruption and the honours system by no means began with Lloyd George; indeed they have had a long and tortuous relationship even though the sale of honours did not become a criminal offence until the Honours (Prevention of Abuses) Act 1925. In the United Kingdom the honours system has a delicately calibrated scale of awards from ennoblement down to the humble MBE (Member of the Order of the British Empire). The selling of honours is long established in England, stretching back at least to the Stuart monarchs, for whom the practice, which fell within the royal prerogative, constituted a vital means of raising extra-parliamentary finance. Under the influence of Lloyd George, however, honours sales became excessive, not to say vulgar, a means of securing both party funding and personal wealth.

Searle notes that whereas prior to 1885 few businessmen were honoured on grounds of social class, the practice of widening the honours list was, rather improbably, adopted by Lord Salisbury, who gave 23 per cent of his honours to businessmen (Searle 1987: 84–85), a practice accelerated by his successor, Balfour. This uncharacteristically unpatrician behaviour on the part of Salisbury appears to have been provoked *first* by the consequences of the Corrupt and Illegal Practices Act 1883, which ended such traditional electoral practices as vote buying (anyway now impracticable following the Reform Acts) by restricting constituency electoral expenditure. *Second*, in 1886 came the abolition of the Secret Service Fund, traditionally a clandestine election pot for the governing party (Searle 1987: 85). Unfortunately these two squeezes occurred as the extended franchise, improvements in transport and literacy levels, the intensity of party competition and unpredictability of popular voting behaviour all invited increased expenditure. Manipulating the honours system was an obvious way out.

A number of scandals occurred from the mid-1890s onwards. For example the notorious swindler Hooley paid the Conservatives £50,000 for a baronetcy (which he never received) in 1897, the negotiator, Marriott, the former Solicitor-General, no longer an MP but still a Privy Councillor, demanding an additional £10,000 for himself (Searle 1987: 88). The number of honours awarded increased steadily under the Unionists with 81 peerages and around 150 baronetcies created between 1895 and 1905. Accordingly, the relationship between honours and party donations became a source of intense interest, though because both main parties were using the system for party purposes neither was in a position to exploit the problem for political gain. The situation was further complicated following the death of Queen Victoria. On succeeding to the throne Edward VII acquired the habit of approving honours lists subject to the inclusion of members of his circle, described by a contemporary aristocrat as 'a bevy of Jews and a string of racing people' (cited in Searle 1987: 21). This circle included the newspaper baron Alfred Harmsworth, widely thought to have been generous to one of the King's mistresses, Mrs Keppel, whom Balfour, under pressure from the King, ennobled in 1905. At the time his chief whip, Acland-Hood, had noted privately:

> obviously the King means Harmsworth to have a Peerage. If he doesn't get it now he will get it when [Campbell-Bannerman] makes his Peers on taking office – we should then lose all his money and influence – I very much dislike the business, but as we can't stop it in the future why make so handsome a present to the other side? . . . I think in this case we might allow our virtue to be raped.
>
> (cited in Searle 1987: 93)

The number of honours granted continued to rise during Asquith's prime ministership from 1906, when honours were increasingly awarded to party donors of dubious reputation. In 1910 to 1912, 47 peerages and 68 baronetcies were announced, and rumours were rife that Elibank, as government chief whip, had introduced a scale of charges and attempted to poach Conservative sympathizers (and hence potential donors) with the offer of an honour.

Following the First World War Lieutenant Colonel Henry Croft MP spoke with distaste of the ennoblement of men who 'would have been blackballed by any respectable London club'. Indeed a tradition developed in some such clubs for members to congratulate newly ennobled members by singing heavily ironic renditions of 'Lloyd George Knew my Father' to the tune of 'Onward Christian Soldiers'. Music hall comedians nicknamed the Order of the British Empire (OBE), created primarily to acknowledge the wartime achievements of civilian non-combatants but seized upon as a convenient cut-price honour, the Order of the Bad Egg (Low 2001). Other notorious cases included Sir Roland Hodge, a wartime black marketeer, sold a baronetcy for public services in 1921 (Searle 1987: 354). Sir Joseph Robinson, a fraudster who had made a fortune from South African gold, was given a baronetcy in 1908 after donating £30,000 to the Party, and sold a peerage in 1922 which only public pressure forced him to decline (Searle 1987: 350). Sir William Vestey, a tax exile held in popular contempt following the relocation of his meat-packing business to Buenos Aires during the war at the cost of thousands of jobs, was sold a barony.

Protests increased, from radical literati such as Hilaire Belloc and Cecil Chesterton, from the newly formed National League for Clean Government and from establishment figures, notably the Irish MP Lord Selborne, whose high-minded campaigning embarrassed his party leader, Bonar Law, who was well aware of his party's complaisance in the matter. This complaisance was to increase during Bonar Law's involvement in Lloyd George's wartime coalition government when, at the end of a lengthy period in opposition, numerous pledges made to benefactors over the previous decade were inevitably called in. The 1916 Birthday Honours List which, to strong opposition from the King, ennobled Law's (and subsequently Lloyd George's) allegedly crooked friend, benefactor and business associate Max Aitken, the Canadian owner of the *Daily Express*, attracted widespread political criticism, not least from the Canadian High Commissioner, who had not been consulted in advance.

More generally the necessity of wooing press barons was well understood. Two years after his ennoblement as Baron Beaverbrook, and eight years before being satirized as Lord Raingo by Arnold Bennett, Aitken was created Minister of Information by Lloyd George. Also in 1918 Lloyd George's supporters took control of a number of provincial papers as well as the hostile *Daily Chronicle*, which was virtually turned into a prime ministerial mouthpiece (Searle 1987: 341–342). The implication is clear: the press exercises a vital function in a democratic society[14] but is a necessary but not sufficient means of ensuring probity in public life. The media can (literally and metaphorically) be bought by the powerful, their owners and editors being as much part of as outside the political process.

In the face of continuing political pressure Lloyd George, shortly before resigning in 1922, instituted a Royal Commission to investigate the honours system. The Commission, which recommended reform rather than abolition, proposed instituting a small advisory committee to scrutinize the names of nominees and the reasons for the recommendation, and creating the new criminal offence of offering money for a title or acting as an intermediary in such a transaction (Searle 1987: 372–374). Lloyd George's successor, Bonar Law, endorsed these proposals, a new Political Honours Scrutiny Committee was charged with examining nominations and vetoing unacceptable ones, and the Honours (Prevention of Abuses) Act 1925 made the sale of honours a criminal offence. Ironically an early victim of the Act was Lloyd George's former 'fixer' Maundy Gregory, apprehended trying to sell a knighthood to a retired naval officer for £10,000.

The question arises as to why, in a reformed House of Commons now representative of most of the adult country,[15] such corruption should persist, and why in particular the Liberal Party, nothing if not high-minded (not to say priggish) in its public statements, should have been so cynical. Clearly the primary motive was securing party funding and the secondary one personal rent-seeking by a new breed of national politician. In addition, however, Searle notes that the Liberal Party, unlike the Conservatives who had quickly appreciated the folly of relying on small funders in the new political context, had failed to adjust to the new funding realities. Securing corporate donations was now necessary, but the Liberals continued to rely excessively on rich individuals. As Searle notes, while the scope for the growing links between the Conservative Party and business to be corrupt is self-evident (Searle 1987: 416), the very personal nature of Liberal leaders' association with their backers signalled more immediate political danger. And it was in the honours arena that any fall-out was most likely to occur.

The Civil Service

The process of achieving Civil Service reforms, which began with the Economical Reform movement in the 1780s, continued with legislation in 1816 to provide a coherent salary structure to replace fees and gratuities and to increase the Service's political independence. By the time of Queen Victoria's succession most sinecures had been suppressed, a uniform system of superannuation had been introduced, offices could no longer be bought and sold and the Treasury had began to exert control over administrative probity (Doig 1984: 49). This process did not prove decisive, however, until the path-breaking (if rather opinionated and unfair) Northcote–Trevelyan Report (Northcote and Trevelyan 1854), the institution in 1855 of the Civil Service Commission and the political fall-out from scandals following administrative and logistical failures during the Crimean War (1853–1856).

Northcote–Trevelyan advocated entry by public examination, promotion on the basis of merit and a bipartite system of superior intellectual (First Division) and inferior mechanical tasks. These innovations, though not decisively implemented until Warren Fisher's tenure as Head of the Civil Service after the First World War,[16] created a framework still recognizable today. Under Fisher a unified Civil Service ethos (aided by new social and sporting facilities) gradually replaced earlier departmentalism;[17] inter-departmental transfers became the norm, and recruitment strategy favoured Oxbridge generalists over technical experts (Pyper 1995: 7–8). Above all the Treasury was strengthening its grip over other departments, developing Service-wide terms and conditions of service and imposing restrictions on both external appointments and the handling of public funds by bankrupt or insolvent individuals. It was also beginning to address the sensitive issue, over which it had no powers of enforcement, of Civil Servants' retirement moves to commercial organizations with government connections. It has been reported, for example, that very recently 60 per cent of senior Civil Servants and armed forces officers held up to six directorships within six months of retirement (Pyper 1995: 86). In addition, the *Estacode* of conduct, first published in 1944, deals with a wide range of issues from gifts and hospitality to liability for customs duty and VAT. It subjects Civil Servants to far stricter rules than those governing the conduct of MPs, and corruption, very rare in the British Civil Service, is virtually unknown at the most senior levels.

Since the days of Northcote–Trevelyan step-changes have occurred in Civil Service recruitment, and in terms and conditions of employment. This process began with the radical Fulton Report of the 1960s (Committee on the Civil Service 1968). Fulton recommended removing the Treasury's strategic management function, introducing management training, ending

Northcote–Trevelyan's preference for arts-educated generalists, introducing an integrated pay and grading system, widening the Service's social and educational recruitment base, hiving off certain executive functions and introducing new systems of accountable management, devolved budgeting and planning units. Many of Fulton's proposals were strongly resisted by the Service and few were enthusiastically adopted by government, though several were to re-emerge almost a generation later in the work of Sir Derek Rayner, Head of the Efficiency Unit in Mrs Thatcher's Private Office. Rayner's tenure led to the creation of Next Steps agencies, conceived of along Fultonesque lines (Efficiency Unit 1988), undertaking former Civil Service functions but without the same restrictions:

> Policy formation would take place in small, core or parent departments, but these would be very different from the conventional departments of state, which would effectively be broken up into executive agencies and cores . . . the agencies should be headed by Chief Executives, who would be given significant managerial freedom (over recruitment, salaries and gradings) and made accountable to Parliament as well as to their departmental ministers.
>
> (Pyper 1995: 71–72)

More recently still, the government's determination that First Division recruitment should embrace broader social strata and second-career appointments has begun to challenge the cultural homogeneity which has continued largely unbroken since Northcote–Trevelyan. While there is no reason to believe this will lead to increases in Civil Service corruption, the period since the 1980s has seen a diminution in the Civil Service's size and role. This has been brought about by the introduction of the Next Steps agencies, the increasing proliferation of special advisers from outside the Service and the tendency of successive prime ministers to seek policy advice from sympathetic 'think tanks' rather than seconded Civil Servants. Should these changes reduce the traditional attractiveness of a First Division career to the best graduates, however, any resulting repositioning of the Civil Service in the political formation would have consequences it is currently impossible to predict; though it is unlikely that they would be beneficial.

Local government

Local government, where a party system has been imposed much more recently than at Westminster, and where, powers of patronage being slight and councillors for the most part unpaid volunteers, whipping is less effective, has always presented problems of corruption. Until a reform process beginning with the Municipal Corporations Act 1835 got under way local government was structured around some 15,000 vestries or parishes and 200 towns, and closely associated with poor law administration (Loughlin

1992). In both the potential for corruption was great, and many vestries were indeed institutionally corrupt. Even after the mid-century reforms abuses continued. London was chaotically and corruptly run, and as late as the 1870s members of committees of the Metropolitan Board of Works were engaged in systematic contracting frauds, particularly relating to the rebuilding of Shaftesbury Avenue in the West End. Central government increasingly attempted to control the metropolitan authorities, and the Public Bodies Corrupt Practices Act (PBCPA) 1889 was the result. Under this Act giving, promising or receiving gifts, inducements or rewards to or from members or officials of public bodies became a misdemeanour for both parties (Doig 1984: 79).

In 1898 a report of the London Chamber of Commerce claimed secret commissions were both endemic and inevitable. Repeated but abortive attempts by successive Lords Chief Justice to pass an Illicit Secret Commissions Bill followed before such a Bill passed into law in 1906. The Act made it an offence to accept an inducement or reward for showing favour or disfavour in matters of business, or to give or use an incorrect document to mislead or deceive. Ten years later the Prevention of Corruption Act 1916 shifted the onus on to defendants charged under this Act or the PBCPA 1889 to prove that any money they were proved to have received as an inducement had not been received corruptly (Doig 1984: 79–80).

By the turn of the century parliamentary supervision of local government was developing through a committee structure which included the Public Accounts and Estimates Committees, whose powers to investigate and determine responsibility were, however, limited and unsatisfactory. More generally successive governments responded to the corruption endemic in local government by attempting to impose a uniform national structure under central control. The Local Government Act 1933, which increased uniformity and, through a strengthened District Audit, accountability, contributed to this, though the policy's logical conclusion lay in the *Scheme of Conditions of Service*, or 'Purple Book', of 1946, a nationwide charter of salaries, conditions of service and conduct for local government employees. More significant still was the increasing dominance of the Treasury over local government finance. The Treasury was the ideal vehicle for both expressing and ensuring the subordination of the local to the central state so characteristic of the British polity. We return in the next section to the consequences of this approach for political corruption.

From the 1960s to the twenty-first century

Local government

There is little doubt that in the nineteenth century systematic central attempts to address the problem of high corruption in local authorities were necessary. Nonetheless one consequence of the perpetuation of centralization has been a flaccid and uncompetitive ethos among many authorities which, for many, means that the immediate word association with 'local government' remains 'red tape'.

The subordination of local to central government in the United Kingdom means that historically the responsibilities of the former have been largely restricted to administering local services, and for strategic planning or major investment recourse to central government, for permission as well as funding, has been necessary. By the same token the imposition of national negotiations of terms and conditions of employment has restricted competition among local authorities in staff recruitment and retention, encouraged the growth of trade unions dedicated to developing a supplier-led service and had an inhibiting effect on promotion by merit. This subordination has been maintained by a funding mechanism which, by imposing severe restrictions on direct revenue-raising powers, ensures that central government remains local government's main revenue source, and by legislative restrictions on local authority discretion as regards spending plans in particular.

The consequent marginality of local authorities has caused problems in attracting elected members and senior officers of adequate quality. Local government service offers few rewards, material or social, voter interest is low, and with certain exceptions elected members' service is unpaid other than by expenses, recompense for loss of earnings and a modest attendance allowance. In some areas where opposition is weak, a single party is able to remain in power almost indefinitely. In such situations not only is the quality of debates often poor but the act of debating is self-evidently futile; and for members of the ruling party collusion with officers and local interest groups is an ever-present temptation. Additionally, the fact that local government has seldom proved attractive to high-quality officers means that many authorities have been, at best, barely competently managed. Few authorities have, at least until recently, had any tradition of customer care. Departmentalism has been strong, with competition for resources, favour and prestige, and staff morale and loyalty levels seldom high. In such a context it is not surprising that corruption at many levels has traditionally been a problem.

Nor has the impact of press freedom been significant in attacking such corruption, at least outside London where the national press is based, and where stories have appeared about corruption in several boroughs, including Lambeth and Westminster. The national press takes little interest in provincial stories: investigating costs and the risk of libel suits are high and the impact on advertising or circulation figures at best minimal and at worst negative. In addition few senior investigative journalists are willing to spend months going through the books in distant locations where local government corruption has been endemic, such as Glasgow, parts of the north-east, south and east Yorkshire, South Wales and the West Midlands. The local press, on the other hand, whose editors are anyway significant figures in local communities and seldom wish to damage their town's image, has few resources and fewer skilled investigative journalists. Naturally, too, the continued cooperation of local dignitaries, including local councillors and officers, is essential to their continued existence. The local press also depends for advertising revenue on the support of local companies which may themselves be commercially or personally associated with local ruling groups, and therefore anxious to avoid negative local publicity. In fact the co-option of the local press by the very interests it would, if wholly free and financially sound, be investigating constitutes a severe restriction on the media's capacity to expose local corruption.[18] A few national publications (notably the satirical magazine *Private Eye*) have devoted journalistic resources to such matters and have been used by whistle-blowers as a vehicle for publicizing individual scandals, but resources generally are limited, and whistle-blowing cannot be relied upon to yield systematic or reliable information. In addition, what does emerge from whistle-blowing is, though sometimes of considerable importance, at other times petty, unbalanced and *ad personam*.[19]

While UK local government as a whole is by no means institutionally corrupt, a small number of localities may still be exceptions to this generalization. But while institutionalized local government corruption, notably in contracting, was a main justification for the introduction of the centralizing approach, the approach itself has subsequently contributed to the problems of uncompetitiveness, low morale and corporatism which have themselves permitted corruption intermittently to flourish. In this sense centralism is both cause and effect of the problems local government has traditionally presented.

Local government corruption became of particular public concern in the 1960s and 1970s. At this time massive residential and commercial redevelopment was taking place in many parts of the country, with local authorities deploying compulsory purchase orders for slum clearance purposes to construct what were then considered state of the art city centres and housing estates. But poor design, lack of artistic vision, late completion and the use of substandard materials, the results of which remain all too visible today, were caused by a combination of corruption and incompetence. So the City Council of Birmingham, a city not widely regarded as the zenith of post-war urban planning,[20] awarded contracts worth £267 million between 1961 and 1973.

Of these contracts 34 per cent were awarded to one firm, Bryant's, which was later found to have bribed the city architect, said at his trial to have turned Birmingham into a (presumably metaphorical) 'municipal Gomorrah'. By 1969 Bryant's gift list had extended to 575 people, including 175 councillors or officials, 70 of them in the Architect's Department and 58 in Public Works (Doig 1984: 182–185).

The Poulson affair was more significant because less localized, more complex and considerably subtler.[21] John Poulson was an unqualified Yorkshire architect, and a devout Methodist and Freemason whose cultivation and exploitation of contacts in different local authorities stretching back to the 1950s created a network of corruption probably unparalleled in Britain. It embraced the Home Secretary (Reginald Maudling), three MPs (Herbert Butcher, Albert Roberts and John Cordle), a senior Civil Servant (George Pottinger), the head of a major building firm, Bovis (Harry Vincent), high-profile city leaders (T. Dan Smith and Andrew Cunningham) and numerous councillors and officers hired as contract scouts.

In the late 1950s Poulson had begun setting up a string of companies which, by providing an invaluable 'one stop shop' of architect, engineer and surveyor, had enabled him to progress from jobbing architect to deliverer of entire building contracts. Poulson's original company, Ropergate Services, entailed a partnership of Poulson and Vincent, with Smith (former Leader of Newcastle City Council and Chairman of the Northern Economic Planning Council, a charismatic and dominating figure in north-eastern politics) as consultant. Smith's job was to extend Poulson's network of contacts on a commission basis, for doing which his payments between 1962 and 1970 totalled £155,000. Smith also recruited another key member of Poulson's team, Cunningham, the dominant figure on Durham County Council. Cunningham's local power base was the stuff of local legend:

> He also chaired the Durham Police Authority, the Northumbrian River Authority and the Newcastle Airport Authority. As well as his official posts he was Chairman of the Northern Area of the Labour Party and of the regional General and Municipal Workers' Union . . . industrial relations at Newcastle airport were conducted from the management side by Cunningham as Chairman of the authority, and from the union side by Cunningham wearing his GMWU hat. Local investigations into his activities were hampered by fear that he would, in his Police Authority role, learn what witnesses were saying.
>
> (Baston 2000: 94–95)

Between them Smith and Cunningham operated a network of corruption centred in the north-east but extending to the Midlands and Wandsworth. Companies fronted by Smith dealt with smaller players, particularly councillors on key committees where major builds were under consideration, without the targets necessarily being aware of Smith's involvement with Poulson. So Poulson's company entered legitimate tenders while Smith ensured Poulson won the contracts by hiring the councillors, either as consultants or advisers or by overt bribery. Poulson was not, of course, wholly dependent on Smith for his contacts. A genuinely affable, plausible and clubbable man, he initiated many of his own contacts, some of them, apparently, on trains. Whether this was by chance or, as has been suggested (Baston 2000: 91), through intelligence provided by a corrupt contact in Leeds City Station ticket office as to who was travelling to London on what day has not been established. Either way he exhibited truly impressive networking skills.

In spite of numerous rumours, the extent of Poulson's activities only came to light following his bankruptcy hearing in 1969. The bankruptcy followed over-expansion: the complexity of his activities had been such that Poulson, more attracted to entrepreneurship than administration, had failed to monitor his empire sufficiently to identify and eliminate its loss-making elements. Cash flow problems stemming from excessive front-loading of costs, a large Inland Revenue bill, bank pressure for loan repayment and a boardroom coup that saw him removed from power constituted his nemesis. The bankruptcy hearing took place in January 1972, initially with little press interest. In July, however, now in a welter of national publicity, the papers were sent to the Director of Public Prosecutions. Criminal trials followed in 1973, resulting in the imprisonment of Poulson and his main collaborators – for seven years in Poulson's case, a sentence upheld on appeal.

Police investigations continued after Poulson's imprisonment, though they were hampered by the numbers of suspects, their geographical spread and the self-protective refusal of some councils which had hired him to cooperate. Hence in 1974 the Director of Public Prosecutions scaled down the investigations, though even this more limited operation came to little. As a result, many of Poulson's 'small potatoes' were never brought to justice, and in some cases their local government careers continued with impunity.

Poulson always claimed that his corrupt activities were simply gift-giving: introductions, golfing and racing trips, money, houses, champagne and fine wines, architectural designs, clothes and cars were unconditionally given, any reciprocity simply following the rules of the universal if unspoken practice of networking. While Poulson's guilt was manifest, it is hard not to have some sympathy for his trial comment that 'Someone is going to have to sit down and work out just what is entertaining and what is corruption so that everyone will know where they stand'. In this sense Poulson's corruption is, like that of others we have encountered, better seen as a crossing of the line between normal business practice and deliberate and systematic corruption than as an act of distinctive criminality. While some might say that in this case the line was crossed especially decisively, others might take the view that it was the tempted even more than the tempter who were guilty of betraying trust; the tempter was simply making a business proposition to people who should have declined. But by the end it is probably correct to say that Poulson could no longer be plausibly regarded as inhabiting the interstice, the grey area, between entertaining and bribery in a manner akin to, say, a small Chinese *guanxi* relationship. Rather he had become a serial tempter of public servants whose manifestation of a combination of vanity, cynicism, naivety and avarice made them, irrespective of what their reaction *should* have been, putty in his hands.

It was, however, precisely this interstitial area which he had occupied twenty years earlier, and from this position that the incremental growth of his corrupting occurred. Poulson's career amounted to a systematic conspiracy to divert public money for his own benefit by subverting the contracting processes of numerous elected bodies. In doing so he discovered, doubtless to his own surprise, how easy and cheap it was to corrupt public officials and elected members, how easily their vanity was flattered and how innocent many of them were as to the significance of what they were doing. In short, local government was not exactly in the hands of outstanding or perspicacious public servants. These findings were, of course, both interesting in themselves and invaluable to subsequent legislation.

No inquiry into the structural conditions underpinning Poulson's activities was ordered, probably both on cost grounds and to avoid overlapping with police enquiries, though others have seen conspiratorial motivation. Nonetheless the government did commission two broader inquiries, the Prime Minister's Committee on Local Government Rules of Conduct, 1973–1974, chaired by Lord Redcliffe-Maud (Redcliffe-Maud 1974) and the Royal Commission on Standards of Conduct in Public Life, chaired by Lord Salmon, 1975–1976 (Salmon 1976). In addition, following pressure from the Commons, a Select Committee to examine the activities of MPs associated with Poulson was instituted in 1976 after the publication of the Salmon Report.

Maud's limited brief was to consider questions of conflict of interest and qualifications in relation to council membership, and his report made recommendations on tightening standards, transparency, probity and press vigilance. More significantly the Royal Commission's brief was to examine standards of conduct in public life and recommend safeguards. Salmon's recommendations included forfeiture of corrupt gifts, criminalizing the corrupt use of official information, increasing police investigative powers, strengthening conflict of interest disclosure rules, tightening rules on gifts and hospitality, permitting public access to council committee minutes, suspending councillors charged with corruption and restricting the chairmanships of any one councillor. In addition, in two addenda Salmon noted, *first*, the dangerous coexistence of a grudging electorate, inadequately rewarded and trained councillors with increased powers, one-party rule in some areas, the weakness of chief officers' tenure, the lack of central government action on standards and the escalation of competition for work. *Second*, he noted the need for improved detection of private sector bribes in the public sector. These, Salmon believed, were especially tempting to councillors given their patchy quality and the fact that many saw themselves making financial sacrifices only to assume an increasing workload and ever more onerous responsibilities. Any sense of resentment created by such a mindset might lead to the thought that as one was working voluntarily such peccadilloes only constituted one's moral due, albeit necessarily claimed through the back door.[22]

Since the 1970s local authority accountability has grown greatly in quantity and complexity, and a plethora of local government legislation as well as the transfer of the responsibilities of District Audit to the independent Audit Commission in 1983[23] have made it among the most heavily regulated parts of the state. In addition to several major reports, central government has issued numerous circulars and publications ranging from prohibitions on multiple chairmanships, requirements to declare conflicts of interest and procedures for internal audit to provisions covering officers' off-duty activities, job canvassing for relatives, procedures for electing committee chairs and dealing with dominant individuals in one-party authorities, and rules on disseminating information. The Local Government Association and central government currently face items including corruption in a small number of specific (and well-known) localities and communicating effectively with, and hence being practicably accountable to, predominantly apathetic voters.

Political corruption has, however, been mainly subsumed or submerged in a welter of broader priorities, and is no longer high on the agenda of local government reform. An enhanced legalism stemming mainly from European legislation and the deregulation of advertising by the legal profession in the 1980s, policies to encourage and protect whistle-blowers, the increasing deployment of judicial review of administrative decisions and the enhanced role of the Local Government Ombudsman have all provided recourse for complainants. So while residual and appellate powers continue to be vested in the Secretary of State (for example in relation to planning applications, traditionally a major source of corruption), the courts and the national Commissions for Local Administration have become increasingly central. The Audit Commission has a broader brief and higher profile than District Audit, and is active in monitoring, comparing and publicizing local authorities' effectiveness, efficiency and economy. With devolution and regionalization both under way and more in prospect, leading to larger units of local government emerging in an increasingly integrated and regulated sector, most conditions conducive to high corruption in local government have probably been removed. Accordingly, while doubtless minor 'fiddles' will continue there as elsewhere, high corruption appears unlikely to re-emerge in the short term as a major political concern within local government.

Central government

In addition to its recommendations on local government, the Salmon Commission suggested that bribe-taking by Members of Parliament should fall within the ambit of the criminal law (Salmon 1976). In particular the Director of Public Prosecutions is said to have believed there would have been sufficient evidence to bring charges against Roberts, Cordle and Maudling had it not been for this exclusion (Baston 2000: 107).

The Select Committee considered Cordle in contempt for raising a matter in the House for financial reward. It was more mildly critical of Roberts and

Maudling, Home Secretary and effectively Deputy Prime Minister, whose four letters to the Maltese Government, including one to the Prime Minister of Malta, had been a central plank of Poulson's attempt to secure a hospital building contract in Gozo. The House proved reluctant to endorse the Committee's report, though Cordle had resigned his seat by the time the debate took place. Roberts apologized for his 'shallow waters' activity. Maudling, in his rather self-serving *Memoirs* (Maudling 1978: Chapter 14), continued to deny all wrongdoing, attacked what he perceived as the injustice of parts of the Select Committee report, and twice claimed that, even with hindsight, he could not see what he had done wrong or could have done differently. He was restored to the shadow front bench, though he was to die suddenly and prematurely three years later, having, in Baston's view, fought in the meantime to prevent the full case against him reaching the public domain (Baston 2000: 109).

The Select Committee on Members' Interests, instituted in 1969 following reports that Gordon Bagier, a Labour MP, had been hired by a public relations firm to improve the image of the ruling junta in Greece (Riddell 2000: 133), had never been effective. This was not least because the question of the suitability of interests (as opposed to the declaration of interests) lay outside its remit. The House responded to this inadequacy with new rules on disclosure in 1974 and a Register of Members' Interests, proposed at the same time, was introduced in 1975. The Register, however, was weak and vague; and, largely because Enoch Powell, then Unionist MP for Down South, refused on principle to complete it, not published for five years. This weak approach was short-lived mainly as a result of fall-out from the fact that during the 1980s increasing numbers of MPs were hired by lobbying organizations. This led to mounting press and public concern about standards in public life (or, more precisely, about the catch-all onomatopoeic word 'sleaze'), and in 1994 the Register of Members' Interests eventually, though not bloodlessly, achieved bipartisan acceptance as a necessary part of that process. So from a situation in which MPs openly and sometimes jocularly manoeuvred to conceal ambiguous interests or exploit loopholes or accidental omissions, failure to register even minor interests rapidly became sensitive, with whips leaving Members in no doubt as to the likely consequences of concealment.

Also in 1994 the Prime Minister, John Major, instituted an independent Committee on Standards in Public Life, chaired by a senior judge, Lord Nolan. The shock waves from Nolan's first Report (Nolan 1995) profoundly affected the political process. The Report enunciated seven principles of public life (selflessness, integrity, objectivity, accountability, openness, honesty and leadership) and made fifty-five recommendations, addressed to MPs (1–11), Ministers and Civil Servants (12–32), and Quangos (Quasi-Autonomous Non-Governmental Organizations) comprising Non-Departmental Public Bodies (NDPBs) and National Health Service Bodies (NHS bodies) (33–55).

So far as *MPs* were concerned, the Committee accepted that they should be permitted to earn income from extra-parliamentary activities, but with 30 per cent of MPs holding consultancies Nolan proposed prohibiting multi-client lobbying or participation in commitments that effectively restricted their freedom of speech. The Committee recommended the compulsory declaration of all income from external sources in £5,000 bands and an estimate of the value of benefits in kind. Next it recommended expanding the existing rules and guidance on avoiding conflicts of interest, reviewing the bribery law and introducing a new Code of Conduct for MPs. Finally it recommended appointing a Parliamentary Commissioner for Standards. The Commissioner would maintain the Register, advise MPs on matters of conduct, advise on implementing the Code, investigate allegations of misconduct and decide 'like a French examining magistrate' (Riddell 2000: 148) whether a prima facie case had been established. Where this was so the Commissioner passed the cases concerned to a sub-committee of the Committee of Privileges for further investigation, with the full Committee operating in an appellate capacity.

On *ministers and civil servants* the recommendations, though more numerous, were less radical as there was less cause for disquiet. Nolan's *first* concern was to protect the independence of the Civil Service from the executive. The appointment of growing numbers of political advisers charged with developing and implementing government policy had, since the 1980s, reflected the frustration of successive prime ministers with the Civil Service's traditional detachment and seemingly bottomless capacity for obfuscation. Nolan's *second* area of concern was the familiar one of retired Cabinet ministers parachuting into lucrative private sector employment relevant to their former responsibilities. Here the Committee proposed extending to them the existing restrictions to which permanent secretaries were subject.

On *quangos* Nolan expressed concern at party political appointments to governing bodies. Both main parties had deployed this practice, particularly in the National Health Service, since the 1980s. The appointment system was clearly open to abuse, was designed, by politicizing the policy-making functions of arm's-length bodies, to achieve the opposite of open and independent debate, and was by definition guaranteed to lead to the appointment of political placemen rather than the best candidates for the job. To address this and other potential sources of corruption the committee recommended instituting an independent Commissioner for Public Appointments to 'regulate, monitor and report on the public appointments process', recommend best practice and head the Public Appointments Unit. It also made a number of relatively uncontentious recommendations concerning propriety and accountability (including financial accountability, which was to be reviewed by the Treasury) in public bodies.

After a hostile and predictably self-interested debate a Select Committee was instituted to advise on implementing Nolan. The Committee initially, and rather ineptly, sought a compromise which replaced statements of earnings with a prohibition on paid advocacy, a proposal defeated following strong media pressure. Accordingly the Register was introduced and the first Parliamentary Commissioner, Sir Gordon Downey, was appointed in November 1995. Downey's successor, Elizabeth Filkin, appointed in 1999, quickly busied herself with high-profile investigations into the conduct of ministers, investigations about which some MPs believed the press to have been disturbingly well briefed. Controversially the House of Commons Commission did not offer Miss Filkin automatic reappointment at the end of her contract in 2002, and, though guaranteed shortlisting if she applied for reappointment, she concluded that what she considered her assiduity had been otherwise interpreted, particularly by the government. The circumstances of Miss Filkin's departure and the fact that the Commissioner's future employment, terms and resources were all determined by MPs invite reflection as to the nature and extent of the Commissioner's independence. Certainly the procedure raises the legitimate question of how to deal with future situations, particularly where genuine dissatisfaction with an appointee's performance exists, in a manner which avoids any suggestion of *parti pris* decision-making. Certainly it appears improbable that the present arrangements will or should prove enduring.

In 1997 the incoming Labour Government revisited the issue, raised twenty years earlier by Salmon, of extending the corruption laws to MPs by means of the creation of a new offence of misuse of public office. The government also, following a Nolan recommendation, proposed tightening the Code of Conduct for ministers following a series of salacious but mainly minor scandals which had proved highly damaging to the previous government. More significantly the government decided to face head-on the longstanding problem of party funding, passing the issue to the Committee on Standards in Public Life, now chaired by Nolan's successor Sir Patrick Neill. The one hundred recommendations in Neill's first report aimed to dispel what Neill called the 'tradition of secrecy' surrounding both donations and General Election expenditure (Neill 1998). The Committee recommended full disclosure of donations in excess of £5,000, a ban on overseas donations, a limit of £20 million on campaign expenditure, the end of blind trusts and the institution of both an Election Commission and a special court with powers to fine wrongdoers. The Committee also made recommendations concerning the long-running problem of honours manipulation. It recommended that the (renamed) Honours Scrutiny Committee[24] investigate all cases in which recommendations were made for an honour at or above CBE level in respect of individuals who had made a party donation of at least £5,000 in the previous five years. The Committee's duty was to satisfy itself that the donation 'made no contribution to the nomination for an honour', as well as to conduct an overall scrutiny of the list to ensure that no pattern of favouritism existed in respect of donating organizations or individuals associated with them.

The main legislative outcome of these recommendations was the Political Parties, Elections and Referendums Act 2000, a substantial piece of legislation which came into effect in 2001. *First*, and most fundamentally, the Act established an independent Electoral Commission, charged, inter alia, with overseeing the management of individual elections and referenda, making more general recommendations concerning electoral law, procedure and boundaries and seeking to promote public understanding of local, national and European electoral systems.[25] Most subsequent provisions fell under the aegis of the Commission.[26] *Second*, the Act imposed restrictions on donations in cash or kind amounting, individually or in total, to over £5,000 in the first instance and £1,000 subsequently. In the case of repeated small donations, mainly to avoid evasion through anonymity or pseudonym, the reporting obligation extended to the donor; company donations were to be declared in the annual directors' report. Parties had the duty to report donations quarterly (weekly during general election periods), with services in kind costed at commercial rates. *Third*, the Act imposed restrictions on campaign expenditure, all of which had to be approved by party treasurers or their nominees. Included in this was expenditure by a third party, to discourage the use of this device to circumvent the Act.

The Act contains provisions that reflect the importance, in corruption control, of independent scrutiny, transparency and criminal sanction. It would be naive, however, to believe it will eliminate all forms of electoral malpractice or be adequately funded to discharge its wide-ranging duties effectively. So long as parties have access to funding which they are not permitted to deploy in elections they will doubtless continue to exploit the interstices between what is permitted and what is not:

> one senior Labour Party source, looking forward to a General Election destined to take place 5 months later, observed: 'The Electoral Commission . . . are dealing with hardened professionals and, as they try and work out what this legislation means in the course of a campaign, I suspect there will be several rings run around them. We are all experts at creative accountancy'.
>
> (Baldwin 2001)

Only a shortage of funds, which has emerged as a real possibility following, *first*, a sharp decline in party membership, *second*, high levels of debt and, *third*, increasing negative publicity attaching to corporate donors, is likely to have such an effect. Such a possibility has in fact caused the government tentatively to raise the possibility of central funding. So many problems, technical as well as political and constitutional, are associated with this, however, that it appears only slightly more of a short-term possibility than the idea of global standards for party financing optimistically, but hopelessly unrealistically, advanced by Transparency International (Ewing 2001).

Conclusion

The story of this chapter is of the United Kingdom's transition from high to low corruption and of the contemporary management of corruption. While, like all case studies, this one is in some respects historically specific, aspects of the British experience may have rather broader relevance.

While the moment of the abandonment of the institutionally corrupt Stuart Court in 1688 and the consequential shift of power to Parliament might appear to have been timely for reform, for a number of reasons this was not so. In fact governance passed from monarchical to what was arguably oligarchic rule with many of the characteristics of the Stuart Court simply transferring to Parliament and the Civil Service. This is not surprising, since for the most part the aristocratic heirs of the Stuart courtiers retained responsibility for the affairs of state largely untroubled either by external scrutiny or by any sense of *noblesse oblige*. In the absence of an effective party system, never mind any notion of politics as a profession, parliamentary politics was predominantly *ad personam*, with loyalty secured through various combinations of bribes, threats, favours returned and family or clan loyalty. As a result Parliament largely reproduced the factionalism of the Stuart Court, and in the early eighteenth century the main challenge to its legitimacy came not from any pressures to democratize but, on the contrary, from Jacobite attempts to raise an army and reinstate the Stuart monarchy. In spite of periodic popular unrest and the best efforts of intellectuals and satirists, therefore, the main political preoccupations of the day lay in foreign and imperial policy.

It was not until the late eighteenth century that it began to be clear that the removal of institutional corruption was a precondition for the continued legitimation of the existing social order. A new political context had emerged, which combined social, demographic and economic transformations at home with the impact of the American and French Revolutions and the French Wars abroad. At home the economic changes and unparalleled levels of social mobility brought about by the collapse in agricultural land values, the new bourgeois industrial class, urbanization, changes in agricultural tenure and methods and exponential increases in population were transformational. The *louche* conduct, protectionist policies, extravagance and incompetence of the ruling elite became unsustainable as Britain transformed into an industrialized capitalist economy in which time became money and free trade a realistic demand of the new bourgeoisie, and in which a new work ethic permeated social, political and economic relations.

These transformations were buttressed by a new instability in the social order, as the rejection of British rule by the American colonists (1775–1783) and the overthrow of the French monarchy (1789–1793) signified the translation into political reality of the philosophical liberalism of Locke and the rationalism of the *philosophes*. If Britain escaped the revolutions which affected much of Europe in the early- to mid-nineteenth centuries it was in part precisely because its power elites had demonstrated a greater willingness and ability to absorb its 'third estate' than had its counterparts in much of Catholic Europe. This process of absorption, which occurred during the early nineteenth century, is in good part the story of the death of old corruption. In fact so conducive to the decline of old corruption were the social, political and economic changes of the ensuing half century that while numerous *manifestations* of corruption continued to exist, by the mid-nineteenth century the underlying *structures* of British governance were sound.

The Klondike mentality of the early Industrial Revolution gave way to a political process in which the merchant classes increasingly assumed political power in both central and local government. Factors including strong party competition, bureaucratization, fear of armed revolt, the need for a fit labour force, the influence of Protestantism on social reform, the rise of worker combinations as prototypical trade unions and a compassionate middle class (including many women) combined to change the face of public policy. Part of this change involved increasing pressure for government to be cheaper, more accountable and less corrupt; demographic changes and the extension of the franchise removed the conditions in which traditional forms of electoral corruption thrived. Accordingly, legislation such as the Corrupt and Illegal Practices Act 1883 was pushing on an open door.

But as we have argued or demonstrated throughout this chapter, while these changes undoubtedly reduced the *incidences* of corruption they also heralded the emergence of new *forms* of it. The extensions of the franchise, while they certainly signalled the end of rotten boroughs and vote buying on the village green, were associated also with an intensification of party competition, the emergence as powerful leaders of men lacking private means, and exponential increases in the costs of election campaigns. The shifts in party funding from small private donations to large corporate ones, whether from business and commercial interests or trade unions, led to vote buying being replaced by policy buying. Successive Honours Lists were manipulated for party and personal gain. The rise in popular literacy led to the emergence of newspaper magnates as power brokers to be wooed and bought by political parties. The attractiveness of London to successful businessmen from around the world during the unsettled period during and after the First World War led to an influx of 'new money'. This proved a temptation which the increasingly impoverished elites, many of whom were more than happy to trade social class and prestige for hard currency, saw little reason to resist.

But while corruption transformed itself it also declined dramatically. Though there are exceptions to this rule, normally the political conditions conducive to successful democracy are not conducive to high corruption. These include a strong, or at least potentially strong, civil society with constitutional safeguards on the use of coercion, a wide franchise, healthy party competition, free press, independent judiciary, accountable and transparent executive, free trade policy, competitive economy, rule of law, social mobility, a strong middle class and an educated and well-fed electorate. In Great Britain, where these characteristics all exist, corruption is now the exception, not the rule. Nonetheless any complacency would be misplaced, for maintaining low corruption entails identifying pressure points where the potential for disequilibrium exists; and it should be apparent by now that in some areas of the polity, notably local government, system integrity remains both recent and fragile. *Domestically* these pressure points include, *first*, the culture of secrecy, and the lack of robust, independently monitored freedom of information legislation; *second*, regionalization and devolution, likely to be transformational for local government, which will, however, still be managed by some of the people currently in charge of it, and which will provoke new turf wars with central and supranational governments which will offer scope for ambiguity and manipulation; *third*, changes in Civil Service size, recruitment, functions and terms and conditions stemming from factors including the bipartisan political popularity of Next Steps agencies and the proliferation and status of special advisers, which are impacting on the culture and conduct of some (not all) parts of the Service.

Internationally the UK is by no means exempt from the pressure points identified elsewhere in this book – organized crime, human trafficking, large-scale smuggling, legal migration and the international drug and weapons trades. In addition, problems with the weakening of border controls, particularly following the Schengen Agreement 1995, will be exacerbated by the European Union's proposed extension of its eastern borders in 2004. Finally, as a net contributor to the EU, the UK is also a victim of international corruption. As we have seen already, and shall see again in Chapter 7, subsidy and grant fraud is now a major source of income for organized criminals. But the EU's internal accounting mechanisms lack robustness and are vulnerable not only to this but also to peculation by bureaucrats and politicians. With the increasing integration of the United Kingdom into the European Union it may well be that the unit of attention in corruption studies will shift eastward. This, however, is not an aspect of the topic addressed centrally in this book, not least because the post-2004 transformations of the Union itself will render anything we can say about EU corruption out of date almost as soon as it appears. For a detailed study of this subject another book, probably by another author, will be needed.

Notes

1 Though entitled 'the United Kingdom' this chapter is predominantly about England. The story of political corruption in Northern Ireland is, though both interesting and instructive, better reserved for a full-length study. Nor do we address banking probity in the UK's off-shore tax havens in the Channel Islands and the Isle of Man.

2 Party whips are executive postholders charged with ensuring discipline and bringing potential sources of dissent (and individual dissenting members) to the attention of the chief whip. The chief whip's capacity to damage (and in extreme cases end) the careers of both corrupt and troublesome MPs is considerable. Another traditional function of the chief whip is to oversee the Honours List; we shall encounter chief whips in that capacity later in the chapter.

3 Parliamentary privilege also provides other rights and immunities, including freedom of speech, freedom from arrest in civil actions and exemption from compulsory jury service and witness attendance. The topic has been under review since 1997, when both Houses established a Joint Committee on Parliamentary Privilege which reported to both Houses during Session 1998–1999.

4 For ministers the rules have been tighter since Balfour (1895) Campbell-Bannerman (1906) and Asquith (1913) laid down restrictions, albeit more to prevent ministers being deflected from their duties than to discourage corruption.

5 There have historically been stronger rules with regard to voting; and while with today's strong party system it is rare for voting to be contentious this was not always the case. For example in the nineteenth century individual members frequently had financial interests in the success of individual railway Bills. This is discussed in greater detail later.

6 Lloyd George introduced the payment of MPs in 1911, not to make the job a salaried profession but to enable low-paid workers to enter the Commons. In 1964 the salary of £1,750 was lower in real terms than it had been at £600 in 1911. Since the 1980s parliamentary salaries have been subject to review by an independent body, the Review Body on Top Salaries (now the Senior Salaries Review Body (SSRB)). Nonetheless the sight of MPs voting themselves a salary or pension increase remains a matter of political sensitivity, especially in times of economic recession or when Parliament is for some reason in bad public odour.

7 Such economy was legitimated in the case of Civil Servants by the Osmotherly Memorandum, which guided their answers to questioning by Select Committees.

8 It knew not least because MI6 was allegedly running an agent inside the company. The supposed agent, Henderson, was to be a defendant in the ensuing trial (Leigh 1993: 9).

9 In his evidence to the Scott Inquiry in 1994 the Head of the Civil Service, Sir Robin Butler, defended ministerial statements to Parliament on the ground that 'half the picture can be true' (Pyper 1995: 162).

10 The phrase 'akin to' is chosen carefully. No such conspiracy occurred, though it is just possible that in the absence of parliamentary privilege – see discussion above – a prima facie case that one existed could have been established.

11 Mr Major did not address the more difficult problem of the democratic accountability of these services, a matter which remains unresolved. The possibility of corruption in MI5 and MI6 naturally exists, but is not addressed in this book.

12 *The Life and Strange Surprising Adventures of Robinson Crusoe of York, Mariner*, published in 1719, was set in the seventeenth century.

13 Cordite is a form of smokeless explosive, essential in the manufacture of certain kinds of weaponry.

14 For example, during the Lloyd George administration an anti-corruption campaign launched by the *Morning Post* brought in nearly £22,000 as a fighting fund, 'so that the forces of good could combat the forces of evil on more or less equal terms' (Searle 1987: 360).

15 Not entirely representative: women aged 21–29 were not enfranchised until 1928.

16 Controversies over Civil Service recruitment in 1911 had led to pressure for a Royal Commission to investigate aspects of the Civil Service, including recruitment. Further controversies had followed the wartime appointment, without open competition, of over 2,000 established Civil Servants and almost 10,000 temporary ones, many of them to administer Lloyd George's new social welfare provisions. Some of the new recruits were former Liberal MPs; one, employed in the Port of London Authority, was Lloyd George's own son (Searle 187: 222–226).

17 As late as the mid-nineteenth century, 'government departments were largely independent fiefdoms, recruitment methods varied, there was great scope for patronage and corruption, and favouritism rather than competence tended to be the main determinant of promotion' (Pyper 1995: 6).

18 For a helpful discussion of the various constraints on the practical freedom of the press see Doig (1983).

19 *Private Eye*'s success in highlighting corruption cases should not, however, be underestimated. The magazine was the first national publication to take an interest in Poulson in the 1970s – see discussion below – when the interest among national dailies was minimal. The magazine also tenaciously reported a long-running corruption saga in Doncaster (South Yorkshire) in the 1990s, which led to the imprisonment of several councillors and officials.

20 Birmingham is the United Kingdom's second city. So poor was the work undertaken in the 1960s that its city centre was at least partly rebuilt once again in the 1990s, naturally at great public expense.

21 For fuller accounts of the affair see Doig (1984: Chapter 5) and Baston (2000: Chapter 6).

22 The author's mother once informed him that this technique of neutralization was employed by volunteer staff in a charity shop who considered themselves justified in stealing any gifts that took their fancy. Like Queen Victoria, Mrs Harris was not amused.

23 The Commission was created under the Local Government Finance Act 1982, implemented on 1 April 1983.

24 Previously the Political Honours Scrutiny Committee.

25 This last duty reflects the government's wish to address voter apathy by promoting 'active citizenship' from school onwards. It will be clear that we believe such an approach, when associated with the literacy and economic well-being that can be taken for granted in advanced industrialized democracies, constitutes, in principle, a potentially significant contribution to corruption control. How achievable it is in practice remains to be seen.

26 There are, however, specific (and sometimes significant) exclusions, notably relating to Scotland, in respect of matters under the jurisdiction of the Scottish Parliament. The impact of devolution on national corruption control may prove an interesting research topic in about a decade's time.

5 Transnational political corruption (I): international finance

It is by no means evident that the chancelleries of the donor governments fully understand that the Africa with which they maintain relations is often no more than a decor of *trompe-l'œil*. . . . Discourses concerning 'good governance' . . . intended by donors as therapeutic remedies, are more surreal than real when considered in relation to what is happening in Liberia, Sierra Leone, Chad and the Central African Republic, where the only effective law is frequently that of the various armed bands whose political and moral codes, informal though they may be, are certainly not those of the World Bank.

(Bayart *et al.* 1999: 19–20)

Contemporary political corruption and its criminal accretions are global in scope, and to understand them it is necessary to understand also something of the changing politics of international, transnational and supranational activity (see Beare 2000b). The delicate multiculturalism which has characterized much western intellectual thought since the 1960s is relevant to the 'real world' transactions of politicians, bureaucrats, economists, entrepreneurs, banking and commercial corporations and aid donors and recipients mainly to the extent that an awareness of it is good for business. The world of action's counterpoint to the intellectual push towards cultural, social and political pluralism is a pull towards international standardization and harmonization, and a sometimes selective preference for international free trade over cultural constraint or nation state mercantilism.

From the point of view of corruption control this is, in spite of the unavoidable short-term turbulence attendant upon economic liberalization discussed in Chapter 2, on the whole probably beneficial. Few things are better designed to perpetuate political and bureaucratic corruption than the unquestioning acceptance of traditional relations and customary authority. Whether the elites are village elders, tribal chiefs, hereditary aristocrats or military dictators, customary authority elevates them almost to the role of Hobbesian Leviathans, insulated from the disciplines of the market, devoid of obligation and above external scrutiny. Such models of governance are, irrespective of cultural provenance, palpably unsuited to the contemporary world. Rose-Ackerman's comment that economics 'cannot answer cultural problems, but it can help one understand the implications of a society's choices' (Rose-Ackerman 1999: 92 has its parallel in politics also).

Nonetheless, this pull towards international standardization and harmonization is heavily qualified by the absence of any universally legitimated supranational authority. For example the International Criminal Court, eventually inaugurated in 2002, lacks superpower recognition and has residual functions only, while the jurisdiction of the World Court is limited to the resolution of disputes between sovereign states. Nor, so far as corruption is concerned, and in spite of work undertaken under the auspices of the OECD in particular, does there exist any comprehensive international treaty on corruption of the kind sought by the idealist President Carter. Nation states, for all the battering they have received from international and supranational organizations, multi-national corporations and subnational, including terrorist, organizations, remain key players in the international system.

Nonetheless, a number of structures and arrangements have come into place, including the cautious extension of some legal jurisdictions to embrace crimes committed by nationals overseas, predominantly in spheres of criminal law outside the scope of this book. Attempts to deal with the intrinsically transnational problems associated with sex tourism, for example, include the British approach to overseas child sexual abuse by UK citizens (the Sex Offences Act 1997), and the broadly similar Australian Crimes (Child Sex Tourism) Amendment Act 1994. Australia has also entered into a bilateral agreement with Fiji, a popular location for Australian paedophiles, while there have, in addition, been developments, mainly in the field of police and intelligence cooperation, related to trafficking in narcotics[1] and human migrants. These crimes have in common the fact that their perpetrators, because they attract widespread opprobrium from the left, are soft targets for jurisdictional extensions which would otherwise be vulnerable to attack by civil libertarians.

So far as corruption is concerned, the most significant among such moves remains the US Foreign Corrupt Practices Act 1977 (FCPA), which criminalizes bribes paid by American nationals to public servants abroad. Corrupt practices were sensitive in the United States in the 1970s for a number of reasons. *First*, the US Administration had been embarrassed by investigations by the Securities and Exchange Commission (SEC) in the middle of the decade, revealing that over 400 US companies admitted making questionable or illegal payments in excess of $300 million to foreign government officials, politicians and political parties. *Second*, the legislation may have been motivated in part by US concern to ensure that its own courts dealt, so far as possible, with crimes committed by US citizens. There had been periodic jurisdictional disputes (notably with Japan), between the USA and host countries to US military and airforce bases concerning criminal offences committed by US service personnel, and there was no wish in Washington to extend this problem into such a sensitive area as corruption. *Third*, the unravelling, in the course of Watergate, of revelations about slush funds and internationally laundered illegal contributions to the President's re-election campaign had become of great political significance. And *fourth*, new revelations about US foreign policy escapades in Cambodia and Laos were contributing to a press and public disenchantment not only with US politics but with the democratic and capitalist economic system itself:

> An American aircraft manufacturer owns a European subsidiary that makes passenger seats for its line of jet aircraft. It orders 5000 seats from its subsidiary in Europe but pays for them at a prearranged artificially high price. The difference between the real price, which has already been agreed upon through secret communications, and the fictitious high price, as represented in the invoice, is untaxed gravy. It is deposited by the subsidiary in a special Swiss or Caribbean account and used by the corporate executives as a slush fund, to make illegal political contributions, or to pay bribes. . . . A 'corporation' incorporated for a few hundred dollars in an offshore country can double-invoice nonexistent products just as easily as American Airlines, which used double invoicing to make illegal campaign contributions to President Nixon's 1972 campaign.
>
> (Clarke and Tigue 1976: 105–107)

The Act itself was precipitated by the Lockheed Aircraft scandal, which in turn was a by-product of Watergate. During the Nixon presidency, Lockheed, a near-bankrupt US-based aircraft manufacturer with strong presidential support, bribed senior Japanese, Dutch, Italian, Turkish and other government officials to buy their planes. The case was sensational in almost all the countries concerned, and led, inter alia, to the criminal conviction of the popular former Japanese Prime Minister, Kakuei Tanaka and the disgrace of Prince Bernhard of the Netherlands (Boulton 1978; MacDougall 1988). Such outcomes, associated as they were with widespread publicity and prolonged criminal trials, caused the United States acute diplomatic embarrassment.

On the same principle, the Money Laundering Control Act 1986 involves extraterritorial jurisdiction in respect of overseas money laundering by US citizens, while developments in international banking regulation now feature regularly as part of an attack on organized crime and money laundering.[2] Similarly the intervention of law enforcement agencies in areas such as customs and excise, the intelligence services and the army has become more assertive, reflecting a growing international trend towards prioritizing national security over individual liberty (Naylor 1999; Sheptycki 2000b; Bigo 2000; for a Canadian case study, Brodeur 2000). This is seldom a straightforward process. Sheptycki suggests that action against drug money, for example, is a 'Trojan horse', with surveillance systems designed to identify money launderers being capable of targeting the much larger sums concealed by tax evaders (Sheptycki 2000b). And:

> when law enforcement and foreign policy are mixed together, on the ideological justification of meeting a new threat to national security, all too often the first gets twisted to serve the independently-derived requirements of the second.
>
> (Lupsha 1996: 52)

Any contemporary analysis of political corruption must set its subject in the context of a network of activities which includes negotiating and developing policies to develop, and administrative machinery to implement, a transnational response to these global trends in criminal activity. In Europe this has included the creation of data centres such as the Schengen Information System, European police liaison officers (Bigo 2000), Europol[3] and, more broadly, the virtual merging of policing and military functions in some UN peacekeeping operations and the diversification of Interpol.

Nonetheless, globalization has ramifications for domestic law enforcement agencies too, both because transnational corruption normally requires the corruption of a range of domestic officials and because the availability of overseas bolt-holes for illicit money reduces disincentives to common criminality. Nonetheless, the challenges facing the necessarily cooperative international responses should not be underestimated. Investigating transnational corruption is often highly technical, complex and costly, making heavy demands on law enforcement agencies' intelligence and investigative resources, which often have to be deployed for long periods and at high cost before a successful prosecution can be mounted. Hence the thought, near universal in collaborative enterprises, that some of what is being investigated is someone else's business or that other partners are not contributing equally to the task inevitably occurs periodically to domestic politicians. Political support for funding investigations in areas such as international fraud and money laundering, particularly when more visible forms of crime cause far greater public concern, will always be limited. For the foreseeable future the likelihood of transnational political corruption featuring prominently on any country's fear of crime indices remains modest; and fear of crime has a decidedly greater influence on voting behaviour than does the control of international corruption.

Yet while international cooperative activities are often described as manifestations of global interdependence, this concept, in that it implies an equality of dependence belied by the economic and political imbalance between developed and less-developed worlds, invites analytic sloppiness and is used parsimoniously here. It is not, however, a concept that can be ignored. At a banal level it has force in environmental and cyber politics. Self-evidently, faulty nuclear reactors are no respecters of national boundaries, US greenhouse gas emissions are unlikely to be deemed a purely private matter by the countries affected by them, and a computer virus hatched in a Manila tenement can cause chaos in the Pentagon or on Wall Street. Nonetheless, the 'dependence' of developed world countries on exploiting less-developed world labour markets and natural resources is of a lesser order than that of the less-developed world on the economic strength and political benison of the west. This asymmetrical interdependence (Keohane and Nye 1989) ensures that emerging transnational and supra-national legal, political, intelligence, communications, commercial and trad-ing formations reflect developed world (particularly US) interests, culture and values.

A consequence of asymmetrical interdependence is that less-developed nations are encouraged to conduct themselves in ways most likely to bring US approval. It is scarcely novel to comment on the role of superpower influence during the Cold War as a surreptitious prop for corrupt less-developed world regimes (see for example McCoy 1991). Indeed superpower support for such regimes was understandably deployed by the Jubilee 2000 Coalition[4] as a response to the argument that political corruption in less-developed countries justified delays in debt rescheduling or remission. *First*, the Iran–Contra affair is a well-documented instance of the use of laundered money to fund sympathetic organizations (Walsh 1997). *Second*, the extraordinary conduct of the Bank of Credit and Commerce Inter-national in moving hidden money round the world, defying all regulators until it was shut down in 1991 owing a still unknown number of billions of dollars resembles a Hollywood blockbuster (Adams and Frantz 1992). *Third*, the US role in attempting to suppress opium-growing and heroin manufacture in Pakistan's wild and lawless North-West Frontier Province was considerable (Asad and Harris 2003).

Especially significant among emerging transnational and supranational structures have been around 500 regionally negotiated common interest groupings, particularly intergovernmental organizations (IGOs). While they operate in significantly different ways, these bodies all entail aspects of national autonomy being traded for the benefits of operating within more powerful political and economic blocs. Some of these organizations com-prise groupings of aid-dependent nations subject to conditions imposed by the World Bank and IMF, increasingly pressed to enforce western standards of non-corrupt behaviour as well as sympathetic economic systems on their member states. Although not all such bodies have proved exemplary on their own count in this respect, creating vast new rent-seeking opportunities for their staff and clients, it seems likely that there will emerge in the longer term a simultaneous simplification and complication of transnational politi-cal corruption: simplification as globalizing forces and superpower pressure gradually diminish the cultural and governmental quirks of less influential member states; complication as new corrupt and criminal opportunities burst through to accompany those same globalizing forces.

Hence the latter part of the twentieth century saw the realignment of the international system under pressure from changes which followed the end of the Cold War and which were achieved by technological advances in electronic communications. Globalization is better comprehended politically than technologically, however, with the present unipolar international system the end, and technology a central part of the means, of this realignment. While the electronics revolution, by permitting technological transformations such as global round-the-clock banking, has enabled globalization to take the form it has and therefore helped shape its nature and character, technology alone would not have achieved globalization in different political circumstances. Globalization is, therefore, essentially a post-Cold War phenomenon.

The end of the Cold War, however, while it permitted certain transformations *within* the existing international system, did not effect any transformation *of* that system. *First*, as part of an overall restructuring of military expenditure yielding a peace dividend of over $100 billion in the 1990s, the US largely ceased supporting anti-communist regimes in former client states such as Chile, South Korea and Indonesia. Only Taiwan, which has strong support in the Senate and continues to provide useful leverage in Sino-US relations, continues to enjoy significant political clout in Washington, being awarded periodic diplomatic coups and being permitted to purchase quite high-level military hardware. Similarly the US lost interest in supporting rebel factions in former Soviet client states such as Nicaragua, Angola (an African oil-producing country containing strong US oil interests, taken over by a Marxist regime in 1975) and, until 2001, Afghanistan. The loss of superpower support has been economically devastating for many less-developed countries, not only on the US side but also for such former Soviet client states as North Korea and Cuba, which currently lack the infrastructure to survive in a competitive global economy.

Superpower withdrawal has had complex consequences, for example the ending of the First Republic in Italy, while the Soviet collapse has led to domestic instability in much of the former Soviet Empire. This has transformed some countries, such as Tajikistan and Moldova, into privatized predatory states, and permitted others, notably Azerbaijan and Armenia, to engage in armed conflict – in this case over a longstanding border dispute concerning Nagorno-Karabakh, an Azerbaijani territory with an Armenian population. In short, the informal rules of international conduct, built up over the forty years of the Cold War, have been, if not torn up, at least found in need of major revision. This has thrown up new challenges and opportunities, both for nation states and for criminal elements, to exploit new vacuums and create new interstices.

Second, this change in the international climate has seen a shift away from the dominance of Cold War realpolitik towards the liberalization of international trade and new forms of collaboration through regional supranational groupings and cartels such as OPEC. This new framework allows that a state's interests, political, economic and military, may be better secured not by a zero-sum game in which both sides compete for the same slice of cake but by collaborative activities geared to securing the Pareto optimal condition of increasing the size of the cake. This involves regarding other nations as prospective trading partners which can safely be strengthened, rather than prospective enemies to be weakened at every opportunity. It also reflects a change from the traditional assumption that war is good for the economy to the view that, while war does indeed provide a temporary fillip, ultimately it is a costly and dangerous activity best regarded as a last resort. This perceptual transformation entails permitting international trading agreements designed to enhance global efficiency and wealth generation, not an arms race, to fuel the global economy; though in a unipolar international system the ambivalent attitude of the remaining superpower to such agreements and treaties inevitably restricts their effectiveness and authority.

Third, however, as trade barriers come down, whether through removing import tariffs or through the free movement of goods and people within regional free trade zones such as the European Union, new challenges have arisen. International law remains, with qualified exceptions, more akin to the rules of a club of independent sovereign states than a domestic legal system: Hedley Bull's 'anarchical society' (Bull 1977) remains an apposite paradox. If the United Nations in particular is to retain its near universality it can exercise the option of suspension or expulsion only rarely, for if it loses members it also loses status and authority by dint of the jurisdictional contraction involved. So the General Assembly operates by mediating the frequently conflicting interests of different members and voting blocs, while conflicting interests within the Security Council's permanent membership of the USA, Russia, China, Great Britain and France mean that speedy and decisive military action is authorized only in exceptional circumstances. Accordingly, powerful members periodically undertake foreign policy adventures such as the invasion of Grenada and Iraq the Kosovo intervention without Security Council endorsement (for further discussion see Cusimano 2000b) on the formal basis of their own assessment of their position under international law.

Fourth, when developed countries contain less than 25 per cent of the world's population but 70 per cent of its goods and services, economic pressure from potential migrants in less-developed countries will inevitably continue to be a source of friction. The criminal networks instituted to facilitate it will consolidate and expand. Hence they will continue to meet the developed world demand for prostitutes, of whom the supply in LDCs appears almost limitless, and drugs, grown in LDCs and distributed by organized criminals like the Chinese Chiu chau syndicates (McCoy 1991: 389–390).

In this chapter and the next we try to untangle some of these complexities. We proceed by focusing on those aspects of globalization dependent on, predictive of, or productive of, political corruption. Accordingly this discourse moves us away from the study of political corruption in action and towards the conditions associated with it. We have stressed throughout that political corruption cannot sensibly be perceived as a battle between good guys and bad guys, even though there is no shortage of the latter in particular. But bad guys always exist in politics, and they are able to express themselves criminally only in the right conditions nationally and, preferably, transnationally. The transformations in international relations which began in the final decade of the twentieth century constitute part of the opportunities currently available to corrupt politicians.

We begin with the international banking system. In high-corruption countries this is characteristically subordinated to the executive, members of the ruling elite using it rather as a private bank account. But the corruption endemic in such situations also, naturally, makes such banks attractive to international organized criminals as well as to a whole range of smaller potatoes in the criminal world. Accordingly, here and elsewhere political corruption and organized crime exist symbiotically.

International banking

> On signing a four-year, $4.8 million contract with the Boston Red Sox baseball team in 1985, a 30-year-old relief pitcher came up with one of the more memorable tax-related quotations. Said he: 'I guess I'll have to get one of those Swedish bank accounts.'
>
> (Walter 1985: 52)

The architecture of the international and transnational banking and financial systems, put in place at Bretton Woods, New Hampshire in 1944, is normally attributed to John Maynard Keynes and Harry Dexter White, respectively UK and US economic planners during the Second World War (for a fuller account, see Williamson 1977). A key achievement of Bretton Woods was the institution of the International Bank for Reconstruction and Development (or the World Bank, actually a financial intermediary, not a bank) and the International Monetary Fund (IMF), complementary institutions charged with promoting economic reconstruction, stability and growth in a devastated Europe. Today both the Bank and the IMF are situated at the tip of a complex array of public and private banking structures of which they are in no sense in control but with which they attempt to achieve increasingly close liaison. These structures include public and private banks (including the all-important Export–Import Bank of the United States, the official US export credit agency)[5] and commercial operations, and transnational fora such as the Bank for International Settlement, (BIS)[6] and the Institute of International Finance (IIF).[7] In addition, an informal consortium of creditor governments, the Paris Club, formed in 1956, comprises creditor governments from major industrialized countries and meets monthly, often with debtor countries, to negotiate debt restructuring.

The World Bank now has three main arms. *First* there is the original International Bank for Reconstruction and Development (IBRD), which borrows money in the international markets and lends it to middle-income countries and creditworthy poorer countries at an attractive rate. *Second*, the International Finance Corporation (IFC), established in 1956, invests in private enterprises without government guarantee. *Third*, the International Development Association (IDA), established in 1960, receives funding from international donors (mainly governments) and lends it to poorer countries at such low interest rates that the loans in practice contain a substantial grant component. The three institutions together are known as the World Bank Group. Members are required also to be members of IMF.

The International Monetary Fund, effectively a credit cooperative, acts as both agent of member states and intermediary between the collective membership and individual countries, its Board of Governors comprising one senior financial controller from each member country. Like the United Nations, the Fund lacks coercive power over members, though unlike the UN it operates with a weighted voting system under which voting rights are proportional to quota payments. Hence the Group of Seven major nations,[8] charged with policy coordination, remains especially influential in the Fund's Byzantine committee, group and club structure (for an overview of which see International Monetary Fund 2001a). The Fund's twenty-four-strong Executive Board chaired by the Managing Director (by convention a European) meets at least three times a week to supervise policy implementation.

From the first IMF was charged with promoting international monetary cooperation, facilitating the expansion of international trade in the postwar era, helping establish a multilateral system of payments, advising members experiencing balance of payments problems and reducing any disequilibrium stemming from such problems. The Bank, meanwhile, was mandated to provide longer-term strategic developmental funding. Nonetheless these functions were to become blurred during the 1980s, when vastly increased levels of debt following the oil price rise of 1979 posed insoluble balance of payments problems for less-developed countries in particular. At this time the Bank began to emulate the Fund's practice of policy-based lending, making loans to address immediate balance of payments problems and facilitate structural readjustment on the ground that it was removing institutional elements prejudicial to development.

Since the abandonment of the Bretton Woods gold-based system of pegging exchange rates in 1971, the Fund has made loans in the form of Special Drawing Rights (SDR), a meta-currency used, if a tactless analogy can be forgiven, rather as a gambler uses chips. SDRs are exchanged for currency from the country's reserve, with the result that IMF's reserves, which derive mainly from members' quota subscriptions, are never depleted, though their composition varies depending on what loans are outstanding. Countries pay back loans by buying back their own currency. Traditionally each IMF loan *tranche* has entailed increasingly severe obligations. These typically involve an adjustment programme including austere economic measures such as devaluation, public expenditure reductions, privatization, the abolition of price control, demand management through wage caps, credit restrictions and tax and interest rate increases to reduce inflation.

The last quarter century, however, has seen transformations in international political economy. These have included the end of the Cold War, the South-East Asian debt crisis and the stock market crashes of 2001–2002 following the collapse of technology shares, the World Trade Center attack and the exposure of accounting irregularities among major US corporations, some of them boasting the involvement of politicians at the most senior level. In particular, however, the debt crisis following the oil price rise of 1979 meant that Fund policies had to adapt to the fact that levels of LDC debt were no longer curable by traditional prescriptions. Naturally the fact that for some years the USA, economically weakened by financing the Vietnam War, was the largest international debtor, and that between 1968 and 1972 Japan was the only G7 country not to draw on the Fund (Bird 1995: 8), exacerbated the less-developed world's economic problems.

Many debtor countries were at this time experiencing major structural upheavals untreatable by the Fund's usual approach to controlling aggregate demand. To the Fund's critics, 'administering the familiar medicine in larger doses and with a thinner sugar coating' (Killick 1995: 6) could only tip debtor countries into recession, turning them into 'aid junkies' (Payer 1974). Certainly in the 1980s the Fund was increasingly embarrassed to find itself no longer a net contributor to less-developed countries but a net recipient of return flows from them (Killick 1995: 3). In addition it was aware that any perceived weakening of the economy by debt conditions was likely to accelerate capital flight. This was to prove especially so in Eastern Europe following the end of the Cold War, when corrupt capital was exported and laundered by former nomenklatura, KGB personnel and organized criminals with the necessary contacts and language skills, while official governments turned a blind eye (Shelley 1994: 347).

The exponential growth of less-developed world debt, then, occurred between 1978 and 1982, accelerating around the time of the second oil price rise in 1979. At that time, aided by aggressive selling techniques and a less cautious approach to unstable overseas governments than to domestic loans, US private bank exposure among non-oil-producing LDCs quadrupled from $110 billion to $450 billion, with some banks left dangerously short of liquidity. In fact the strategic shifts of several private banks, notably Citicorp, from conventional to money-centre banking (under which they act as brokers, lending money they have themselves borrowed on the international markets) exacerbated this problem. Hence in squeezing debtor nations IMF became vulnerable to the criticism that it was a publicly funded conduit for protecting the interests of private banks, enabling them to make reckless new loans which they immediately reclaimed as interest payments on previous ones. George, a radical critic, remarked acerbically that because in principle this entailed funds being lodged in the very banks that had made the loans in the first place it enabled the latter to 'defy the adage about cake. It turns out the banks *can* both have and eat it' (George 1988: 19).

Another radical critique pursued the logic that accumulated debts were illegitimate because they were instruments of political oppression, and that Latin American countries therefore had a moral duty to default (Branford and Kucinski 1988. For a more balanced analysis of the complex impact of IMF programmes on Latin American countries in the 1980s, see Pastor 1987). In fact the possibility of a debtors' cartel to default had already been mooted in 1982 by Mexico, Brazil and Argentina but rejected as unrealistic for all except the very few countries with the potential for future economic self-sufficiency (Korner *et al.* 1986: 162). The possibility resurfaced in 2002, when, at the height of its economic crisis, Argentina gave active consideration to deploying the same tactic, this time on an individual basis.

Overall, evidence was increasingly emerging that IMF programmes were failing either to secure compliance with loan conditions or to effect the liberalization of trade. Consistently with our arguments in Chapter 2 it was increasingly being acknowledged that liberalization was not the right solution for less-developed countries lacking the legal, political, social and financial frameworks and western economic cycles to support it (Korner *et al.* 1986). But when, as sometimes occurred, IMF loans became a lucrative source of corrupt capital for ruling groups, three problems arose. *First*, they worsened the debt problem by failing to create the liberalized economies they were designed to stimulate; indeed the consequences were more often forms of pseudo-liberalism sustaining inefficient and corrupt political and economic infrastructures that might otherwise have imploded. *Second*, they were saddling debtor countries' economies with new interest payments on capital which included sums already clandestinely exported by the ruling elites. *Third*, pressure on the Fund from powerful creditor countries to avoid slippage and ensure repayment was increasingly encouraging it to turn a blind eye to those governments of debtor countries which achieved repayment by unorthodox and sometimes undesirable means, so causing yet further infrastructure damage.[9] In Sierra Leone, for example, requirements attached to a loan in the 1980s were so stringent that the Government was able to claim it had sold off nationalized corporations to corrupt Lebanese traders (who transpired, happily, to be close associates of the ruling group (Hibou 1999: 92)). Inevitably such situations increase states' vulnerability to effective privatization by criminal elements.

Clearly for the Fund to survive (and, both in 1971 following the abolition of the Bretton Woods system and between the 1980s and the mid-1990s, this was by no means certain)[10] change was necessary. Above all the Fund had to show sufficient flexibility to respond to the comments of its critics by ensuring that programme administration fell into line with the rapidly developing norms of international commerce. These included ever stronger adherence to free trade, a heightened awareness of the likely unintended consequences of trying to buck the market (a charge to which IMF and the Bank were naturally vulnerable) and increased transparency and accountability. The criticisms were fundamental:

First, during the Cold War both the Bank and the Fund had been heavily criticized for acting politically (and therefore inconsistently) in relation to the problem of states whose debtor status had largely been caused by the profligacy and corruption of unaccountable political elites. Undoubtedly during this period both institutions used development aid to restrict the spread of communism and to support US client states. In Nicaragua, George archly wondered, 'Was the Fund acting frivolously when it made a sizeable loan to the Somoza regime only weeks before the Sandinista victory in 1979? Or was it gently but firmly encouraged to do so?' (George 1988: 55). In Zaïre, Mobutu's kleptocratic rule was extended, in spite of previous defaults, by discreet loans on the back of the country's rich mineral deposits in copper, cobalt, diamonds and rare strategic metals (Wrong 2000). World Bank loans to Zaïre totalled over $1 billion in all, with $375 million between 1984 and 1986 alone made in the wake not only of a currency devaluation but also of draconian expenditure cutbacks imposed by the IMF in 1983.

Second, the problem of sovereignty, intrinsic to the activities of organizations such as the Bank and the Fund, emerged as a sensitive issue around this time, particularly given the political corruption endemic in many debtor countries. George, for example, was dismissive of IMF's claim to respect national sovereignty, arguing that its function was precisely to modulate sovereignty on behalf of creditor banks and nations. She argued that IMF should be more, not less, interventive in the political economies of debtor countries, to ensure that loan money was deployed in socially progressive ways, not in a manner designed to enhance rent-seeking opportunities such as unnecessary arms deals and construction contracts:

> economic growth can also result from greater social equality, access to education, health care and other basic services, fairer income distribution, etc., it could perfectly well make such objectives part of its programmes. On the contrary, exactly those countries that have most insisted on maintaining social objectives (for example, Tanzania and Jamaica . . .) have had the greatest difficulties in coming to terms with the IMF.
>
> (George 1988: 53)

Such a goal could most obviously be achieved by boosting the Fund's existing methods of surveillance and increasing both the frequency of review missions and the number of permanent in-country representatives. This, however, would have funding implications for an organization under strong pressure from members, notably the United States, never a country to encourage the ambitions of international organizations to challenge the principle of national sovereignty, to hold and if possible reduce its running costs. Nonetheless both the Fund and the Bank are currently exploring ways of improving the retrospective monitoring of loan expenditure. The Bank, for example, rather than being satisfied with paper promises, is increasing the number of physical inspections and on-site reviews it is undertaking.

While George's line of argument was disingenuous, or at least unrealistic, in implying that improved macroeconomic management could be combined with massive increases in social spending without inflationary risk, and unfair in being aimed at the Fund, not its member states, it had political resonance. From the late 1980s, under the influence of James Baker the policy of the USA, uniquely influential given its 17.5 per cent quota payment and a voting arrangement effectively giving it a veto, became to press the Fund to support programmes aimed at enhancing sustainable growth, placing less emphasis on short-term deflationary measures. This latter approach, normally involving pay cuts, government expenditure reductions, currency devaluation and the removal of import barriers, had so many unintended consequences, in the form of prolonged recession and spiralling debt, that it was detrimental to strategic financial management.[11]

Consistently with this new approach, and under widespread pressure, the Fund experimented with programmes which, while consistent with its traditional emphasis on macroeconomic management, also acknowledged the relevance of social development. Accordingly the Heavily Indebted Poor Countries (HIPC) Initiative of 1996[12] and the Poverty Reduction and Growth Facility (PRGF)[13] of 1999 signalled a cautious venture into social policy. The Fund's delicacy reflected a history of demarcation sensitivities with the World Bank, doubtless sharpened by the suggestion from the Fifty Years is Enough group on the left and monetarist economists on the right that the two organizations might be ripe for merger. In particular the Fund began expressing concerns about levels of military as against social expenditure and environmental protection in debtor countries (both coded language for an intention to address political corruption) and began monitoring debtor government expenditure in far greater detail than would previously have been acceptable. In 2001, for example, the IMF reported itself cautiously encouraged by average falls in military spending during the 1990s of 1.2 per cent of GDP in low income countries, and average increases of 0.8 per cent of GDP in social spending with IMF supported programmes (International Monetary Fund 2001b: 2).

Similarly, successive World Bank Presidents and IMF Managing Directors, goaded by public attacks, made high profile criticisms of their own members, reminding them of their UN pledges:

Debt relief under the HIPC Initiative will remove a critical obstacle to poverty reduction and growth from the path of poor countries, but it is no panacea. Without renewed growth, these countries could once again fall into a debt trap. . . . More outside help is also essential. IMF Managing Director Horst Kohler, and World Bank President James Wolfensohn have called in no uncertain terms for rich countries to meet the UN target for development assistance of 0.7 percent of GNP.[14] Even more important, by removing trade barriers, the rich could also help to provide a livelihood for millions in the poorest countries by benefiting themselves.

(International Monetary Fund 2001c: 2)

By the mid-1990s cross-border lending was running at more than a quarter of GDP of all industrialized nations, and international bank assets stood at twice the value of world trade (Hutton 1995). This gave the banks such political clout as to place them beyond the control of any nation or international organization. At this time both IMF and the Bank were becoming increasingly confident about confronting corruption directly, rather than euphemistically alluding to the need for transparency and accountability. In 1997 both bodies announced plans to use their influence to curb corruption in less developed countries (World Bank 1997), placing greater emphasis on the 'internalization' of the reform process in the polities of recipient countries. In the same year OECD approved the landmark Convention on Combating Bribery of Foreign Public Officials in International Business Transactions, an initiative actively supported by the Bank. The Bank, meanwhile, revised its own procurement guidelines to include corruption and fraud as grounds for contract cancellation, announced an anti-corruption policy framework and offered to advise countries attempting to reduce corruption. The following year the Fund produced its voluntary Code of Good Practices on Fiscal Transparency and was instructed by its Executive Board, stung by periodic complaints about excessive secrecy, arrogance and insensitivity among IMF staff, to increase its own transparency. This was greatly in the Fund's interests: not least, it had recently been embarrassed that its public endorsement of Soeharto's economic achievements in Indonesia had concealed the very brisk nature of its private dealings with the regime (Hill 1998: 98), and clearly a transparent approach would shield it from such criticism. The Bank, meanwhile, made a virtually identical commitment in the same year, instituting a special unit in its Internal Audit Department and recruiting external consultants to monitor the probity of *its* activities.

The Fund's attempts to address corruption included attacks on fiscal incentive distortions, governmental support for inefficient public sector corporations offering rent-seeking opportunities to ruling elites, public subsidies, price controls, and structural deficiencies such as poor management and political manipulation in the banking sector. An example of the kind of problem the Fund had in mind was the Kenyan Government's success in 1994 in persuading two private banks to deposit funds with the central bank on its behalf to raise the balances to the eligibility level for a new loan facility. This deception, combined with subsequent scandals, led the Fund to consider that Kenya had failed to take promised steps against corruption and to suspend a proposed $220 million loan in 1997.[15]

These attempts came also in the wake of the 1997 devaluations and stock market collapses in East and South-East Asia. In that year financial speculators successively attacked South-East Asian currencies, helping precipitate an economic meltdown affecting also South Korea (where the won, currency of the world's eleventh largest economy, was savaged) and even Japan, with serious global consequences.[16] Rapid economic growth among inherently unstable South-East Asian economies buttressed by irresponsible lending stemming from the subordination of the banking sector to corrupt political leaders had seen those countries' stock markets rise to unsustainable levels. When currency speculators began selling off the currencies a loss of confidence among investors led to an epidemic of crashes followed by devaluation and economic chaos. These hits were most successful in countries whose political and economic superstructures were insufficiently robust to sustain their own currencies, and where corrupt political systems impeded economic transparency and propriety. Hence first to be attacked was the Thai baht, followed by the Indonesian rupiah, countries governed, respectively, by a succession of variably weak and corrupt civil administrations interspersed with military ones, and by the institutionally corrupt Soeharto dictatorship.

The Fund's role in relation to this crisis had some success in addressing the acute problem, if not the underlying chronic vulnerability, of weak South-East Asian states. Thailand secured a $16 billion loan after initially rejecting IMF conditions, agreeing to close dozens of indebted banks and accepting tough structural reform conditions which led to the fall of the government. The Philippines, having lost $1 billion in unsuccessfully trying to prop up its own currency, agreed to tough conditions for a $1 billion loan which included tightening government control of private banks, some of them openly corrupt. In South Korea, recipient of the biggest loan, $60 billion, the economic squeeze had an overall positive effect. The country was facing a 20 per cent currency devaluation and a stock market crash. Its banks held $50 billion bad debts resulting from years of chronic political corruption, politically motivated economic decision-making and interference in the banking system (Kang 2002). A reformist president, Kim Dae Jong, was elected, and, as in Thailand, the economic squeeze, precipitated by currency speculators but predisposed by underlying economic weakness and corruption, had at least a medium-term positive effect.

Indonesia, however, facing national bankruptcy, accepted a huge IMF loan but failed to meet its stringent conditions. That country's remarkable economic development over more than thirty years had been accompanied by increasingly embedded corruption. In particular General Soeharto had ensured that the political and banking systems were so inextricably intertwined that as a matter of course the latter's main function was to meet the demands of the former. In addition, his Leviathan status meant the system also provided more then generously for his family (including his deeply unpopular and rather unIslamic playboy son, Tommy), supporters and clients. Now, however, the chickens had come home to roost and the banks, sources of direct revenue for Soeharto's clique during the fat years, faced bankruptcy, in part as a result of the very non-performing loans that had made them rich.

Naturally other predisposing factors also existed. Particularly significant were the maintenance of artificially high lending rates and the accumulation of around $30 to $40 billion in foreign debt, the currency flotation and the panic caused by the sudden and unexplained closure of sixteen banks (for a fuller discussion of the crash see Hill 1998). Additional underlying social and economic factors included capital flight among the economically successful Chinese community whose members had been experiencing mounting racial violence for some years, and poor rice harvests associated with the El Niño phenomenon. So while political corruption is not a sufficient explanation for the Indonesian economic collapse – after all many corrupt regimes elsewhere have not suffered the same fate – Soeharto's fall was precipitated by student revolts against this and other aspects of his regime (Forrester and May 1998). In particular, the public reaction to the killing of four students from Trisakti University in Jakarta in May 1998 in the riots following Indonesia's failure to secure the IMF loan provoked the anarchic conditions which led to the deaths of 1,000 people on 14 May 1998. It was this in turn that, a week later, provoked the resignation of Soeharto, now bereft of the support of even his closest political allies (Bhakti 1998).

Money laundering

> The Mafia man telephoned his *capo di tutti* back in the old country and said: 'OK, we have the cocaine sourced in Bolivia, we have the courier system to bring it in to Britain together with all the forged import documentation; we have the concealed containers produced and we have various customs officials on the payroll. We have a distribution network developed on a cell basis, impossible to track back, and we have all the offshore accounts in place. We have opened various shell companies and are able to implement all the placement and layering to legalise the funds. But we have just hit a major snag. The British anti-money-laundering rules say we have to produce a gas or electricity bill before we can open the trading account. How can we possibly organise that?'
>
> (Hilton 2000)

Money laundering normally involves three key phases – placement, layering and integration. These are not always distinct, and each can, unsurprisingly in a world where obfuscation is the key to success, take multifarious forms. For example, any of them can be subcontracted in return for generous commission payments or delayed for lengthy periods of time during which the money is transacted within such illicit markets as those in stolen art and antiques.

Placement entails depositing the funds in a local or foreign bank. If the local bank is compliant with the Financial Action Task Force's (FATF) Forty Recommendations (see below), senior staff are incorruptible, the launderers are insufficiently well connected and corrupt political leaders cannot exert political leverage on the banks, placement risks are high and wise launderers will look elsewhere. One possible option is to make use of less reputable domestic outlets such as independent *bureaux de change* and casinos, where relatively small sums of money can be 'buried' at relatively low risk, though a number of countries are currently attacking the *bureaux* option with regulatory legislation. A more paradoxical method is to declare dirty money as a business profit and pay capital gains tax on it – at a stroke laundering the remainder (Clarke and Tigue 1976: 134).

For larger sums launderers might consider it prudent to make their deposits, simultaneously or sequentially, in corrupt foreign banks or in those non-compliant with the Forty Recommendations. This tactic, however, exposes launderers to risks associated with physical transportation as well as to the high transaction costs of courier expenses, commission and insurance in the form of bribing officials along the way.[17] In the case of corrupt banking regimes in weak or predatory states, the fact that enforcement is a perennial problem in criminal transactions means there is also a risk of losing money through double-crossing by bank officials or their political patrons.

The existence of informal and criminal networks often permits dirty money to stay dirty for a prolonged period of time. This can be done by investing in stolen goods including gold (especially useful as it can be melted down or disguised without loss of value), jewellery,[18] works of art and such prohibited goods as ivory or protected species, or paying other criminals for services rendered. In many less-developed countries, particularly in Africa, launderers will place their funds in informal or underground 'banks', many merchants and local 'big men' openly providing such a service by offering a commission-deducted voucher exchangeable at a specified alternative location (Bosworth-Davies and Saltmarsh 1994: 74–77). Dirty money's heavily discounted market value, reflecting the fact that the receiver, not the purchaser, is exposed to the laundering risk, makes permitting or participating in such activity an attractive additional income stream for predatory politicians and bureaucrats in countries whose financial structures are effectively an arm of politics.

Layering, a battle of wits between launderer and auditor, involves, as the name implies, creating complex layers of financial transactions to separate the money from its illicit source until the money is 'lost' in the system. Funds can be wired across jurisdictions, split, placed in numerous (legitimate) accounts in different names where they can be disguised as payments for goods or services, transferred, withdrawn and redeposited with such rapidity and over such a wide area that tracing them is almost impossible. Otherwise the money can be placed in loss-making shell companies offshore, channelled through the purchase and sale of investment instruments such as securities or used as collateral for loans (Sheptycki 2000b). Tracking it down is, for two main reasons, more difficult than looking for a needle in a haystack: that quest may at least ultimately result in the location of an identifiable object; and doubtless it is also undertaken by dedicated needle hunting personnel. Effective layering, however, makes dirty and clean money indistinguishable, as though, while the haystack were undergoing the search, the needle had been by alchemy transformed into a piece of hay. In addition, those hunting the dirty money are not part of a single investigative force working within a single jurisdiction with a unitary command structure. Rather they are officials seconded by different nations, but not always adequately trained, funded or supported, trusting of their international colleagues or working to the same priorities. And the quest takes place in a system which is itself variegated and uncoordinated. There is scope for confusion as to the jurisdictions and practices of bodies mandated to tackle the problem, with consequent duplication, omission, bad feeling and competition. And ultimately, though the main private banks are increasingly moving towards accepting a common approach (the so-called Wolfsberg Principles, following a key meeting in the eponymous Swiss town in 2000) success is dependent on the cooperation of officials whose enthusiasm for the task may be variable.

Integration involves reinvesting the separated funds in legitimate enterprises. At this point, and assuming layering has been successful, the launderers can spend the money as they wish, ensuring only that dramatic changes of lifestyle do not attract the attention of law enforcement agents. Stashing, historically common among organized criminals with a distaste for banks, is seldom wise in view of the vast sums of money involved since the emergence of heroin as a profitable commodity and the possibility of theft, detection, betrayal, inflation, note deterioration and new issue banknotes. Nor, indeed, is stashing any longer necessary, given the new technical options afforded by the global free market in financial transactions.

Popular integrating techniques include borrowing funds from front companies in the control of the launderer's associates or from foreign banks which accept the newly clean money as surety, and producing false invoices for goods supposedly sold across borders. Much laundered money is invested in property, the sports or entertainment industries, bearer bonds in cooperative less-developed countries (especially in the Indian sub-continent), life assurance (cashed in shortly after inception), blank airline tickets, business enterprises in emerging markets and luxury goods likely to increase in value. In addition, gambling activities with high cash transactions such as vending, video and pinball machines and gambling on a wide and increasing range of sporting events are attractive propositions, even though expenses are inevitably incurred, whether as gambling losses or corruption costs.[19] In other situations laundered money offers commercial advantages in bribery of commercial operators and politicians and in high-risk-for-high-return business activities such as venture capitalism. In relation to the former, dirty money can support clean money precisely because it does not have to be buried in company accounts. Launderers are free of large public corporations' need for caution, and untaxed criminal money can substantially shorten the odds against success. By such means newly laundered money can make clean money, and for this reason the Mafia, to whom laundering has long been a vital income source,[20] is now widely believed to make more money from legitimate than from illegitimate enterprises.

Recent decades have seen a phenomenal increase in transnational financial transactions, estimated in 1995 (though caution is indicated about such estimates) at a level of $1.3 trillion a day. Such a level of financial activity has been made possible mainly by the currency floatations which followed the abandonment of the Bretton Woods system in 1971 and the technological changes associated with globalization. The Financial Action Task Force estimates that of the $120 billion thought to be made annually from sales of cocaine, heroin and cannabis to the USA and Europe, around $85 billion is available for money laundering. In 1996 IMF estimated that in total between $590 billion and $1.5 trillion was being laundered annually, though criminal transactions are extraordinarily hard to detect because the mechanisms are in key respects identical to those of legitimate ones. Indeed the very purpose of such transactions is to integrate them seamlessly into legitimate outlets. The involvement of many weak, not to say criminally privatized, states in international banking, their numbers increasing following the break-up of the Soviet Empire in the early 1990s, naturally accelerated and expanded such possibilities. For example, of around 1,000 new banks in Russia, probably two-thirds are financed or heavily influenced by criminals.

Though the widespread economic liberalization of the 1980s played a part in facilitating this, it is only partially correct to regard such criminality as an unavoidable outcrop of the intrinsic properties of the market. Of greater significance is the fact that that from the first the fox has had better legs than the hounds, the technologies of surveillance lagging behind those of criminality. Even more significant, however, was the assumption, widespread in the 1980s, that the deregulation of trade and financial services associated with economic liberalization necessitates less rather than more state supervision of financial transactions and border controls. This problem, which has developed since the 1960s with the rapid increase in off-shore banking facilities, has been compounded since the 1990s by the strengthening of supranational regional groupings. There have been reductions in border controls in several Latin American countries, including Panama, Mexico, Colombia and Brazil, while border controls between NAFTA countries (Canada, Mexico and USA) are politically very sensitive.

Some of the main concerns, however, have centred on the European Union, where, following the Schengen agreement, implemented in 1995, most border controls between mainland member states (including quotas and permits and air cargo capacity) effectively ceased to exist, and the free movement of all road cargo transported by EU companies is now permitted. This facility has provided criminals with a single entry point to a huge continental European market for illicit goods and services, while the political transformations in Eastern Europe have, virtually simultaneously and as if for that very purpose, created new supplies of both drugs and women. Polish amphetamines currently account for 25 per cent of the European market; Poland, the Czech Republic and Romania are key sources for the illegal transportation of women and children; and many Western European money launderers have moved east to take advantage of inadequate legislation, weak enforcement and endemic corruption. It is for reasons such as this that the eastward extension of the Union's boundaries, scheduled for 2004, will inevitably transform the face of corruption on the continent, rendering it untimely to say much here about the subject.

Since the 1980s international pressure from developed world governments, particularly through IMF, the World Bank and OECD, has heightened political sensitivity surrounding money laundering. The Financial Action Task Force (FATF), an intergovernmental body associated with but organizationally distinct from OECD and charged with assessing and proposing reforms to the anti-money-laundering regimes of its twenty-nine member countries, was founded by the G7 countries in 1989. It operates within a framework containing four main enactments and many subsidiary ones. *First*, it prohibits back-to-back loans designed to deceive. *Second*, it requires banks to establish the name and identity of beneficial owners (the 'know your customer' rule). *Third*, it requires the decision to enter into a business relationship with a high-ranking public official to be taken at the highest management level. And *fourth*, it requires the rejection of deposits known to derive from corruption (Hauri 2000). One of its early achievements was to develop a strategy based on Forty Recommendations (revised in 1996), translated into legislative form by most members and designed to ensure that banking secrecy laws do not impede money-laundering investigations. The Recommendations include extradition (Recommendation 3), implementing the Vienna Convention (see below) (4), confiscation of proceeds (7), providing the authorities with customer information without warning the customer (17), developing a global currency tracking system (30) and bilateral and multilateral agreements of cooperation (34).

Numerous developments based on regional cooperation have followed these Recommendations. One example is the path-breaking EEC Directive of 1991, in England and Wales substantially incorporated into the Criminal Justice Act 1993, requiring the reporting of suspicious financial operations. This in turn led to the institution by member states of Financial Intelligence Units (FIUs),[21] known collectively as the Egmont Group after the location of their first meeting, the Palais d'Egmont in Brussels (Egmont Group 1997). FIUs have independent and specific relationships with banks, central banks and law enforcement agencies, and are charged with collecting and disseminating financial information of possible criminal significance (Council of the European Communities 1991a, 1991b).

FATF has also supported and encouraged a wide range of bilateral and multilateral treaties. The Council of Europe's PC-R-EV Committee (Committee of Experts on the Evaluation of Anti-Money Laundering Measures) has been significant (Council of Europe 1990). So have initiatives from the Organization of the American States (Inter-American Drug Abuse Control Commission (OAS/CICAD)) and the European Union, all of which bodies established anti-money-laundering standards for their member countries in the early 1990s. Newer initiatives include the Caribbean Financial Action Task Force (CFATF), the Asia/Pacific Group on Money Laundering (APG); the Eastern and Southern Africa Anti-Money Laundering Group (ESAAMLG); the Intergovernmental Task Force against Money Laundering in Africa (ITFMLA) and the Financial Action Task Force on Money Laundering in South America (GAFISUD). The Interpol agency FOPAC (Fonds Provenant d'Activités Criminelles) also participates in these organizations and, like other bodies, contributes to maintaining the Imolin (International Money Laundering Information) Database originally developed by the UN Office for Drug Control Crime Prevention (UNODCCP). More recently FATF has introduced the Non-Cooperative Countries and Territories Initiative of 2000–2001. This Initiative, supported by strong member states in the form of the threat of economic sanctions, is an attempt to persuade fifteen problem countries (subsequently reduced to three – Russia, The Philippines and Nauru) to adopt the Forty Recommendations in furtherance of FATF's aim of establishing:

> a world-wide anti-money laundering network through an appropriate expansion of FATF membership, increasing support for FATF-style regional bodies, and closely co-operating with international organisations involved in the combat of money laundering, particularly the international financial institutions.[22]

Increasing concern at the scale of money laundering and its facilitation of organized crime led the United Nations, in 1988, to approve the Vienna Convention against Illicit Traffic in Narcotic Drugs and Psychotropic

Substances, under which the scales balancing secrecy and disclosure were recalibrated to prioritize the latter. The Convention called on member states to criminalize money laundering and, among a range of prophylactic and investigative measures, pressed for improved transnational collaboration, the confiscation of criminal proceeds, the introduction of improved police liaison and the acceptance of proactive policing.[23] Shortly after the Vienna Convention, the Basle Statement of Principles was implemented (Bank for International Settlements 1988). This statement, while heavily criticized by law enforcement professionals for its breadth and ambiguity (Bosworth-Davies and Saltmarsh 1994: 136), laid the groundwork for reforms which included the prohibition of numbered accounts. UN involvement continued with the Palermo Convention against Transnational Organized Crime, ratified by the General Assembly in November 2000, requiring signatories to establish in their domestic laws four criminal offences: participation in an organized criminal group, money laundering, corruption and obstruction of justice.

National banks and money laundering

> the Swiss numbered bank account is not a part of any country's traditional culture.
>
> (Transparency International)

National banks face increasing demands from both governments and international banking organizations to address corruption and money laundering through a developing regulatory framework, while also having to compete commercially in this sensitive and confidential field. In the absence of supranational governmental authority with dedicated law enforcement officers working within a coherent legal and political framework, the regulatory system can only emerge from and in practice be enforced by the industry. But in a liberalized and competitive international money market it is hard to see how self-regulation can be effective: the banks' primary duty of care is to their customers, and the regulatory framework effectively forces them to hunt with the hounds and run with the hare. So, given the distinctly unenthusiastic approach of much of the industry and the cost and complexity of implementation, it would be unrealistic to have great confidence in the capacity of self-regulation to solve the problem. In characteristically dramatic language one Canadian commentator notes:

> Those rules and regulations are so complex and frequently changing that they are virtually impossible for smaller private sector institutions, which cannot afford the luxury of 'compliance officers' and high-priced legal advice, to understand, let alone to properly implement.

Simultaneously, it takes privatization of public functions one step further, forcibly recruiting bankers as police spies if they themselves do not wish to end up in the dock with their clients.

(Naylor 1999: 45)

Along similar lines the Chairman of the Swiss Federal Banking Commission sharply observed that financial supervisors are suffering from a '"Christmas tree" effect, in which government offices are gradually divesting themselves by adding new decorative tasks to our already widespread functions' (Hauri 2000). Hauri's own Federation, set up in 1935 in response to the economic crisis affecting Switzerland and its banking system, is naturally mandated to be protective of both. Switzerland's popularity as an international banking centre has always lain in its combination of political stability, neutrality and security,[24] financial strength, convertible currency, the integrity, range, variety and sophistication of banking services, the personal liability of private bankers and, especially, banking secrecy regulations. Switzerland's stability and neutrality have been especially important at times of international tension and overseas domestic uncertainty or instability. For example, following the freezing of Egyptian assets by British and American banks at the time of the Suez invasion in 1956, a number of Middle Eastern companies transferred their assets to Switzerland, some setting up special Arab–Swiss banks as a means of doing so (Clarke and Tigue 1976: 26). In addition, following the election to the French presidency of the socialist Mitterrand in 1981, capital flows from France exceeded all previously known levels, much of it in defiance of French tax and foreign exchange regulations (Walter 1985: 103). Further, the fact that secrecy regulations are buttressed by the criminal law (in particular Articles 47, 159 and 273 of the Swiss Penal Code) is decidedly more reassuring for international investors than a mere ethical code.

In the 1980s, however, as the Swiss Government, its own scope for action hampered by cantonal autonomy, came under international pressure, the Federation acquired the additional duty of preventing criminal abuse of the Swiss banking system. This pressure reflected widespread international ignorance of the sums of money involved: deposits by overseas customers (estimated at around $4,000 billion) do not appear in Swiss Government statistics, are excluded from GDP and have been consistently under-reported by the banks. In addition, international investors' concerns about the system mounted following the collapse (sometimes in criminal circumstances) of several foreign-owned private banks, awkward publicity about Nazi gold hoards and the use of numbered accounts by organized criminals and corrupt politicians, including former President Abacha of Nigeria and the family of ex-President Marcos of the Philippines. Under strong international pressure the Swiss Government froze Marcos's assets in 1987, while an internal investigation into Abacha's affairs in 2000 reported that nineteen banks had been involved in accepting $600 million of corruptly acquired funds. Although the Swiss Government eventually agreed to participate in FATF, the central role of banking in the Swiss economy makes it unsurprising that historically Switzerland has not been one of FATF's more enthusiastic members (Bosworth-Davies and Saltmarsh 1994: 209–211). And though there are indications that its approach is now increasingly compliant, such is the secrecy surrounding international banking that it is hard to establish to what extent system reform has occurred and to what extent claims to this effect are window-dressing. For example, while the Federal Government set up a Money Laundering Reporting Office (MROS) in 1998 to implement an extremely tough law against money laundering, it funded only six staff, all of whom resigned in 2000, frustrated at their lack of power and resources.

Any reforms that may have occurred in Switzerland have certainly not been replicated in all the weaker states which offer off-shore havens, and whose main qualifications are a favourable tax regime, a benign regulatory framework and a political elite that values secrecy and discourages inquisitiveness. Such havens include Panama and Liberia, where the US dollar is accepted as a parallel currency, Mexico, a member of NAFTA and the most substantial money-laundering country in Latin America, and Pacific islands such as Vanuatu, Tonga, Nauru and the Marshall Islands. Such countries lack a central bank or independent monetary authority, while poverty and corruption mean that the proceeds of domestic taxation would be minimal. Accordingly no other income source can offer gains equivalent to those deriving from financial entities such as trusts set up by highly taxed developed world individuals and corporations. In Panama in 1983 for example, even under the corrupt Noriega an attractive target for US off-shore funds, the 1.8 million population contained 3,000 lawyers, many working in the 'secrecy trade' associated with the £38 billion held in bank deposits (Walter 1985: 22, 115–118). While all dollarized economies provide attractive havens for money laundering, Panama offers the added benefits of proximity to the USA, a traditionally strong US military presence combined with an influential National Guard, a business-friendly political and military regime, high economic dependency on honest international banking and tight secrecy laws.[25]

In the United States, anti-money-laundering legislation began during the Nixon presidency with the federal Currency and Foreign Transactions Reporting Act (better known as the Bank Secrecy Act, or BSA) 1970. This Act introduced record keeping requirements in respect of most domestic cheque transactions, to permit effective audit trailing for anti-tax evasion purposes and Inland Revenue Service (IRS) notification requirements for full details of all overseas bank holdings. In particular it obligated banks to verify the identity of all persons wishing to export sums in excess of $10,000. The Act proved unworkable, however, partly as a result of the limited enthusiasm of both banks and law enforcement agencies for implementing it. In addition, high-profile court cases involving the Bank of

Boston, the Chemical Bank and other financial institutions demonstrated that the system was more successful in prosecuting the negligent or careless than the criminal, while fines were anyway set at too low a level to be an effective deterrent. From the 1980s the banks began to improve their systems and training in order to emphasize the importance of detecting suspicious money movements, and banks' compliance with BSA requirements was increasingly closely monitored by the Federal Reserve Bank. The Money Laundering Control Act 1986 criminalized many aspects of money laundering itself as well as failure to report transactions, further expanding the circumstances permitting forfeiture. In 1997 the reporting threshold for wire transfers out of the US to named countries (notably Colombia and the Dominican Republic) was set at $750 and a requirement to report smurfing[26] was enacted.

Naylor writes of the Money Laundering Control Act that:

> Though supposedly a Drug War measure, in fact the very act of attempting to hide money, even if its origins were strictly legal, was criminalized. Almost every federal offense became an occasion to also lay money laundering charges. What would previously have been considered fairly minor administrative offenses (failure to fill out forms or attempting to evade reporting thresholds by making small deposits etc.) became major crimes. And the penalties for handling criminal money in many cases became far more severe than the underlying offense.
>
> (Naylor 1999: 17)

The increased mobilization of transnational responses to transnational crime of the 1990s caused civil libertarians like Naylor to express concern as to the impact of these responses on human rights. The American Civil Liberties Union (ACLU), conscious that investigating tax evasion in particular would yield additional revenue for national treasuries, questioned the legitimacy of cross-border undercover operations and what they considered the excessively harsh treatment of minor criminals. ACLU argued that the political problems surrounding not only money laundering but also high-profile organized criminal activities such as drugs, prostitution and illegal immigration were acquiring the status of 'moral panics'. Moral panics are minor problems which attract disproportionately strong public feelings which are then used to justify inappropriate and excessive responses. In this case these would include unjustifiably intrusive intelligence gathering and sharing among law enforcement and financial authorities in the public and private sectors. In addition, new investigative and forensic procedures stemming from transnationalism were utilizing such tactics as jurisdiction hopping, whereby arrests were made under jurisdictions most helpful to the prosecution, and where sentencing was likely to be the most punitive

(Sheptycki 2000b). Other writers (Beare and Naylor 1999), questioning 'sting' policing methods and forfeiture policies, suggest including civil liberties on the debit side of any economic cost–benefit analysis of dealing with money laundering and organized crime. Naylor, sceptical as to the logic as well as the propriety of forfeiture policies, and noting the wide discretionary powers exercised by the IRS, claims that the pursuit of money laundering involves:

> the undermining of traditional presumptions in favour of financial privacy, the opening of tax records to police probes . . . the muddling of civil and criminal procedures, and, in extreme cases (the U.S. is the most notorious example) the impairing of the right of an accused to due process.
>
> (Naylor 1999: 1)

Naylor and other civil libertarians rightly point to the absence of proper checks and balances when agencies whose main functions are not to do with thief taking are co-opted into such a role. Nonetheless it can be replied that if the fox is now bionic only a bionic hound can catch it; and balancing that exigency with considerations of civil liberty may well prove one of transnationalism's future political challenges. At present the dominant perspective is that, given the cost and complexity of pursuing laundered money and the vast resources allocated by launderers to evasion, and since criminal proceeds by definition entail tax evasion, to approach the problem from this end is both proper and sensible. If in the process some smaller fish are caught, that is scarcely an injustice since they are hardly innocent passersby:

> In law enforcement investigations into organised criminal activity, it is often the connections made through financial transaction records that allow hidden assets to be located and that establishing the identity of the criminals and the criminal organisation responsible [sic]. . . . Without a usable profit, the criminal activity will not continue.
>
> (http://www.oecd.org/fatf/Mlaundering_en.htm)

In fact since the use of the US mail to further fraud is a criminal offence, postal inspectors have long acted as law enforcement agents (Clarke and Tigue 1976: 82); similarly the Inland Revenue Service has for many years used armed agents to monitor disparities between the lifestyle of suspected criminals and their declared income (Clarke and Tigue 1976: 16). Such activity is also routine in other countries where unexplained wealth often features in political corruption trials. Following the 1991 coup in Thailand (for which political corruption was a key justification), for example, the new regime instituted an Assets Committee to investigate twenty-five ministers and their associates for unusual wealth. The Committee found thirteen of these ministers, including the former Prime Minister Chatichai Choonhawan, to be 'unusually wealthy' (Pasuk and Sungsidh 1994: 13).

Conclusion

> keeping an average Nigerian from being corrupt is like keeping a goat from eating yam.
>
> (Nigerian newspaper, cited by Agbese 1998)

We have seen in this chapter that it is a characteristic trait of high-corruption countries for the banking system, like the legislature, bureau-cracy and judiciary, to be subjugated to the demands of a Leviathan-like executive. Typically this occurs in countries lacking an independent central bank, where control of public banks is therefore in the hands of politicians or their surrogates. In such situations banks are effectively available for use like a private account, with funds drawn in the form of 'loans' never intended to be repaid. At the same time account manipulation permits the laundering of dirty money and the deception of overseas donors by false accounting as to the use of previous loans, or in connection with the country's eligibility for new ones. Normally also such countries contain numerous private banks, some set up for overtly criminal purposes, some the property of members of the ruling group, and some lacking genuine liquidity, being created only to fail at propitious moments. Such banks, many of which lack any resemblance to the institutions familiar to westerners, being small and transient operations run not by bankers but by corrupt businessmen and organized criminals often from post office box numbers, naturally form alliances with similar entities overseas. Such alliances multiply the opportunities for predation on the part of the politician-bankers by making the tracing of funds more complicated for the various international organizations.

This blurring of the interstice between politics and banking helps create the obfuscation which makes such banks attractive to international criminals. They, as well as a host of tax evaders and small-time crooks, therefore join reputable individuals and corporations as customers, the latter attracted by selectively high interest rates offered to enhance the banks' reputation. For this attractiveness to continue, naturally investor confidence that international investment banks will not default needs to be maintained, and successful tax havens, mainly small, isolated countries heavily dependent on the financial service industry, take pains to boost this confidence. In a paradoxical example of honesty being the best means of sustaining criminality, so great are the economic benefits accruing to tax havens that bank collapses are rare: where golden eggs are plentiful nothing is to be gained by killing the goose that lays them. The international hard currencies passing through tax havens, once secured, are available for deployment in a host of predatory ways. Some of these are themselves criminal or corrupt, others are themselves legitimate but permit tax or customs revenue, international loans or aid money to be siphoned instead.

Opportunities for such activities have multiplied with economic liberalization and technological advance. With $1.3 *trillion* a day estimated to be involved in transnational financial transactions and the estimated annual profits from sales of cocaine, heroin and cannabis to the USA and Europe totalling $120 billion of which $85 billion is available for money laundering, the sums involved defy comprehension. Accordingly we have outlined some features of the international banking system in which such activities flourish, as well as the attempts by governments and their law enforcement agencies to control them. Such attempts face major obstacles. These include, *first*, the legitimate claim of criminal states to national sovereignty. As we have seen, transnational policing and regulation are beset with difficulties, with transnational organizations having no right to intervene in the internal affairs of such states; and only very rarely will individual nations do so. *Second*, the tradition of banking confidentiality means the banks' independence, which is not only commercially necessary but vital to restrict the power of politicians in the sector, ironically contributes to the problems faced by anti-money-laundering efforts. *Third*, the imbalance of resources between hunters and hunted means the criminals are fortified by the very money that the law enforcement agencies are attempting to confiscate, while the latter seem always to be playing catch-up. And *fourth*, the problem of proof is exacerbated by the self-evident fact that the purpose of money laundering is precisely to turn dirty into clean money: and once clean as well as dirty money is to be the subject of inquiry, the scope of any investigation becomes potentially limitless.

We have focused in this chapter on banking because political corruption contributes significantly to the perpetuation and expansion of money laundering. Corrupt political systems permit corrupt banks to exist, to engage in a wide range of non-banking practices (such as the purchase and exploitation of the overseas shell companies essential to layering) and to be shielded from legal sanction. Of course by no means all FATF non-compliant countries are so because of political corruption: some simply regard non-compliance opportunistically, as a chance to benefit by sustaining an uncontrolled banking market in the face of the regulatory and therefore counter-competitive endeavours of others. But while without political corruption money laundering would doubtless continue to exist, detecting it would be a more manageable forensic activity, unencumbered by the relative insulation of political leaders from the legal processes of their own country.

Notes

1 Such developments are not necessarily conventional. In a dramatic and illegal intervention in 1989 the US military invaded Panama, arrested its corrupt dictator, Manuel Noriega, and put him on trial in the United States for complicity in drug trafficking. The US then oversaw the swearing in of his (legitimate) successor in a military base in Panama.

2 See the International Money Laundering Information Network's website on ⟨https://www.imolin.org/⟩.

3 Europol, formed in 1995 under the European Council Convention on Establishing a European Police Office, succeeded the European Drug Unit.

4 Now Jubilee Research.

5 Ex–Im, created in 1934 to stimulate economic activity following the Depression, becomes involved in transactions attractive to the national economy but not to private lending banks. It provides guarantees of working capital loans for exporters, guarantees the repayment of loans, makes loans to foreign purchasers of US goods and services and provides credit insurance against non-payment by foreign buyers. For more details see ⟨http://www.exim.gov⟩.

6 BIS, established in 1930 and based in Basel, was created by the major central banks to foster cooperation with other agencies to achieve monetary and fiscal stability. It functions as a bank for central banks, to which it provides a range of financial services, as a centre for monetary and economic research and as an agent or trustee facilitating international financial agreements. BIS has become increasingly stern in relation to money laundering, in 2001 pressing members to accept a tougher regulatory framework to avoid reputational damage. For more details see ⟨http://www.bis.org⟩.

7 IIF, created in 1983 by thirty-eight banks of the leading industrialized countries in response to the post-1979 crisis, is now a global association of financial institutions. It represents the private sector in discussions with governments, international banks and debtor groups. Its present membership of around 320 includes banks from less-developed countries and many financial and commercial houses in insurance and investment management, multinational corporations, export credit agencies and fund managers. For more details see ⟨http://www.iif.com⟩.

8 G-7 comprises Canada, France, Germany, Italy, Japan, the United Kingdom and the United States.

9 The problem of slippage also faces the World Bank: on a strict interpretation of the rules, slippage has been calculated at over 40 per cent, with debtor countries' behaviour ranging from Turkey (almost entirely compliant) to Guyana and Ecuador (barely compliant at all) (Mosley *et al.* 1991: 300–301).

10 The Fund's 50th birthday in 1994 was hi-jacked by the Fifty Years is Enough group, including a number of international NGOs, which drew support from a range of liberal opinion (Danaher 1994). Critics from the right, meanwhile, regarded IMF as having outlived its *raison d'être*, having become, in the words of Milton Friedman, merely 'a junior World Bank' (quoted in Killick 1995: 157).

11 Such an approach was, however, to re-emerge in emergency loans granted to western Pacific Rim nations following the East and South-East Asian currency crisis of 1997.

12 Eligible countries were those engaging in sound economic policies, facing an unsustainable debt burden, with a sound record of reform involving IMF/World Bank policies and with a year's progress in implementing a Poverty Reduction Strategy Paper. In 2000 IMF and the Bank approved debt reduction packages for twenty-two countries, eighteen in Africa, under HIPC, lifting half

their debt and entailing a 30 per cent drop in debt service. All twenty-two countries are now spending more on health than on debt servicing and all have shown an increase in health and education funding.

13 PRGF was initiated following a 1999 mandate to 'integrate the objectives of poverty reduction and growth more fully into its operations in our poorest member countries' (IMF 2001b). The Fund stresses that surveillance will focus on the impact of such policies on macroeconomic performance, that collaboration with the Bank will be close and that it will not stray into areas beyond its remit or expertise.

14 In 1998 the figure stood at only 0.24 per cent, a figure heavily criticized by former IMF Managing Director Michel Camdessus. In an observation unthinkable a decade earlier Camdessus commented: 'The excuse of aid fatigue is not credible – indeed it approaches the level of downright cynicism – at a time when, for the past decade, the advanced countries have had their opportunity to enjoy the benefits of the peace dividend' (IMF 2000: 7).

15 The government's response was memorably reported as follows: 'The Government has this morning formed an anti-corruption squad to look into the conduct of the anti-corruption commission, which has been overseeing the anti-corruption task-force, which was earlier set to investigate the affairs of a Government ad hoc committee appointed earlier this year to look into the issue of high-level corruption among corrupt Government Officers' (*The Daily Nation*, 28 October 1997).

16 These attacks, while precipitating the crisis, could not have done so without the underlying weakness of the currencies. Attributing political or religious motives to speculators such as George Soros, as Malaysian Prime Minister Mahathir Mohammed attempted to do, is clearly absurd: the speculators simply saw an economic opportunity in overpriced currencies and took it. The present point, however, is that the interrelatedness of international trading and financial systems is such that the impact of the ensuing meltdown was quickly experienced globally.

17 One outcome of increasingly determined attempts to control money laundering has been a steep rise in transaction costs, which can now exceed 20 per cent, as against around a quarter of that figure a decade ago.

18 The fake purchase of Colombian emeralds was so useful for concealing cocaine money that the Colombian Government suspended the issuance of export licences (Transparency International, n.d.) Nonetheless, according to Bowden, the same Government was not slow to offer high interest rates to overseas (mainly US) speculative investors in the 1980s, whose 'investments' were known to be in cocaine shipments (Bowden 2001: 34).

19 Cricket has become an improbable source of such gambling because, as a team game immensely popular in India and Pakistan and with measurable individual contributions, it facilitates betting on personal as well as team performance. Hence individual players can be bought without the expense and risk of bribing an entire team. In addition there is the popularity of gambling on incidental aspects of the game, such as the number of fielders who will walk on to the pitch wearing caps for a specific session of play. Supposedly innocent opportunities such as this permit the purchase of players keen to make some money but unwilling to go so far as to throw a match. Much more could be said about corruption in sport; but this topic justifies a book in its own right.

20 For an account – journalistic in tone but well researched – of the famous 'Pizza Connection' of the 1980s, in which Mafia families bought a range of pizza parlours, used pizza ingredients as code words for narcotics trafficking and

shipped or telexed the proceeds to numerous overseas locations as ostensible profits of the (remarkably lucrative) pizza parlours, see Sterling (1993).

21 The US equivalent is the Financial Crimes Enforcement Network, or FinCEN: see ⟨http://www.treas.gov/fincen/.⟩. In Canada the Financial Transactions and Reports Analysis Centre of Canada, established in 2000, fulfils a similar function.

22 ⟨http://www.oecd.org/fatf/AboutFATF_en.htm⟩.

23 An example of such proactivity was Operation Dinero. This was a joint US–UK operation in 1995 set up to deal with criminal banking activities in Anguilla, a British colony just off the Puerto Rican coast, where the investigating forces set up their own bank as an undercover operation (for further details see Sheptycki 2000b).

24 New dwellings in Switzerland are by law provided with their own government-subsidized nuclear fallout shelters, a fact which helped make the country an attractive location for US money in particular during the Cold War era.

25 More recently, however, US pressure on countries such as Panama has increased significantly. So following its inclusion on the 'non-cooperating list' in 2000 a new administration passed legislation which both expanded the list of financial crimes and permitted the sharing of certain forms of information with other countries. It would be premature to judge the impact of this legislation on Panama's haven status.

26 Smurfing refers to multiple transactions just below the threshold imposed on banks – from smurf, the name given to couriers hired to perform this task.

6 Transnational political corruption (II): organized crime, smuggling and the global political economy of drugs

I regularly end up giving money to the non-European immigrants who offer to wash the windscreen of my car when it is stationary at traffic lights in Bologna . . . at least half the coins I give them end up in the pockets of the organised criminals who control the racket of 'illegal windscreen washers'. These same criminals also run a large part of the distribution of illegal drugs, again making use of the forced labour of illegal immigrants. But in order to be economically viable as players in the drugs market, such criminals need to have large supplies of capital at their disposal. Such funds will be provided from the world of illegal economic activities by those specialised in running prostitution rings or in the hijacking of lorry loads or in bank robbery. In turn, criminals specialising in bank robbery will need access to costly technology such as thermic lances and sophisticated weaponry. These can be bought or hired only from those who in practice have a monopoly over the supply of these materials and these same criminals are frequently those engaged in international drugs and arms trading. The enormous profits that are made in this trade are regularly recycled in the banking system and the money, finally 'laundered' clean, is then invested in absolutely legal activities. It is in this way that, link after link, the great 'net of the illegal economy' is stitched together and its complicated pattern interwoven with that of the legal economy.

(Pavarini 1994: 58–59)

Increasing globalization and the collapse of Eastern European communism have had a profound impact on the political economy of organized crime, while the internationalization of organized criminals such as the Mafia (Sicilian and Russian varieties),[1] Camorra, Triads and Yakuza has been of great significance in the development of transnational crime. Russian organized criminals are heavily involved not only in arms trafficking in Russia itself but also in arming combatants in former Soviet territories such as Chechnya, Armenia and Azerbaijan, as are Latin American drug traffickers. The Sicilian Mafia is entrenched not only throughout Western and Eastern Europe and the United States but in much of Latin America and Canada. There members engage in criminal activities such as smuggling, and invest in quasi-legitimate businesses such as ownership of casinos (notably in Germany, France, Spain and the Caribbean) and travel agencies, the former doubling as a conduit for money laundering, the latter as a front for alien smuggling.

Opiates have had a transformational effect on the political economies of many South-East and South-West Asian countries including Vietnam, Cambodia, Thailand, Myanmar, Pakistan, Iran and Afghanistan, while at non-governmental levels drug money has been vital in the funding of para-military forces. For example, links between the Provisional IRA in Northern Ireland and other terrorist organizations have been, though clandestine and surreptitious, longstanding and mutually beneficial. Such organizations are typically funded by criminal proceeds, sometimes, as in the case of drug money, still dirty, sometimes laundered. Alternatively drugs themselves may be used as currency between criminal organizations, as when in 2001 cocaine was used to pay IRA experts to train Colombian terrorists from the Marxist Fuerzas Armadas Revolucionarias de Colombia (FARC) organization in techniques of explosives manufacture. The cocaine was then recycled in Northern Ireland for military and criminal purposes as a means of sustaining the IRA as a combined criminal and military organization and, presumably, its leading officers, some of whom are predatory criminals thinly disguised as political idealists, in a comfortable lifestyle.

Elsewhere in Europe criminal opportunities involving the fraudulent conversion of EU subsidies have so multiplied over the last quarter of a century that subsidy fraud is now a major (if not the major) income source for some criminal gangs operating in Europe (Fiorentini and Peltzman 1995: 16). Counterfeiting, already a lucrative activity which causes many governments to change bank note design with hitherto unparalleled frequency, is almost certain to become more so since the introduction of the Euro in 2002.

In this chapter we consider drug trafficking, human migration and illegal arms dealing (including nuclear weapons). Organized crime, problematic concept as it is, is the cement binding together these seemingly disparate examples of criminal entrepreneurship, so it is that with which we begin.

Organized crime introduced

Since the beginning of the post-colonial era, there has been an unparalleled growth in the number of state actors in the international system that lack the institutional capacity to exercise sovereignty over much of their territory. Actors within these new states have virtually unrestricted access to the global economy as a result of the worldwide trend towards economic liberalization. Wholesale privatization and deregulation within national economies has diminished the capacity of all states – developing, post-communist, and developed – to exercise control over production and distribution activities within and across their borders. As a result, the global economy has slid increasingly into a status of laissez-faire, creating little practical distinction between engaging in legitimate and illegitimate commercial activities.

(Flynn 2000: 54)

Organized crime has already featured in this book and the following comments for the most part develop information already provided.

First, economic crime, and all organized crime is at heart economic, thrives in situations where law, custom or product availability impedes free commerce between a willing buyer and a willing seller. Such situations are attractive to criminals both because the proceeds are free of tax and regulation and because illegality forces up prices. Organized criminals are normally available to meet demand for:

- *illicit products*, often involving a combination of money, drugs, sex and gambling. Organized crime is also a vehicle for providing health and sexual products based on prohibited species for the Chinese market, prohibited luxury goods such as fur and ivory, and products such as antiques and some jewellery, where export licences are hard to obtain;
- *licit products* which bear heavy customs and excise duties, such as petrol, alcohol and cigarettes;
- *human migration* resulting from the combination of global economic inequality and curbs on a global free market in labour imposed by nation state immigration controls;
- *weaponry*, including nuclear devices, from terrorist groups and rogue states. Weapons and the means of manufacturing them, often involving quantities of enriched uranium for nuclear warheads, have become increasingly available following the end of the Cold War. In some of the former Soviet republics in particular organized criminals have found little difficulty in purchasing the necessary equipment, either from politicians or from disaffected or impoverished members of the former military or security services, though most of it is a decade or more out of date. Such vendors typically possess the foreign networks and language skills necessary to make contacts with organized criminals, negotiate and complete the deal, and launder and export the funds, as well as being sufficiently well connected to ensure that the state turns a blind eye;
- *hazardous waste disposal* is an increasing source of income for organized criminals, especially the Neapolitan Camorra, which largely controls solid waste collection in the Naples area. Legitimate waste disposal companies are purchased as fronts, and undertake hazardous waste dumping for their clients. It has been estimated that Italian organized criminals make up to £6 billion annually from all forms of environmental crime.

Second, for commercial, self-protective and status reasons most successful organized criminals are ambitious to demonstrate their membership of respectable local power elites by insinuating themselves into legitimate business and political activities. At a simple commercial level this enables local criminals to manage such matters as brokering public, especially construction, contracts between corrupt local politicians and favoured or criminally owned local businesses, and to head off, whether by presidential diktat or violence, potentially awkward investigations. Likewise, legitimate businesses may on occasion hire criminal organizations to undertake 'dirty work' such as informal contract enforcement and debt collecting.

Such matters pale into insignificance, however, when set against the broader political opportunities offered by the crossover between organized crime and political corruption. In particular the veneer of respectability deriving from networking with elite groups (not only politicians and business leaders but celebrities such as television personalities, movie and sports stars) is as vital to organized criminals as it is to legitimate business-people and politicians. This need for respectability also necessitates investing some of the power and influence laundered money has yielded in political, populist and charitable donations as well as in developing legitimate businesses, supporting the cultural milieu as well as the economy. In fact, in good part thanks to money laundering, organized criminals can actually cease to be involved in criminal activity at all except in the self-evident sense that their legitimate investments include (but, unless they are unwise, never solely comprise) criminal proceeds. If they are clever enough they can become, rather, pillars of the community. Naturally, however, acquiring and sustaining this veneer of respectability necessitates effective, indeed ruthless, information control, not only within their own organization but also over such interested outsiders as police and journalists. This control may be exercised by any combination of bribery, blackmail[2] and threats to targets and their families, and as a last resort, by physical coercion up to and including elimination. So however respectable one may be, one's murky past can seldom be finally buried, a fact which itself can make the friendship of powerful politicians worth the investment.

Conversely, for politicians the everyday job involves brokering trade-offs, protecting the interests of influential groups, trimming beliefs and voting practices according to the exigencies of the moment, securing adequate election funding and presenting such activities publicly as consistent and honourable. This unspoken dark side of politics can make access to unrestricted and clandestine resources irresistible, but the price to be paid can, in some places, be at least some involvement with criminals. It becomes important, therefore, for politicians also to do what they can to make their business associates respectable. Hence at a certain point successful organized criminals and local 'big men' become conceptually and empirically almost indistinguishable; and there is a strong mutuality of interest between them. So even where direct influence is not secured, subtle but still substantial benefit may accrue to corrupters, as Mafia leaders – and not only Mafia leaders – are well aware:

> after the man has won, and is in office, he is rarely asked to exercise blatant influence on behalf of the Syndicate. . . . Good associations, being seen with the right people, and having important contacts are as vital to organized crime as they are to an ambitious businessman, politician, or social climber. In the political area, Syndicate men's activities are designed to secure power, or the appearance of power, which is almost as good as having it.
>
> (Salerno and Tompkins 1976: 311)

Third, this process of merging reaches its logical conclusion when organized criminals actually seize control of the state, an entire country effectively being run as a criminal enterprise. In parts of Latin America, the Caribbean, Eastern and Southern Europe, South-East Asia and sub-Saharan Africa this is precisely what has occurred. It has led in some cases to the privatization not just of specific utilities and public companies but of key elements of governance, ranging from the police or military to the presidency itself. In such cases the criminals either operate under unofficial licence from the civil authority or are indistinguishable from it. In the latter instance beneficial stakeholders are largely restricted to the ruling group and their clients, their sole ambition being to maximize the rent-seeking opportunities obtainable from running the country. This entails neutering potential obstacles such as an independent judiciary and a free press. It constitutes a model of governance based on the acquisition of power as a means of self-enrichment.

In Jamaica, for example, the two main parties, the People's National Party and the Jamaica Labour Party, established their Kingston power bases in the 1970s with the aid of local gunmen, and since that time each has been associated with, and supported by, geographically distinct gangs. These gangs, subsequently enriched by the drug trade but still closely associated with the parties, have weapons including Glock semi-automatic pistols and Uzi or Mac 10 sub-machine guns. Between them they have committed numerous murders in Jamaica, the United States (where the FBI holds one gang alone, the Shower Posse, responsible for 1,400 East Coast murders) and Great Britain (Campbell 2001). Institutionalized high-level political, bureaucratic and judicial corruption is very helpful to organized crime, while, concomitantly, the existence of organized crime multiplies the rent-seeking opportunities available to politicians, bureaucrats and judges.

We should not, however, restrict ourselves to considering institutionally weak and corrupt countries such as Jamaica and Indonesia. *First*, for example, the Allies made use of Mafia personnel as the basis of post-war anti-communist administrative machinery in Southern Italy (Behan 1996: 33–35).[3] Many Mafia personnel were already well known to Allied leaders from the assistance with the 1943 Sicily invasion provided by the mobster

'Lucky' Luciano from his US prison cell. Luciano, imprisoned in 1936 on sixty-two counts of forced prostitution, provided the US Navy with both topographical information to aid the Sicily landing and the names of trust-worthy mafiosi to aid the resultant Allied Military Government (AMGOT) (McCoy 1991: 30–33). This led to the appointment of Sicily's Mafia leader, Don Calogero Vizzini, as Mayor of Villalba, an acknowledgement that Mafia rather than the official *carabinieri* could guarantee national security. The occupying forces turned a blind eye to political and revenge assassi-nations[4] and the predatory conduct of the island's new ruling elite, which quickly spread beyond Sicily through alliances with other organized crim-inals (particularly the Neapolitan Camorra), the Church (as ruler of the Vatican State) and the Christian Democrat party. The US, meanwhile, increasingly concerned at the rise of popular support for the communists, provided covert CIA funding for the Mafia locally and the Christian Demo-crats nationally.[5] Naturally the Christian Democrats and the Church, though itself suspected at the time of exploiting its control of the Vatican State for money laundering purposes, gave the Mafia legitimacy and influence. The covert CIA funding, however, enabled Luciano, now safely home in Sicily, together with Don Calogero to develop an international narcotics trafficking syndicate. This involved moving morphine from the Middle East to Europe, transforming it into heroin and, then, ironically, exporting it to the United States. This they did by exploiting their links (nurtured by Luciano's hench-man Meyer Lansky) with both the corrupt pre-revolutionary regime in Cuba and the Trafficante mobster family, a dominant force in Florida's political machine. So successful was the syndicate that it reportedly helped increase US addict numbers from 20,000 to 150,000 between 1945 and 1965 (McCoy 1991: 38).

Second, in Northern Ireland the de facto surrender, by British forces and the former Royal Ulster Constabulary, of the policing of parts of West and East Belfast to Catholic and Protestant paramilitary forces respectively is a further example. In both cases the paramilitaries enjoyed the support of local community activists, and enforced a brutal form of retributive justice involving punishing common criminals according to a tariff which pro-gressed from a stern warning through beatings-up to knee capping, exile and execution. Since traitors were dealt with equally firmly there was little incentive to express reservations about what Nationalists in the Falls Road called the appointment system, after the procedure by which victims were given an appointment to report to a particular location at a certain time to receive their punishment. *Third*, we have noted the impact of globalization on organized crime and the increasing tendency of criminal networks to form alliances and, effectively, operate a franchising system using methods almost identical to those of legitimate business. *Fourth*, the corrupting power of drugs, which has a crucial impact on leading actors in weak states, also has a considerable impact on lesser actors in strong ones. In 1960s New York, for example, the Bureau of Narcotics and Dangerous Drugs agreed with a Mafia drug syndicate to arrest only those dealers nominated by the syndicate. The agreement yielded a steady flow of names, which gave the agents a regular source of bribe income and an extremely impressive arrest rate, while offering, from the syndicate's perspective, an elegant and effective way of eliminating competition (McCoy 1991: 14).

Mafia, the state and society

> the criminals mobilise their considerable electorate around specific candidates, invest large parts of their illegal profits in legal activities which create desperately needed jobs, and create a climate of fear and intimidation, keeping the lid on a society that often resembles a pressure cooker. The politician repays the favour in three ways: by awarding public sector contracts to companies controlled by professional criminals; guaranteeing a considerable amount of legal protection through applying specific pressure within the judiciary and the police force; and often allowing gang leaders to control the allocation of resources and personal favours to ordinary people.
>
> (Behan 1996: 4–5)

The image of organized crime, popularized through media representations and underlined by the Special Committee to Investigate Organized Crime in Interstate Commerce (the Kefauver Committee)[6] (United States Congress 1951) and the President's Commission (President's Commission on Law Enforcement and the Administration of Justice 1967), is controversial. The view began to gain ground among sociologists in particular that this Mafia 'myth' conveniently ignored the criminogenic aspects of acquisitive, capitalist society. This view is clearly expressed by Findlay:

> If society countenances violence, considers personal gain to be more important than equity, and is willing to bend the law in the pursuit of wealth, power and personal gratification, then society itself will always be receptive to illicit enterprise.
>
> (Findlay 1999: 150)

Hence, the argument went, if Mafia flourished in the United States it was not because Mafia was an alien movement deriving from the migration of Sicilians but because the US provided fertile territory for economic crimes. So naturally an underworld existed, naturally there were Sicilians and naturally there were rudimentary forms of organization; but to move from these self-evident truths to the claim that respectable society was therefore under attack reflected an untenable view of both Mafia and US society. If Mafia was anything, it was more a symptom of a corruption already embedded in American society and culture than a cause of it.

To deny that capitalist societies are receptive to organized crime would, as our discussion of China has already shown, be to stand logic and experience on their head. Since the mainly rather elderly sources used by Findlay appeared, however, much has happened in the world of organized crime. The social organization of the Mafia changed following the mass arrests of the 1960s and 1970s as it abandoned many of its patriarchal, formalized and introspective traditions in favour of an approach more attuned to the international opportunities then opening up (McCoy 1991: 72). In addition, empirical investigations have increased our knowledge of linkages among hitherto relatively disparate groups of criminals. We now know, for example, *first*, that high-level contacts have taken place among such criminal groups as Mafia, Camorra, Triads and the Colombian drug cartels, with world trade in illicit substances and activities increasingly managed on a global basis. *Second*, terrorist groups, including ETA, the IRA, the Contras and numerous groups in sub-Saharan Africa and Muslim countries, look to criminal organizations for commerce in equipment, training, drugs and hard cash, the latter sometimes being raised by political supporters in covert operations like Iran–Contra, through corrupt banks like BCCI. *Third*, through methods such as money laundering, organized criminals' infiltration of society is now so extensive that distinctions between criminal and straight businesses are increasingly blurred.

To say this is not to feed on the fictional images of Mario Puzo and inter-war Warner Bros movies. Reuter's measured and cautious empirical New York study, which Findlay, surprisingly, does not cite (Reuter 1983; see also Anderson 1979 for a detailed study of a Cosa Nostra family), does much to demythologize Mafia activity. Reuter acknowledges that in certain places for certain purposes – dispute settlement in New York City for example – Mafia does indeed (or did in the early 1980s) enjoy an empirically verifiable monopoly – a view enhanced by the dramatic but detailed reportage of Sterling (Sterling 1993). Reuter, however, stresses the non-violence of the large majority of organized criminal transactions, the limits placed on violence by the fact that however well organized Mafia families may be a strong state will always be more so, and the competitive tensions within organized crime which militate against monopoly formation.

So unlike its Sicilian counterparts, the US-based Mafia almost never assassinates politicians,[7] law enforcement officers or judges, and historically sought to avoid illegalities falling under federal jurisdiction (Anderson 1995: 44). These conventions obviously stem in good part from the calculation that the costs of raising the ante in a state too large and powerful ever to come under their control would vastly outweigh the benefits[8] (Sterling 1993). They reflect Mafia's respect for the FBI, its institutional non-corruptibility and, in consequence, the high costs and risks associated with attempting to corrupt individual officers or units. They are also based on the assumption that strong states will tolerate Mafia unless and until it engages in activities which threaten the existence of the state itself, or at least significant elements of the state's apparatus of government. Conceptually therefore, if the state surrenders its monopoly on violence it does so partly for practical reasons, partly because it recognizes that in certain situations order can be more efficiently, effectively and economically maintained by criminals, and partly because key agents have been corrupted. But such surrenders are rare and temporary, and therefore, from the criminal's point of view, simply heighten the danger.

In weak states the situation is markedly different: there the organs of government are eminently purchasable, as a result frequently falling into the hands of organized criminals and warlords with the result that government and crime become indistinguishable or identical. *First*, for example, in Albania criminal gangs moved to fill the vacuum created by the collapse of the Stalinist Hoxha regime. Hence the country is now a hub for the smuggling of drugs, people and other contraband, and Albanian criminals pose threats to security in much of the Balkan region, Turkey and Italy and, increasingly, to stronger European states. In the United Kingdom, for example, Albanian criminals have increasingly seized control of London's rich prostitution market from Italian, Maltese and other racketeers. And *second*, in an episode perhaps more dramatic than typical, Pablo Escobar, head of the Medellín cocaine cartel, in his purpose-built luxury prison is in the process of kidnapping the Deputy Minister of Justice. The minister, Mendoza, backed by a 400–strong brigade of the Colombian army, has been instructed to transfer Escobar to a less salubrious institution:

> They sat Mendoza down on a sofa in the warden's living room, and Pablo addressed him. The drug boss now had a pistol in his hand. 'Señor Vice Minister,' he said. 'From this moment you are my prisoner. If the army comes, you will be the first to die.'

> 'Don't think that by retaining me you will stop them,' Mendoza said, believing his argument. 'If you take us hostage you can forget about everything. They have heavy machine guns, loads of them. They'll kill everybody here! You can't escape!'

> Pablo laughed. 'Doctor,' he said, speaking softly, leaning in close to Mendoza. 'You still don't understand. These people all work for me.'
>
> (Bowden 2001: 168–169)

In the United States, Mafia has always suffered from informants and grasses as a result of surprisingly weak internal discipline and resentment among junior members at the expropriation of their 'scams' by more senior colleagues. The risks of betrayal clearly increase with size because both surveillance of, and loyalty on the part of, fringe members will, *ceteris paribus*, diminish as the organization grows. It appears, ironically, that Mafia's sense of internal property rights is a somewhat restricted one.

This is not to deny that attaining monopoly power, particularly over coercion, is a rational objective, or that criminal gangs invest in military weapons and corrupt connections as means of attempting to secure it (Fiorentini and Peltzman 1995: 12). Clearly, however, not all modes of criminal organization which make perfect sense in a small, hierarchical, paternalistic, aristocratic and largely non-industrial island such as Sicily transfer happily to the industrialized north, or, even less, to the transnational arena. When operating on a global scale the last thing any professional criminal should do is to permit life to imitate art to the extent that he transforms himself into a James Bond villain, a 'big fish' whose elimination will save the world from the forces of evil. On the contrary, the layering activities so effective in money laundering are equally desirable for criminal organizations themselves. The more they can obfuscate their character and command chains, and the more they can devolve responsibility, the better they can adapt to rapidly changing circumstances, and the better, therefore, their chances of freedom and prosperity.

Accordingly Mafia families are today best seen not as unified and centralized command structures, but rather as umbrella organizations sheltering a range of variably coordinated entrepreneurial activities among their members. At their most successful they assume the role of a criminal government, at least in selected and lucrative departments, but this level of monopoly is beyond the reach of most *cosche*. Hence they define and enforce rules for members, use threats and violence to secure a geographical monopoly over selected criminal enterprises (often gambling and prostitution), managing or controlling new entrants by protection rackets with a passing resemblance to legitimate franchising operations (Anderson 1995: 40). In fact 'protection' in this sense is not necessarily a euphemism for extortion: it often has strong economic utility for its clients. A key characteristic of protection is the use of organized crime to control entry into a given activity, thereby facilitating anti-competitive practices such as price fixing and cartel formation (Gambetta and Reuter 1995). When they operate in this way protection rackets enable the client/victim to achieve the desirable business aim of reducing competition: enforcement costs diminish to the mutual benefit of protector and protectee, so protection becomes a tax paid to a de facto government for a beneficial service. In situations where this model applies, the protection racket, far from entailing the extortion of the legitimate business by the organized criminal, becomes, rather, an anti-competitive price-fixing conspiracy between suppliers of criminal protection and suppliers of the legitimate service or commodity.

For the most part, people who are today termed organized criminals work collectively over a prolonged period of time and on a hierarchical and professional basis to earn a living through persistent criminal enterprise. They are not necessarily tied by bonds of family or ethnicity. They naturally require access to complementary criminal skills and intelligence, and equally naturally and like any legitimate business they create appropriate organizational hierarchies and functional divisions of labour. The extent and sophistication of criminal networks vary just as do those of legitimate enterprises, the networks being a means to an end, not an end in themselves. Different criminal activities naturally require different organizational models. So a model conducive to running a localized numbers racket would not pass muster as the basis for an international money laundering or drug-smuggling enterprise. This is partly a matter of scale, but partly also reflects the fact that the larger and more sophisticated the network the more numerous the escape routes it offers into legitimate business, and the greater, therefore, the symbiosis between the criminal and the legitimate.

Where criminal and legitimate enterprises differ most strikingly is in their enforcement procedures. In the case of criminal organizations these inevitably reflect the fact that they lack the recourse to law available to their legitimate counterparts. These procedures, ranging from bribing, threatening or blackmailing juries and law enforcement officers to beatings and assassinations, necessitate extensive and ever increasing criminal activity. And while, as Reuter points out, violence may be the exception rather than the rule, the threat of violence and therefore the existence of coercion are omnipresent. Hence crime maintains crime in an expansionist logic characteristic of all successful enterprises as it seeks to diversify its product base, anticipate and meet new consumer demand, exploit competitors' weaknesses and generally stay ahead of the game:

> during the 1970s, the drug trade developed in Italy in the hands of smuggling gangs run by the Camorra which had previously specialized in trafficking in cigarettes. This development took place notably on account of the fact that both activities made use of the same financial channels. In Colombia, drug networks first developed from among structures earlier established in the emerald smuggling trade . . . drug trafficking in Nigeria is mainly in the hands of the Ibo groups, which are well connected to networks engaged in general-purpose smuggling, the illicit manufacture of patented goods, counterfeit currency trading and credit-card fraud.
>
> (Hibou 1999: 84)

There are good reasons for governments to consider adopting more liberal approaches to the victimless prohibited activities where demand is met by international crime syndicates. In a world in which governmental paternalism is regarded with increasing scepticism and individual freedom is as much a *leitmotif* as pursuing the good life was for ancient Athenians, the continued criminalization of suppliers and users of narcotics and commercial sexual services requires justification. Nonetheless, any belief that following, say, the regulation or legalization of heroin or prostitution today's criminal suppliers would quietly disband and seek employment as bus drivers or insurance clerks should have no place among them. On the contrary, like any other resourceful supplier of a redundant service organized criminals would work to diversify their product base. Clearly this would in part entail developing smuggling enterprises, involving both aliens and goods attracting high levels of duty. But it would also involve providing weaponry and mercenary soldiers for rogue states and terrorist groups, building up coercive activities such as hostage-taking and assassination and facilitating the kind of corrupt opportunities for politicians which form the subject of this book.

Corruption and the transnational drug trade

> As long as we are determined to continue our futile efforts by means of the criminal law to prevent people from obtaining goods and services which they have clearly demonstrated they do not intend to forgo, criminals will supply those goods and services. And insofar as the market is of a character in which combination and organization is profitable they will organize.
>
> (Morris and Hawkins 1970: 235)

This is not the place to embark on a full account of the transnational drug trade: this has been very competently done already (see for example McCoy 1991; McCoy and Block 1992). Our aim is to insinuate the drugs issue into a discussion which thus far contains as its main ingredients the contributions made to political corruption by changes in the international system, economic liberalization, transformations in communications (human and electronic) and the expansion and diversification of organized crime. We conclude with case studies of two drug barons/local warlords, Khun Sa and Pablo Escobar, ruthless criminals who used drugs to corrupt national political systems, benefited from those corrupt systems and operated, at least for a time, as successful politicians with large and loyal power bases. The case studies aim to show that, at least in primitive domestic LDC politics, there exist opportunities for criminals to buy both popularity and success. But the continuation of that success is dependent on the acquiescence and sometimes complicity of stronger and more powerful players in the international arena. At the point at which the criminals constitute a threat to the interests of more powerful players they are eliminated as significant political players (Khun Sa) and if necessary killed (Escobar). Their experiences stand as exemplars of a more general principle and remind us again of the necessity of analysing political corruption internationally and transnationally.

The international market in illicit drugs, though subject to wildly different estimates, is vast and growing, and the enormous revenues generated are very significant in the global political economy of crime and corruption. Illegality naturally guarantees the industry freedom from regulation and taxation, though as with any illegitimate enterprise a proportion of the yield has to be reinvested in bribery and coercive enforcement. In some less-developed countries drug income permits local warlords to purchase weaponry with the help of which they can overthrow or co-opt a nation state's government or engage in terrorist activity against strong states in complete disregard of international conventions. In developed countries the cost of drugs to the health, welfare, customs, police, judicial and prison systems is vast, both directly and, because drug use provokes so much common criminality, indirectly. And the sums involved naturally facilitate the widespread corruption and intimidation of the politicians, judges, bureaucrats and multitude of front-line law enforcement officials whose active co-operation or passive acquiescence is necessary for the enterprise to succeed.

The international drug trade, historically maintained by government monopolies such as the East India Company and involving major, legitimate, pharmaceutical companies like Roche and Bayer, was effectively privatized in the early twentieth century following its widespread interdiction. It was around this time that at successive international conferences what we currently term illegal drugs were first defined as illicit commodities rather than legitimate consumer preferences for medicinal or recreational purposes (Braithwaite 1986: 206–207; Asad and Harris 2003).

Myanmar, Afghanistan and Laos account for over 90 per cent of the world's heroin production. Since, however, the border between Afghanistan and Pakistan's poppy regions is fluid and crossed regularly by the Pakhtoon tribespeople mainly responsible for opium cultivation in that area, part of the Afghan yield almost certainly derives from Pakistan. Drugs are grown mainly in interstitial and poorly policed areas: in Pakistan, for example, opium growing and heroin production are concentrated on tribal border territories outside the jurisdiction of federal law where federal agents seldom dare venture (Asad and Harris 2003). Like its predecessors, the junta currently ruling Myanmar regards heroin as a form of both official government and private predatory revenue. Afghanistan is inherently unstable, lacks any effective central government, and its international support is largely dependent on the continuation of threats to western security from Muslim terrorists and rogue states. Laos, a corrupt and impoverished socialist state, was further weakened internally by US bombing in the early 1970s and is now of little strategic superpower interest.

The necessary administration – mainly processing the raw drugs, funding the distribution, ensuring the financial arrangements are in place and ensuring strategic product development (entailing nurturing future target areas for production or distribution by a combination of corruption and coercion) – follows similar principles to those of a legitimate multi-national corporation. Narcotics entrepreneurs identify areas which make geographical sense and where controls are weakest – usually the weakness stems from a combination of incompetence, lack of resources, geographical inaccessibility and corruption – and locate their field activities there. This explains the crucial importance of Colombia, a country which until recently was not itself a significant producer. In fact as recently as 1994 only 20 per cent of Andean coca was produced there, though by 1999, largely as a result of the growing power of FARC, which uses drug revenue to finance its armies in the civil war, the figure had risen sharply to 67 per cent. Colombia is a relatively prosperous (though highly unstable) developing country where cocaine administration was historically in the hands of rival cartels based in Cali and Medellín, supported by Panamanian money-laundering services and smuggling arrangements with corrupt states such as Mexico and the Bahamas. In the 1990s:

> As one observer has noted, 'The Cali cartel operates more like the senior management team at Exxon or Coca Cola. Its transportation, distribution and money laundering networks cover the globe'. It is no exaggeration to say that the Cali cartel is not only the developing world's most successful TCO [transnational criminal organization], but is also its most successful transnational corporation.
>
> (Williams 1994: 103)

This situation was not to endure, however, and since the decline of the cartels in the mid-1990s coca production and distribution have fallen into the hands both of political groupings such as FARC and ELN, and of more fragmented criminal organizations including some from Peru and Bolivia.

Colombia offers a particularly convenient trafficking route to Mexico, a high-corruption country where the capacity of local drug barons to corrupt authority figures has been highlighted by the imprisonment of six generals for drug corruption since 1997 (Bureau for International Narcotics and Law Enforcement Affairs 2000) and the certainty that they are but the tip of the iceberg. For some time the Cali cartel concentrated its efforts in the northern part of Sonora Province abutting Arizona, where it was reported to have had nearly all police, *federales* and government personnel on its payroll (Copher 1997). But in such regions criminals are far from static, distribution administration as well as growing areas moving regularly into new geopolitically suitable regions and countries. So in spite of Mexico's membership of NAFTA, drug and people smuggling across many busy border points, notably Ciudad Juárez/El Paso, well to the east of Sonora, and where the US maintains a large intelligence centre, has been widespread. More than half the cocaine smuggled into the US enters from Mexico across numerous rapidly changing crossing points along the long and unenforceable border. Nor has the corruption involved been restricted to the Mexican side: in the United States forty-six local, state and federal law enforcement officials were indicted or convicted of corruption between 1997 and 1999 (Bureau for International Narcotics and Law Enforcement Affairs 2000).

Attempts at interdiction face almost insurmountable obstacles. *First*, direct 'victims' of illegal drugs are willing participants and therefore unlikely to initiate law enforcement. Indirect 'victims' (particularly of predatory crimes committed by addicts) are seldom in a position to be of use to law enforcement agencies; and even more indirect 'victims', notably the tax-payers who fund health and penal facilities, are of mainly theoretical interest. *Second*, economic liberalization and deregulation have reduced states' scrutiny of activities within their own boundaries. This applies especially to border controls. *Third*, for all the attempts by governments, with UN and superpower support and encouragement, to provide alterna-tive sources of income for impoverished drug-producing peoples, the incomes derived from these activities pale into insignificance when compared with the riches available from opium or coca production (Asad and Harris 2003). *Fourth*, several factors combine to diminish the effectiveness of supply-side control strategies:

- the proliferation of weak states means that many have little control over their more dispersed regions, which frequently remain subject to the rule of local traditional or feudal chiefs. This interstitiality makes them attractive hiding places for political refugees, for whom drugs money is a source of both political and financial aggrandizement;
- many of these regions contain more geographically remote and climati-cally propitious areas for drug growing than are currently used. So it is often possible for farmers to move their poppy fields almost annually; hence even if a crop eradication spray hits its target the best result is the temporary impoverishment of a few expendable local producers who will anyway relocate the following season;
- US supply-side policy has permitted the use of narcotics money to main-tain friendly LDC regimes (McCoy 1991, 1999; Nadelmann 1993) which are dropped when other considerations apply, for example when drugs pose a security threat or there is domestic political fall-out. But whatever its political logic during the Cold War, a policy that locates the source of the problem in supplier countries is inadequate today. During the Cold War the main US foreign policy aim was containing the spread of communism in strategically sensitive areas. There were many such areas, ranging from Italy to Japan, and from the Emirates and Pakistan to Latin America, but many of the operations had unpleasant side-effects and there was considerable global fall-out. In South-East Asia, covert action by the CIA in support of Chinese Nationalists in Burmese Shan and of Hmong tribesmen in Laos facilitated the formation of the Golden Triangle (McCoy 1991: 19) around the Mekong Delta. By the late 1950s this region was producing half the world's supply of illicit opium. Economic and military aid to Pakistan, paid to purchase loyalty and cooperation in the Afghan-Soviet war, contributed to the formation of the Golden Crescent. There the guerrilla commander Hikmatyar, a US appointee, was the channel for more than half US aid, part of which he invested in six heroin laboratories in order to exploit the opium harvest of Afghanistan's Helmand Province (McCoy 1991: 445

et seq.; Asad and Harris 2003). This may or may not have been an acceptable political price at the time, but today Cold War considerations no longer exist, the political leverage obtainable by using drugs as a covert international currency is minimal and there are always the risks of scandalous apprehension.

In addition the USA has long expressed concern about the capacity of narcotics money to corrupt its own politicians and officials. The Drug Enforcement Administration (DEA) was instituted by President Johnson in the late 1960s as a response to just such corruption in its two predecessor bodies. DEA now has a sound international network of agents and appears institutionally non-corrupt, though McCoy claims this was not so during the CIA's covert operations activities in the Cold War (McCoy 1991: 17). More recently, as well as the Mexican border corruption cases already mentioned, widespread drug-related police corruption was reported in Illinois, Ohio and Pennsylvania in 1998; while in the same year in Zapata County, Texas, most political leaders, including the Sheriff, Judge and Clerk, pleaded guilty to drug corruption charges.

Supply-side anti-narcotics policies remain, however, a major plank of US foreign policy. Since 1986 successive Presidents have issued annual certificates of cooperation to countries known to be involved in drug trafficking which are cooperating with the United States in attacking the trade. Cooperation can involve such humiliations as having to permit the State Department's Narcotics Division to attempt the aerial eradication of poppy fields in one's own state (Shelley 1990: 129), but military and humanitarian aid are normally dependent on possession of a certificate. While the six countries cited for failing to cooperate in 2000 – Afghanistan, Burma, Cambodia, Haiti, Nigeria and Paraguay – were mainly ones in which US leverage reduced following the end of the Cold War, such are US power and influence today that few LDCs are willing to risk its displeasure. Hence the US might in the future reasonably expect at least grudging cooperation from many such countries, particularly since its efforts at eradication are unlikely to have enduring effects.

In such wild and lawless conditions the political power of the drug barons and the complex interrelations among drugs, terrorism, money laundering and political corruption can scarcely be overstated. Here we discuss two such barons: Khun (= Lord) Sa and Pablo Escobar.[9] They come from different sides of the world, Khun Sa, self-styled 'King of the Golden Triangle', being a South-East Asian warlord, Escobar a Colombian criminal with origins in the Medellín Cartel.

Khun Sa

Khun Sa was born in 1933 to a Shan mother and a Yunnan Chinese father, this itself being symptomatic of his interstitial character. Geographically

Shan was situated in the interstice of two rival states, Thailand and Burma; politically it was in those of two rival powers, China and the United States. Khun Sa's success, and even survival, depended upon by his ability to exploit these interstices. He joined the Kuomintang (KMT), then occupying Shan, as a teenager in 1951, forming his own militia after the Burmese drove KMT into Thailand in 1961, and increasingly challenging KMT's effective monopoly over Burmese opium exports. In 1967, following his refusal to pay KMT's opium tax, he was attacked with devastating effect, and robbed of his opium supplies by both KMT and a Laotian force whose land and air assault utilized crack paratroops and a squadron of T-28 bombers (McCoy 1991: 355–360). He was arrested by the Burmese in 1969 and imprisoned for associating with Shan separatist movements, but released in 1974 following the mediation of his future patron, the Thai General Kriangsak Chamanan. On his release Khun Sa returned to Shan, where he concentrated on consolidating his position and opening up a sophisticated infrastructure for opium growing and heroin manufacture and distribution.

Khun Sa fell out with Kriangsak, now Thai Prime Minister, in 1978, when he claimed publicly that he controlled and could stop the Shan drug trade. A furious Kriangsak, heavily implicated in the trade and also a KMT client, expelled Khun Sa from the country. He returned to Burma, to his former headquarters, Ban Hin Taek, said to contain a hundred-bed hospital, a brothel, luxurious Chinese-style villas with swimming pools, a holiday home for Kriangsak, and seven heroin refineries (McCoy 1991: 420–421). His army survived Thai bombing raids and intelligence operations until suffering extensive casualties in a raid in 1982. Following this setback, however, he regrouped, and in 1983, having defeated a new enemy in the shape of the Burmese Communist Party, he secured the necessary communication lines to establish refineries capable of processing 75 per cent of Shan opium into heroin. By the late 1980s he had deployed his Mung Tai army, now 40,000 strong and armed with M16s and M60 machine guns, to protect 100,000 square miles of opium fields in the Shan Plateau. He now effectively controlled 60 per cent of the world's illicit opium supply (McCoy 1991: 434).

Khun Sa himself, by dint of living and operating interstitially while enjoying the patronage of successive Burmese governments, was able to form short-term alliances of convenience, fuelled by the drug trade, with virtually any state in this wild, remote and heavily disputed border area. By exploiting the Cold War he helped the CIA when it suited him, offering to help the former CIA Chief, Vice-President, George Bush secure the return of US prisoners held in captivity in Laos fifteen years after the end of the Vietnam war. He played Burma and Thailand off against each other. He supported KMT when it was in his interests to do so and fought them when it was not. In the process he cemented links both with Yunnanese drug lords in China and with the CIA. Even after his expulsion from Thailand he continued to pay lavish bribes in Bangkok to ensure that he had continued use of Thailand's transport infrastructure. He was, in short, a transnational political operator of the very highest quality.

But for all his power and influence Khun Sa could thrive only so long as he could balance the potentially conflicting interests of these sovereign states, and only while he remained useful to their covert aspirations. His fall, to Burmese troops at his Ho Mong (Shan) headquarters in January 1996, was precipitated by his ill-judged and grandiose attempt to confront these powers by creating an independent Shan state, an endeavour which brought him into conflict with, simultaneously, Burma, Thailand, China and the US (McCoy 1999: 156–157). Once Thailand and the United States, for different reasons, united in order to eliminate Khun Sa's supply line his days of power were numbered (Korkhet 1995). The interstices which Khun Sa manipulated and within which he operated were:

- *Myanmar*, its government, wrought by conflict, corruption and incompetence and dependent on drug money for both national and personal economic reasons, gave cover to drug warlords, including Khun Sa, particularly when they were close to the Chinese border;
- *Shan*, a part of Burma/Myanmar given autonomous region status by the British as the Federated Shan States, and divided into sub-states chaotically ruled by corrupt local princes funded by opium money. Shan is hostile mountainous territory bordering China's rebellious Yunnan Province (itself a major opium-growing region controlled at the time by the ousted drug warlord Lung Yun), north-west Laos and western Thailand. Shan's long border with Yunnan Province had made it of great strategic importance following the Chinese revolution, when the CIA, newly instituted by President Truman, was engaged in covert collaborations with Chiang Kai Shek to invade Southern China. Subsequently KMT exploited Shan's geo-politics by exporting raw opium to Thailand, where it was manufactured into heroin before entering the developed world markets. By the 1980s Shan had become an aspirant, if poppy-dependent, nation of eight million people, with Khun Sa its President in waiting;
- *Kuomintang* (KMT) refugees and soldiers remaining in Shan in the 1950s following an unsuccessful attempt to capture Yunnan Province from the communists. These soldiers, with CIA support (the US hoped to stem the southern expansion of communism and draw Chinese troops from the Korean front) and local Chinese collusion, developed and exploited the Burmese drug trade to their own benefit and that of Taiwan. This trade was to prove essential to the survival of the Shan-based nationalist army following the withdrawal of US financial support in 1952. At this time the Taiwanese soldiers began to behave like an occupying force in Shan, assuming such governmental functions as taxation and customs and excise, activities which the Burmese Government, not surpris-

ingly, regarded as an invasion. In spite of a UN-brokered withdrawal, 6,000 KMT soldiers remained illegally in Shan until 1961, when they were driven into Laos and Thailand. From there, having instituted (by brutality and intermarriage) a centralized structure for opium transportation and heroin manufacture, they continued trading, resisting periodic joint US–Burmese attempts at repatriation (McCoy 1991: 162–178);

- *Thailand*, which as a Japanese ally had occupied the Shan states during the Second World War, which possibly had annexation in mind, and which, supported by the CIA, gave covert support to Shan separatists. The fact that the Kingdom of Thailand is the only South-East Asian country to have avoided imperial conquest has always been a source of considerable national pride, but maintaining independence in the face of threats from Burma and China and Vietnam was proving costly. In particular it entailed an unrealistically strong military presence in the remote border regions at a time when the army was needed in Bangkok to protect the government against civil unrest. As a result, Thailand's strategic objectives included a strong intelligence network, mechanisms for ensuring the loyalty of the tribal peoples, and political and military support for KMT soldiers, Shan separatists and the anti-communist drug warlords of Yunnan Province (McCoy 1991: 180). These were all matters in which Khun Sa could be helpful, while in addition, as these objectives were also, happily, consistent with US interests, throughout much of the 1950s Thailand was a beneficiary of the United States' Asia policy.

For much of the Cold War period, certainly between the coups of 1947 and 1973, Thai politics was characterized by periodic military coups interspersed with weak or incompetent civilian governments. The high cost of resisting attempted coups (including the payment of regular loyalty bonuses to all army ranks) necessitated creating and maintaining client networks among rival military and civilian elites, both in Bangkok and in provincial governments. While the dirty money fuelling the economy was produced by such familiar forms of corruption as smuggling, contract procurement and other forms of boundary blurring between the political and business sectors, drug money was also indispensable. Hence facilitating the opium and heroin trading activities of Thailand's client border armies became a central national security concern. Formally the country maintained a legal monopoly of the trade, licensing production in the Golden Triangle area, but opium also became a weapon in the conflicts between two competing military elites, both led by drug lords, which dominated Thai politics (McCoy 1991: 182–185). The Police Chief, General Phao Sayanan, a CIA client awarded the Legion of Merit in 1954, led one faction, the Army's Commander-in-Chief, Marshal Sarit Thanarat, the other. Phao initially gained the ascendancy, exploiting his success by overtly urging Thailand's Chinese population to support the nationalists and covertly using the police to cover and develop the KMT drug business on the northern borders. By such means the production, manufacturing and distribution infrastructure of the Golden Triangle was put in place for subsequent exploitation, and Thailand became the world's leading opium distribution centre. With CIA compliance Phao ran Bangkok in a Mafia-like manner, and by 1955, when Phao was at the height of his powers, his police force was operating as a huge opium-trafficking syndicate. He created a civilian spy network to help him repress all dissent, for example by arresting 104 intellectuals in 1952. He controlled the lucrative sex industry, rigged the gold exchange, collected protection money from rich Chinese businessmen and forced himself on to the boards of over twenty Chinese-run corporations (McCoy 1991: 184–186). By the time of his fall in 1957 Phao had seized control of the ruling political party and was running an election campaign based on large-scale fraud and facilitated by the hiring of gangsters to disrupt opposition rallies and beat up unpopular candidates.

By now, however, Phao had gone too far. His fall followed a successful coup by Sarit's faction, and Thailand entered a phase of corruption which, though subtler in method, was similar in outcome. As well as dismembering Phao's hated police force and neutralizing potentially hostile army factions, Sarit launched a high-profile populist anti-opium campaign which did not, however, prevent him from continuing to offer lower-key support to the trade, from which he continued to benefit until his death in 1963. On his death he left a personal fortune of some 2.8 billion baht, over one-quarter of Thailand's annual budget (Pasuk and Sungsidh 1994: 23).

• The *CIA*, funding KMT in covert operations against the People's Republic of China with the aid of local opium warlords, whose activities were sanctioned in return for intelligence. CIA representatives, including Richard Armitage, who were closely involved with Khun Sa, were themselves apparently engaged in illicit trading,[10] an allegation consistent with official acknowledgement that in the Nicaraguan context:

> In some cases, such as the CIA-Contra-Crack controversy, government complicity in drug trafficking became de facto official policy. In 1982, during the early days of the Contra war, William Casey (Director of the CIA) and William French Smith (Ronald Reagan's Attorney General) drafted a 'Memorandum of Understanding' whereby the CIA would *not* have to report allegations of drug trafficking involving its 'agents, assets and non-staff employees'. . . . by its own admission, the CIA simply ignored or overlooked reports of drug trafficking by the Contras and their supporters.
> (Bureau for International Narcotics and Law Enforcement Affairs 2000: Goal Number Two)

Khun Sa had been helpful to Thailand in making the fortunes and maintaining the power of corrupt senior politicians such as Kriangsak, and in securing the problematic Burmese/Myanmar border. But when, during the 1980s, Thai political objectives changed, with civilian administrations prioritizing trading relations with neighbouring states over armed conflict, his usefulness diminished, and as the costs of supporting him began to outweigh the benefits both Myanmarese and Thai pressure mounted. Khun Sa responded aggressively by centralizing heroin supplies, and, from the mid-1980s, began to promote the political objective of Shan nationalism until, in 1993, the Shan State National Congress proclaimed independence under Khun Sa's leadership. Khun Sa now abandoned the interstitiality which had given him such room for manoeuvre and manipulation, becoming instead prospective head of a state likely to pose major problems for both neighbouring and powerful states. *First*, such a state would have challenged the territorial integrity of Myanmar itself. *Second*, it would have threatened the construction of a major dam jointly conceived by the Thai and Myanmar governments to transport water to meet Thailand's expanding economic needs. *Third*, almost the entire economy of Shan, to the dismay of the western powers, would derive from heroin (McCoy 1999: 143–148).

As pressure continued, Myanmar's military government, the State Law and Order Council (SLORC), decided to change the routes of its drug trade to the Chinese border where it was able to favour drug lords lacking Khun Sa's political influence and ambition. Eventually in 1996 Khun Sa surrendered to SLORC, though on favourable terms which guaranteed his freedom, permitted him to continue in legitimate business, accepted his continuing involvement in heroin, and undertook not to extradite him to the United States. This seeming generosity demonstrated that his influence over leading politicians had by no means disappeared.

Pedro Escobar

Pedro Escobar was born in 1949 to a cattle-farming family in Medellín, Colombia, an unstable, drug-ridden country characterized by clashes between a strong military and almost equally strong Marxist opposition forces. Forty years later he was to be dubbed the seventh richest man in the world by *Forbes* magazine.

After dropping out of school Escobar became a petty local gangster dealing in marijuana, gravitating to car theft and resale, with the associated corruption of licensing officials, protection rackets, kidnapping and systematic murder. At the same time, like other organized criminals he courted public popularity. He espoused populist leftist rhetoric to attack both the Colombian establishment (where 3 per cent of the population owned 97 per cent of the country's wealth) and the United States. Like many other criminals before him he invested huge sums in charitable foundations such as a housing project, Medellín Without Slums, public works, transportation networks and places of sport, culture and entertainment for the poor. He paid his cocaine laboratory workers well above the market rate and nurtured the popular belief that drug smuggling was a patriotic political act. To the elites he portrayed it as morally legitimate (certainly no less so than the slavery and criminality by which their ancestors had secured their wealth); to leftists he presented it as a means of achieving global economic redistribution (Bowden 2001: 42–43). Audaciously, though himself Colombia's most notorious kidnapper, he formed a private militia (Muerte e Secuestradores, Death to Kidnappers) to combat guerrillas who had kidnapped the sister of his partners, and introduced a parallel system of civil justice resulting in a doubling of the murder rate. By such means Escobar became, simultaneously, feared, a popular hero of the poor and rich beyond comprehension. By the late 1970s the Medellín Cartel was shipping loads of up to 600 kilograms of cocaine to feed the seemingly insatiable US market, a figure rising, by the mid-1980s, to 2,000 kilograms by submarine and 10,000 kilograms by private Boeing 727s (Bowden 2001: 47). Escobar was by now above the law and willing to undertake the ruthless elimination of potential rivals.

Increasingly, however, the material benefits of organized crime became insufficient, and Escobar began to develop political ambitions, ultimately for the presidency of Colombia. He founded a newspaper, the *Medellín Cívica*; in 1978 he was elected to the city council as a substitute member;[11] he helped finance the campaigns of both the leading contenders for the Colombian presidency, Turbay (who won) and Betancur (who was to win in 1982). In 1982 he was elected to the National Congress again as a substitute, a post designed to guarantee him immunity from prosecution or extradition to the United States. But his attempt to take his seat in Congress caused a political storm, as Escobar was denounced as a criminal and drug trafficker by the new Justice Minister, Rodrigo Lara, in 1984. A few months later, after supporting joint US and Colombian aerial attacks on cocaine-manufacturing plants Lara was murdered and the armed conflict between the government and the *narcos* began in earnest.

Following an approach from the soon-to-be-President of Panama, Manuel Noriega, Escobar fled there to join other *narcos* acquaintances. Double-crossed by Noriega, he fled again, this time to Nicaragua, where he almost became a victim of a CIA 'sting' when spotted helping the Sandinistas load a drug shipment. He responded by returning home, avenging the kidnapping of his father and launching a prolonged and bloody siege on the Colombian state (Bowden 2001: 68). Supported by an army of lawyers and supporters, Escobar arranged the murders of judges and magistrates, broadcasters and newspapermen, police (including the police chief), legislators, government negotiators and their families. The tens of thousands of assassinations which occurred culminated in the killing of the Attorney General and, in 1989, of the anti-drugs campaigner and prospective President, Luis Galán.

President Barco responded to this killing by declaring a state of national emergency, suspending *habeas corpus* and inviting increased US military support in the war against the cartel. For five years the United States waged a secret war in Colombia, placing intelligence units in Bogotá under the auspices of the CIA's secret intelligence service, ISA (Intelligence Support Activity), now renamed Centra Spike. Centra Spike collaborated with the Colombian Government in a series of covert operations sometimes aided by information from the rival Cali cartel. Eventually, in 1991, Escobar surrendered. So desperate was the Government to end Escobar's campaign of terror, however, that it withdrew from the extradition treaty with the United States, permitted Escobar to build a luxury prison from where he could continue his drug trafficking, and offered him an amnesty in respect of the most serious charges. Having only pleaded to a minor drug offence for which he had been convicted *in absentia* in a French court, Escobar could realistically anticipate early release.

In prison Escobar had little to fear. He was effectively the employer of his own guards. The prison was fitted out like a luxury hotel, complete with 'waterbeds, Jacuzzis, expensive sound systems, giant-screen TVs and other goodies' (Bowden 2001: 153). From there Escobar and his friends hosted lavish parties, entertained women and came and went much as they wished, attending football matches (the police blocking off traffic to give priority to his motorcade), visiting nightclubs and going shopping. Escobar continued, meanwhile, to develop his narco-businesses and authorize assassinations. The arrangement turned sour only when, in the incident we have already noted, the government sought to transfer Escobar to another prison. Escobar, with the collusion of the Colombian army charged with the transfer, kidnapped the Vice-Minister of Justice (who subsequently escaped), and himself escaped from prison. A manhunt ensued. This involved not only the Colombian Police's Search Bloc unit and the CIA, anxious to find a new role following the Cold War, but also Los Pepes, Colombian vigilantes originally associated with Escobar's victims who quickly formed death squads to achieve the slaying of Escobar. The crack anti-terrorist manhunting squad Delta Force was also called in, but any successes achieved against Escobar's forces were paid for in multiple revenge killings. This period of carnage ended only when Escobar was finally tracked down and killed by Search Bloc in December 1993.

Pablo Escobar was both gangster and politician. He used his wealth to enhance his political ambition, terrorize the country and eliminate his opponents, and his political influence to shore up his criminal enterprises – mostly based on cocaine – and to protect himself from extradition to the United States. He bought potentially friendly politicians and eliminated any who were likely to impede his intended path to the presidency. Escobar was a violent and ruthless criminal who possessed an extraordinary combination of unimaginable wealth, tactical and strategic brilliance, media manipulation skills, political astuteness, instinctive grasp of the pressure points in

Colombian society and remarkable oratorical ability. Together these enabled him to take control of significant parts of the army, to buy or to eliminate all opposition through his *plata o plomo* policy (one took Pablo's silver or his bullet (Bowden 2001: 33)), and to inflict a reign of terror which successive governments were unable to counter. His achievement of genuine authority over a semi-literate population aided his rise to the position of the most dominant figure in Colombia's fragile society. Though a known and feared criminal, he was not, for much of his life, a fugitive, but a high-profile and untouchable alternative leader. Hence, though never elected, Escobar successfully propelled himself into the de facto criminal presidency of a country whose inherent instability and corruption he had done so much both to exploit and to augment. It was only when, following the end of the Cold War but at the height of the latest US War on Drugs, the Colombian and US Governments mounted a sustained attack on him that it became clear that this ultimate ambition was to be thwarted.

As with Khun Sa, Escobar was a criminal-politician whose success was based on a combination of manipulation and terror, but who, above all, operated within the available interstices. In Escobar's case these were to be found in the volatile and corrupt politics of his own weak state, his power to buy police, soldiers and prison guards almost at will, to fund and exploit revolutionary opposition forces and to intimidate opponents by destroying them and their families. But for Escobar interstices also existed between Colombia and the USA. These were to be found in part in the US pre-occupation with the Cold War prior to the 1990s. In addition, barriers to cooperation existed as a result of Colombian pride, sovereignty, political instability and corruption, an inadequate and weakly enforced extradition treaty and the corruptibility of neighbouring states such as Nicaragua, from whose leaders Escobar could purchase refuge whenever Colombian interstices appeared likely to close. It was not by chance that Escobar's end came in 1993, shortly after the end of the Cold War. US attention was focusing on the domestic consequences of his criminality, the Colombian Government was able to close ranks in a way that would have been impossible in 1991 and the extent of Escobar's carnage was beginning to weaken his support among the Colombian poor, his natural and necessary allies. This conjunction, temporary as it was, effectively closed the interstices within which Escobar operated with sufficient decisiveness and for enough time for his elimination to become possible.

Human migration

More people became refugees in 1995 than left Spain . . . to colonize the Americas in the nineteenth century. . . . Today's massive movements tell of countries where crime by organized clans or gangs or by individuals is replacing aggression by militaries, where internal conflict is replacing war with neighboring nations, where young people have to look for employment abroad, and where population growth and environmental degradation are making other stresses more acute.

(Kane 2000: 150)

Quite obviously migration has always taken place, and for a wide range of economic and political reasons. Without voluntary migration there would be no Israel, USA or Australia, while compulsory migration to distant and potentially unstable areas has been a feature of authoritarian regimes such as those of the Soviet Union (mainly under Stalin) and China. In the former Soviet bloc the Baltic states of Estonia and Latvia contain sizeable Russian populations. China, from the early days of the People's Republic, sought to weaken resistance in Xizang Zizhiqu (Tibet), Xinjiang Province (formerly Eastern Turkestan) and Inner Mongolia by settling a majority Han population. This has more recently been achieved in part by redirecting some of the several million inhabitants of the Yangzi River basin displaced during the construction of the Three Gorges Dam in the 1990s. Historically, migration has almost always had political causes or political consequences. In Northern Ireland the effects of James I's settlement of London liverymen in what was accordingly to become Londonderry continue to resonate today (Curl 1986, 2000). Saddam Hussein forced many of Iraq's Shiite populations into Iran, and Kurdish populations into Turkey during the 1990s; when Turkey responded by closing its borders, leaving the Iraqi Kurds stranded without sustenance, the western allies sent in a military force to return them to their homelands.

During the Cold War the United States encouraged professionals and scientists to defect from the Soviet bloc and from Soviet client states, and 96 per cent of the 711,303 refugees admitted during the Reagan presidency were from communist countries (Loescher 1993: 21).[12] This was both because their quest for freedom constituted exploitable anti-communist propaganda and because enticing skilled professionals would strengthen the US economy and destabilize and demoralize the communists. Since the start of the Cold War the politics of migration has been fundamental to US relations with Cuba (see Masud-Piloto 1996), and political games have been played by both sides. In 1980 Castro famously encouraged mass emigration from the port of Mariel, ensuring that the numbers included many prisoners and other undesirables. The 125,000 'Marielitos' who arrived in a five-month period caused, as intended, administrative chaos in Florida, committed (or were believed to have committed) numerous violent and sexual crimes and destabilized the Sunshine State's large and vocal Cuban-American community. In the changed international system following the end of the Cold War, however, Cuba lost much of its strategic significance. Hence, in response to a rapid influx of immigrants during a Cuban food crisis in 1994, President Clinton suspended the migration system, interning 27,000 aspiring immigrants in the US naval base at Guantanamo

Bay and imposing an annual quota of 20,000. This was designed to give the United States greater control over immigration, ensuring in particular that future immigrants met US domestic needs and were not 'dumped' by the Castro regime.

Internationally the scale of human mobility since the late 1970s has surpassed all prior experience. In accordance with the UN Convention on Refugees (1951), refugees are, strictly, those who, having crossed a nation state boundary, are permitted to reside permanently in a host country on the ground that they are fleeing persecution (the Convention was drafted with Eastern European Communism in mind). By convention, however, the designation 'refugee' is also given to those fleeing war or natural disaster, though for them refuge overseas is normally in temporary camps pending return. In addition to asylum seekers, normally crossing national borders in pursuit of refugee status, LDCs contain up to 25 million internally displaced persons (IDPs), driven from their homelands by war or famine.[13]

Of course actual or potential migrants are by no means restricted to those fleeing persecution in their own countries and seeking refugee status. Most are economic migrants exploiting low-grade employment opportunities spurned by the indigenous population in developed countries. The opportunities available to this category of migrant, or at least which they believe available to them, far outstrip the possibilities stemming from a counter-vailing product of globalization – job opportunities with multi-national corporations in the land of origin. Migrants also include professionals from the less-developed world recruited to assuage labour shortages in areas of public sector provision including health and education, and individuals legitimately selling their labour within a free trade zone. In addition, and outside the official statistics, innumerable millions of illegal immigrants, mainly economic migrants, have managed to submerge themselves in the black economies of various host nations, on a permanent or temporary basis (Harris 2003).

These exponential increases are more than a transient response to regional or civil conflict or instability in the Middle East, former Soviet republics (where major armed conflicts quadrupled following the Cold War (Cusimano 2000b: 13)), Afghanistan, parts of sub-Saharan Africa or the Balkans. Though such factors help explain recent increases, the effects of continued economic disparities, disruptions to established patterns of existence result-ing from urbanization, ethnic conflict (for example in Uganda, Rwanda, Indonesia, the Balkans and Nagorno-Karabakh), famine, environmental degradation and climatic change will sustain the impetus. And the struc-tures, many of them criminal, facilitating transnational migration are now in place, and demand for their services will certainly not disappear as conflicts diminish. Indeed they receive strong unofficial support from many governments, notably in Latin America where aiding aliens is seldom illegal, and which regard the export of their own citizens to the US in particular as a major economic benefit. In fact several Central American countries act as a hub for prospective illegal immigrants from all over the world, so combining economic utility and significant rent-seeking opportunity for politicians and bureaucrats. In China too, organized criminal rings centred on Fujian Province in the south-east of the country, embrace not only Snakehead gangs but the politicians, police, customs officials and bureaucrats who permit them to operate with impunity. With developed countries containing less than 25 per cent of the world's population but accounting for around 70 per cent of its goods and services, migration is both rational and inevitable. It is unsurprising, therefore, that the proportion of the world's workforces born abroad increased by 50 per cent between 1965 and 1990 (International Monetary Fund 2000: 3).

The problems generated by these changes have defied many of the control efforts of the international system. Hence the need for international co-operation has increased considerably, but problems with informal agreements necessitate the construction of a multi-national framework for their funding and management. For example, according to the United Nations High Commissioner for Refugees the number of international refugees increased from 3 million in 1976 to 21.5 million in 1998, standing at 26 million at the turn of the century (Kane 2000: 150). With the likelihood of prolonged conflict in Afghanistan and the Middle East it seems inevitable that this trend will continue, becoming a distinctive feature of international relations for the foreseeable future.

For legal migrants the potential economic benefits are obviously enormous, but protectionist policies and immigration controls designed to impede the free movement of labour ensure that the benefits for criminals are at least equally so. Where a market of willing buyers and sellers exists or can be created, illegitimate opportunities inevitably emerge, and asylum seekers and prospective illegal immigrants are often transported by, or with the aid of, organized criminals. Illegal immigrants naturally have low market value and face difficulties resulting directly from their illegal status, but, like legal migrants, they are making a rational choice in a disorganized, sometimes illegitimate, and ineffectively regulated global market place where the risk of detection, even for low-level criminals, is nugatory.[14] Such migrants constitute the sharp end of an illicit commercial process originating in and maintained by political or bureaucratic corruption at different levels of seniority in countries of origin, stopping-off points and countries of final destination.

Some migrants are already part of pre-existing networks, including criminal ones, into which, on arrival, they insinuate themselves. Indeed the existence of such networks may be influential in determining an individual migrant's choice of destination. Migrants lacking such a network may be provided with one by others they meet en route or by their transporters. The latter, at least in the case of prospective immigrants from the Far East, are normally Chinese or Vietnamese organized criminals, though not necessarily Triads, whose influence in Europe has diminished in the face of competition from other ethnic Chinese gangs (Chu 1994). Illegal immigrants in debt for their fare will obviously not easily escape their transporters, though, in addition to coercive and extortive activities, such transporters may offer services akin to those provided by Italian, especially Sicilian, gangs to new Italian arrivals in US cities before and after the Second World War. These services, which replicate or complement those provided by the great political machines, include employment (licit or illicit), accommodation, security, cultural companionship, useful contacts, and advice on how to survive in an alien system. Many contemporary illegal immigrants are absorbed into these networks, gradually coming to take on welcoming functions, as well as participating in whatever protection rackets, turf wars, collaborative activities and other forms of criminality are on offer at the time. Hence they in turn help strengthen their network (Chu 1996: 13–15), diversifying its criminality, enhancing its influence and prestige. Conversely, a small number will be instrumental in introducing competing networks, creating new turf wars and increased instability among these criminal groupings.

Nuclear smuggling

> Never before in history has an empire disintegrated while in possession of some 30,000 nuclear weapons, at least 40,000 tons of chemical weapons, significant biological weaponry capability, and thousands of weapons scientists and technicians unsure of how long they will receive salaries.
>
> (Senator Sam Nunn, cited in Lee and Ford 2000: 71)

The world trade in heroin and cocaine and the necessary money-laundering arrangements for managing it are widely believed to have been carved up at a meeting between the Sicilian Mafia and Escobar's Medellín Cartel in Aruba, off the Venezuelan coast, in the late 1980s. A meeting in Prague in 1992 between the Russian and Italian Mafia apparently culminated in an agreement to share ownership of a commercial bank in Yekaterinburg in the Urals. Colombians, Russians and Italians are rumoured, reliably or not, to hold periodic summit meetings, including one on a yacht off Monte Carlo in July 1993, at which Colombian drug traffickers, Chinese Triad members, American Cosa Nostra and Israeli criminals were all present (Lupsha 1996: 25).

While one should not overstate the significance of these meetings, such evidence is hard to come by and the successful transnational organization of crime based on business partnerships has enabled some criminal networks to be in an economically stronger position than many nations. As a result they are in a position to compete for the illicit purchase of weapons, including those with a nuclear capability, offloaded or allowed to fester following the end of the Cold War (notably in Russia, Ukraine, Belarus and

Kazakhstan). In none of these countries were reliable inventories of nuclear stocks maintained, since inadequate state control, corrupt plant management and poor security combined to make the creation of secret caches, for private sale or to make up for subsequent production deficits, a common phenomenon. Since the demise of the Soviet Union, however, the situation has markedly deteriorated. Such security as there was (notably from the KGB and the army, with manufacturing cities closed to foreigners) has disappeared, physical safeguards are frequently unreliable or non-existent, storage facilities are insecure and guards bribable. In particular, the former republics are unable or unwilling to create and support even remotely effective structures to deal with this problem. While ballistic missiles seem likely for the foreseeable future to be well beyond the purchasing power of criminal or terrorist groups, modest quantities of highly enriched uranium and plutonium, the basis of nuclear weapons, are available, and affordable by well-connected and drug-funded criminals and terrorists, and by rogue states. These can be manually delivered to target in the form of an improvised nuclear device (IND) or a radiological dispersal device (RDD),[15] as happened in Osama Bin Laden's first attack on the World Trade Center and Timothy McVeigh's attack on the Oklahoma City Federal Building. Hence the concern today is not simply with rogue states acquiring a nuclear capability or expanding an existing one: constructing an IND or an RDD is also potentially within the grasp of terrorist groups.

This capability has already permitted both criminal and terrorist networks to mount successful challenges to the monopoly on coercive force conventionally claimed by governments. Parts of Russia and some eastern republics, and parts of South-East Asia (for example Mindanao in the Southern Philippines and Aceh in the north of Sumatra), Central America and sub-Saharan Africa are governed by local warlords supported by criminal gangs. Organized crime groups have formed across the former Soviet republics to smuggle stolen materials to the central European market (Lee and Ford 2000: 73), while expertise provided by redundant Soviet physicists is readily available for hire by rogue states such as Iraq or Libya. Accordingly the forces of disorder are dispensing order, not by anything recognizable in the west as good government, but by disposing of rival forces in furtherance of political ambition, commercial opportunity or both.[16]

While, as is to be expected in an unregulated market, instances of fraud are common, with harmless substances passed off as nuclear materials, little reliable information exists about the extent and nature of what materials are available. Both the United States and the United Nations have taken steps to address the problem, but both have in their turn encountered further problems. The joint US military and Department of Energy scheme, the Nunn-Lugar-Dominici Cooperative Threat Reduction Program, aims, by government-to-government and laboratory-to-laboratory contact, to increase security and reduce nuclear proliferation in the former

Soviet republics, particularly Russia itself, where most nuclear sites are located. It does not, however, cover smuggling routes into Iran, Iraq, Pakistan and Afghanistan, nor, for different political reasons, is it in a position to conclude treaties with these weak states, some of which are dealing in, or stockpiling, the nuclear resources themselves. Indeed such is the political sensitivity involved that even in Russia US and UN efforts are largely restricted to advising on improvements in security, safe storage, training and anti-trafficking measures.

UN attempts to stem proliferation through the International Atomic Energy Association (IAEA) similarly founder on problems of funding, inspection and verification (Cusimano 2000c: 67–68), but the IAEA did record 132 confirmed instances of international nuclear smuggling between 1993 and 1996. In Germany, a major entrepôt for the trade, 84 seizures and 576 apparently genuine offers to sell nuclear materials between 1992 and 1996 were recorded, in good part through *agent provocateur* or other 'sting' operations. These included, most spectacularly, the seizure of a large quantity of plutonium in Munich in 1996, stolen following incitement by the Bavarian police. In another key transit country, Poland, 2,045 attempts to import radiation-causing substances were reported between 1991 and 1996 (Lee and Ford 2000: 73).

In Russia, since the end of the Cold War nuclear orders have virtually ceased, $564 million of state debts exist, and $100 million is owed to employees in unpaid wages. Russia has accordingly completed deals to sell technology with nuclear capability to India and Iran, judging that the profits to be made outweigh the risks involved. Unsurprisingly, within the industry itself corruption flourishes at all levels. At a senior level this is 'clouding the lines between criminal behavior and deliberate state policy', with senior MINATOM officials setting up private companies for the purpose of 'undercover export of nuclear materials, technology, and know-how' (Lee and Ford 2000: 82). Nuclear scientists, once the cream of Soviet society, now earn salaries below subsistence level. This is self-evidently unfortunate, given that these are 'people with nuclear bombs in their hands' who are 'stealing not just to make a living, but also because they are angry' (respectively the scholar Orlov and the former nuclear scientist Korolev, cited in Lee and Ford 2000: 81). Hence:

> The real proliferation danger derives from systemic factors: diminished economic prospects in the military-industrial complex (including the nuclear sector), a weakening political control structure, an increasingly corrupt bureaucracy, and widening penetration of the economy by organized crime formations; such an environment increases the likelihood of exports of fissile materials and even weaponry to states or substate groups with goals inimical to the United States . . . controls can be circumvented easily – particularly in scenarios of collaboration between

senior nuclear managers, corrupt officials, and professional underworld elements.

(Lee and Ford 2000: 85)

Such problems permeate the industry, creating a culture of both indifference and institutionalized corruption characterized by a dropping of standards for new recruits, inadequate screening procedures and extensive moonlighting by staff at all levels.

Conclusion

> there are widening holes within the global economy that are facilitating the free trade of an array of nefarious 'commodities'. . . . High-grade plutonium, hazardous waste, counterfeit credit cards and documents, pirated copyrighted materials, stolen vehicles, child pornography, aliens and indentured teenage prostitutes can be found on that list . . . as free trade zones and tax havens proliferate and new and largely lawless capitalist markets gain access to the international economy, global economic activity more and more has come to resemble the kind of capitalism familiar to industrialized countries at the turn of the [last] century.
>
> (Flynn 2000: 61)

This chapter and the last have set political corruption, more often viewed microscopically through case studies, in a changing world of international relations and globalization. As such, we have necessarily painted with a broad brush, and some of the details the chapters *do* contain will quickly be out of date. Nonetheless the two chapters together illustrate that political corruption does indeed need to be addressed within a framework of tensions between national sovereignty and transnational regulation, and between banking sovereignty and transnational regulation. When transactions in global trade and commerce of around $1.3 trillion are estimated to occur every day, the proportion involving 'black' money, though probably fairly small, nonetheless adds up to many trillions of dollars a year, and remains extraordinarily hard to detect.

This money, however, fuels a global illegal economy comprising corrupt politicians (who, Leviathan-like, regard their countries' banking systems as personal fiefdoms) and organized criminals engaged both in the activities described in these chapters – people and arms smuggling, dealing in stolen goods, corrupting officials and so on – and in legitimate business. For unless we rid ourselves of the image of organized criminals operating in closed Sicilian families, centrally controlled and dominating the economy and civil society of a small, socially patriarchal island we misunderstand the issue. Corrupt political leaders, corrupt businesspeople and legitimate businesspeople are almost always interchangeable, and frequently they are the same individuals. We have seen examples of businessmen seeking public office to further their own business interests or, particularly in the case of Silvio Berlusconi, to stop another leader from damaging them. More dramatically, we have seen, in the cases of Khun Sa and Pablo Escobar, the exploitation for both political and criminal ends of the interstices between states and those within an individual state. In both cases their criminal and political methods and objectives initially fed off each other but, as their careers developed, became indistinguishable, each an aspect of the other. And this happened to such an extent that if either the criminality or the politics had been missing these towering, terrifying, figures would have been significantly diminished. Ultimately, in both cases it was over-weening political ambition which so challenged the interests of powerful states as to cause the interstices within which they operated to close, and so to precipitate their downfall. Both men were, though as individuals evil beyond belief, simultaneously tragic heroes, men whose striking qualities would, had they not been so frighteningly misdirected, have been worthy of praise and admiration.

So many of the most corrupt politicians are also organized criminals; and virtually all heads of high-corruption societies may be regarded as such. They create (or exploit pre-existing) structures designed to maximize their predations, normally by means of reward and punishment systems involving violent enforcement. They develop networks of investments at home and abroad, whether in houses, aircraft, land, jewellery or numbered bank accounts. Their overall aim is to appropriate the possessions of others, and in furtherance of this they contract with like-minded criminals when it suits them and eliminate them when it does not. They permit others, in return for concessions or commissions, similarly to engage in corruption, using that corruption to damage or destroy them when it suits them. They invest part of their money in seemingly altruistic ventures – hospitals, schools, sports centres, churches – but these ventures are but a form of vote buying, the purchase of popular support being a necessary investment cost in the maintenance and consolidation of their power. The fact that in the case of corrupt politicians the business organization is a country, and in that of corrupt businessmen it is not is a surprisingly superficial difference. Both organizations serve as maximizing units, and both corrupt politicians and corrupt businessmen aim, by adroit manipulation of their complementary interests, to engage in similar utility-maximizing activities by systematic or *ad hoc* collaborations with their own mirror images.

Notes

1 'Mafia' is now commonly used as a generic term synonymous with 'organized criminals'. This is analytically unhelpful. A more sophisticated approach is to regard 'mafia' as not synonymous with but an advanced subcategory of organized crime, applicable only in situations where organized criminals have also

taken over certain governmental functions. Anderson (1995) mounts an eloquent defence of this approach. In this book as a general rule Mafia refers to Sicilians, though not necessarily working in Sicily. On rare exceptions, as here, for reasons of convention we make an exception; in such situations the word 'Mafia' carries a qualifier.

2 It is said that to facilitate blackmail in the event of treachery only people who have committed a murder may join the Sicilian Mafia. This does not apply in the USA.

3 Mafia probably originated in the mid-nineteenth century, following unification, as a product of the wish of Sicilians to protect themselves against possible alien influences from elsewhere in Italy. Hence the organization was from the first as political as it was criminal, its aim being to prevent the central state securing a monopoly of violence on the island.

4 Don Calogero, for example, wasted little time in consolidating his power base in Villalba by killing his 'overinquisitive' police chief in order to free himself of all restraints (McCoy 1991: 36).

5 The Central Intelligence Agency was founded by President Truman in 1947. In an early covert operation exemplifying the view that any enemy of communism was a friend of the USA, the Agency had aligned itself with Corsican gangsters to attack striking dockers in the strategically important and politically volatile port of Marseilles. The aim had been to prevent communist domination of Marseilles at a time when numbers of communist sympathizers in both France and Italy were expanding alarmingly. Marseilles was crucial to the import of products under the Marshall Plan, which was strongly opposed by the Communists, but also of symbolic importance to the French Communist Party, both as France's gateway to Indo-China and as home to many Indo-Chinese, Algerian and French communists. Following the CIA's withdrawal, patronage of the Corsican criminals was continued by SDECE, the French intelligence service, some of whose senior officers were themselves benefiting from the trade. SDECE, together with a corrupt city government, permitted heroin manufacture to continue undisturbed for a decade under powerful political cover until decimated by a joint DEA–French operation in 1971, as part of President Nixon's War on Drugs (McCoy 1991: Chapter 2).

6 For the Chairman's own dramatic account of the hearings and their effect on him see Kefauver (1952). For a telling methodological critique see Reuter (1983: 185 *et seq.*).

7 Mafia has, however, for many years been suspected by many of orchestrating the assassinations of John and Robert Kennedy (Sterling 1993: 457 is a convenient source of references). The firm delivered Kennedy 200,000 decisive votes in Illinois in the close-run 1960 presidential election against Nixon, but the brothers, in spite of mutually beneficial friendships with a number of high-profile figures with mob connections, repaid their debt by pursuing an anti-Mafia campaign. The rumour continues, however, to lack verification.

8 In good part but not entirely. Any fuller analysis of this phenomenon would point to the greater impersonality of Mafia organization in the USA than in Sicily, where patriarchal relations continue to humanize the activity. But as the US Mafia has increasingly assumed the characteristics of a formal organization it has become, like any formal organization, ever more risk averse. In addition, in contrast with the situation in Sicily, in large US cities there are always sufficient low fruit to provide a feast; so why would Mafia risk its collective neck climbing trees?

9 The following accounts draw heavily on the excellent studies of McCoy (1991, 1999) and Bowden (2001), to which readers are referred for fuller coverage of

these two extraordinary criminal politicians. McCoy's is a remarkable work of scholarship whose Preface alone would pass muster as the basis for a Michael Douglas movie; Bowden's popularly presented coverage, which makes it read like a Graham Greene novel, should not cause scholars to devalue the quality of the research underpinning it.

10 For startling but unproven allegations see ⟨http://www.alternatives.com/crime/CIAOPIUM.HTML#khun_sa⟩.

11 Under the Colombian system both a representative and a substitute are elected, the substitute attending meetings, with full voting rights, which the representative is unable to attend (Bowden 2001: 41).

12 Migration from such friendly but brutal regimes as those in Haiti, El Salvador and Guatemala, however, was always difficult and often impossible.

13 It has been estimated, for example, that 40 per cent of the population of Sudan constitutes IDPs (Cohen and Deng 1998).

14 There are poignant exceptions to this rational choice approach. These include, especially tragically, young women from the less-developed world taken from their homes through parental sale or criminal kidnap and placed in forced marriages or prostitution. These unfortunates, far from exercising rational choice, are victims of rational choices made by others. Other women and girls are intended economic migrants but sorely misled by their transporters as to the nature of the economic activity in which they will be participating. Such personnel too often come to be the poor bloody infantry of the sex industry in the great cities of the developed world (Somerset 2001). The US Government has estimated that up to two million women and children are trafficked across borders each year.

15 An IND, or 'dirty bomb', produces a small nuclear explosion with a high radioactive fallout. An RDD produces a conventional explosion but scatters contaminating radioactive materials (Lee and Ford 2000: 71).

16 For a helpful, if probably dramatized and certainly outdated, account of organized crime's relationship with terrorism and drugs money see Bosworth-Davies and Saltmarsh (1994: Chapter 2).

7 Conclusion

> Because, just as for the maintenance of good customs laws are required, so if laws are to be observed, there is need of good customs. Furthermore, institutions and laws made in the early days of a republic when men were good, no longer serve their purpose when men have become bad. And, if by any chance the laws of the state are changed, there will never, or but rarely, be a change in its institutions. The result is that new laws are ineffectual, because the institutions, which remain constant, corrupt them.
>
> (Machiavelli, *The Discourses*, Book 1, Chapter 18)

This book began by outlining a three-limbed theory of political corruption. *First*, it is a comprehensible extension of normal political life, not a discrete phenomenon. *Second*, it can no longer be viewed simply or even mainly as bounded by the nation state, but needs to be set in an international and transnational context. *Third*, it is an 'interstitial' activity – in other words it exploits and operates within any fractures existing in the polity of a state or between the polities of different states. We rejected the possibility of a unitary definition of corruption: it is such a variegated activity that a single sentence could not encapsulate it, while a comprehensive definition would be too lengthy and have too many qualifications to be useful. Nonetheless we took as a 'signpost' a two-limbed definition by Summers – that it involves 'the use of public position for private advantage or exceptional party profit, and the subversion of the political process for personal ends' (Summers 1987: 14) – though we qualified and glossed this definition quite heavily. This signpost has, however, guided us throughout the book, albeit for the most part silently.

We also distinguished high-corruption from low-corruption countries. High-corruption countries are those where corruption can be reasonably described as having permeated the structures of government to such an extent that being corrupt is normal behaviour. This may manifest itself in different ways. In its pure form it is likely to entail:

- all other branches of government being subordinated to an all-powerful and unaccountable executive;
- a banking system which funds the executive's predatory conduct;
- a series of variably coordinated but symbiotic clientelistic and patronal networks sometimes passing as manifestations of traditional culture;
- a general assumption that to obtain a service one must make a payment;
- a non-democratic or ineffectively democratic political system;
- a heavily controlled press;
- low GDP;
- poor literacy standards;
- high military and low social expenditure;
- heavy IMF debtor status.

A low-corruption country on the other hand is one where:

- the structures of government are basically robust and accountable;
- one would not seriously contemplate trying to bribe a judge or police officer;
- constitutional safeguards against abuse exist;
- whistle-blowing is a practical option;
- where, when instances of corruption emerge, the miscreant is disciplined or prosecuted, an inquiry is held and system glitches rectified. In other words, the system self-corrects and returns to a functioning state.

We begin, *first*, by revisiting the three limbs of our definition in the light of the contents of the book. *Second*, we consider anti-corruption strategies, focusing in particular on the Hong Kong experience which, though in some respects tangential to political corruption, nonetheless offers some clues to good practice. *Third*, we review recent political events in Africa, which, if we are in an optimistic frame of mind, might point the way to a future framework for the reduction of corruption in those states not entirely given over to criminal enterprise.

Political corruption as an extension of normal political activity

> instructing his aides on how to 'stonewall' a grand jury without committing perjury; planning how, with his White House counsel, to 'screw' his political enemies using the FBI and the IRS; developing public relations 'scenarios' to explain possibly illegal actions with the constant and only question being 'will it play?'
>
> (Silverstein 1988: 22 on Nixon during Watergate)

The first limb of the theory, that political corruption is an extension of recognizable political behaviour, is open to criticism from a number of angles. Moralists might criticize the idea that political corruption is an out-crop of political behaviour for abdicating concepts such as honour and decency, and, by implication, for condemning individual politicians who they know or believe to be committed, selfless and honest. Others might point to the excesses, violent as well as pecuniary, of corrupt (and probably crazy) presidents such as Duvalier and Bokassa, and reject as absurd and offensive any idea that their behaviour is indistinguishable from normal political conduct. Others again might pose the problem that to make such a claim is to surrender the right to pass judgement on any one regime or president, or even to compare one political system with another. Obviously innumerable objections along these lines might be raised.

This is not a 'moral' book, however, and while nor, certainly, is it intended to be an immoral one, it aims to analyse the world as it is, not as it should be or might be made to become. It is no part of the theory that as a breed politicians are especially corrupt, lazy, alcoholic, promiscuous, avaricious, cynical or mendacious. Whether or not they are is an empirical question on which we have no view, and while it would doubtless be interesting and instructive to compare politicians with (say) architects, artisans, academics, archaeologists, anaesthetists, astronauts, ambulance drivers or accountants on any of these variables this was not our purpose. What we do know from UK opinion polls is that the public perception of politicians is poor: they are, alongside journalists, regarded as among the least trustworthy of professionals.[1] It is, however, relevant that politicians are, in two senses of the word, public people. They are public, *first*, in that they are in the public eye and, *second*, in that, at least in democratic systems, their careers are dependent on public support. If the public has, or politicians believe it to have, unrealistic expectations of them, this conjunction of expectation and accountability requires them, as a condition of re-election, to juggle appearance and reality, with discreet deception in the form of impression management a necessary part of the professional tool-kit.

The expectations in question are of two distinct and potentially contra-dictory kinds. *First*, electors, disillusioned with politicians as they clearly are, may be assumed to demand not only professional competence but also high standards of moral conduct, normally in relation to personal, financial, religious or sexual propriety. *Second*, they certainly expect politicians to deliver policies which benefit them – as individuals or members of a com-munity – or which reflect and advance their belief systems. Competition in these two areas – being clean and being effective – is the stuff of democratic politics. Naturally electors exert leverage on politicians to endorse their views and interests. In doing so they will be relatively uninterested in their targets' private belief systems, for victory in, say, the abortion debate (in the United States) or the fox-hunting debate (in the United Kingdom) is achieved by changing political behaviour, not private values.

Of course not only individual electors offering their vote in return for such support, but also organized interest groups and commercial corporations offering donations, consultancies and so on will make representations. At a certain point such offers may become corrupt, if not legally then perceptually, but when that point is reached is not always clear. While, as we have seen, the United Kingdom has attempted to be specific by introducing an independent means of specifying acceptable standards in public life and a semi-independent means[2] of determining it, this is by no means usually the case. It also remains to be seen whether the Code of Conduct will address all possibilities popularly deemed corrupt, and whether, in consequence, the framework will meet the political necessity of an anti-corruption strategy in a low-corruption democratic country, which is to bring legal and perceptual requirements into synchronicity. In short, for popular legitimacy to be achieved a close match is necessary between the conduct *actually* proscribed by legislation and what it is popularly believed the law *should* proscribe. Nonetheless it is a promising start, but only a start.

The theory does not question the obvious fact that everyone is different. It does, however, turn on the assumption that when people are faced with a desirable opportunity their conduct will normally be self-seeking, and that this will certainly not always and probably not usually be consonant with their public rhetoric. This is bound to be an especially poignant dissonance in the case of public people of whom genteel expectations exist. So while rock stars may not become less popular for snorting cocaine and trashing hotel rooms the average Secretary of State would be unwise to claim similar licence. Rent-seeking opportunities accrue to politicians because of their possession of, or access to, power. Naturally politicians will make individual judgements about how far to go down the rent-seeking road, but virtually all of them will go at least some way down it. Some will stop at the occasional free dinner or campaign donation; some will accept free flights, family holidays or the paid-for services of lap dancers or prostitutes; some will invite commissions; some will go further. But most will proceed slowly and incrementally, doubtless in many cases looking back, as many of John Poulson's network did when their corruption finally came to light, in genuine shock and surprise at the sum total of what they had taken and what they had done.

A key factor in the minds of politicians contemplating rent-seeking is its probable impact on their career. This is a product of various factors: the likelihood of apprehension, the penalty if caught and the political effect – on electors, the party and the press – of apprehension. Such considerations are then, naturally, weighed against the potential benefits provided by the rent. But these considerations are all rational and political, and certainly not moral.

In high-corruption countries the principle is much the same, but because the political and economic context is different so will be the decisions and so, therefore, the character of political corruption. Where there exist a dominant executive, weak judiciary, state-controlled press, compliant banking system, well-disposed military and an expectation that politicians will act in a predatory manner one should not be surprised when they do. So to hold up individual predators as the cause of the problem is to miss the point that they are actually its products. Equally, however, it would be wrong to regard corrupt politicians anywhere as *only* products of the political system, since this would be to assume both an absence of human agency and that causes and effects are more separate than they are. In the social and political worlds, after all, yesterday's effect is tomorrow's cause, and the decisions taken by predatory politicians have the capacity to perpetuate or diminish political corruption, albeit not always critically.

The international politics of political corruption

> We must tie greater aid to political, legal and economic reforms, and by insisting on reform we do the work of compassion. We must build the institutions of freedom, not subsidize the failures of the past.
>
> (President George W. Bush, Monterrey, Mexico, March 2002)

> You can't blame this tragedy on the poor countries. It wasn't they who conquered and looted entire continents for centuries, nor did they establish colonialism, nor did they reintroduce slavery, nor did they create modern imperialism. They were its victims.
>
> (President Fidel Castro, Monterrey, Mexico, March 2002)

The second limb of the theory locates political corruption in the international and transnational arena, and conceptualizes transnational political corruption as a series of geographically unbounded transactions involving exchanges of money, power, influence and status. While this approach denies neither that most political corruption targets domestic objects nor that its direct victims are for the most part domestic too, the nature, scale and consequences of the problem have global ramifications and hence demand both global analysis and a global response.

If political corruption were purely a matter for the country concerned, no one else would need to be unduly concerned about it and the sovereignty principle would be unproblematic. But while the domestic political turmoil in numerous and increasing numbers of weak states has naturally been critical to the exponential increase in political corruption since the late twentieth century, this is no longer a sufficient analysis. The effects of money laundering, the international trade in drugs, people and weapons, and the growth of organized crime and terrorism are no more the private business of a single state than are those of carbon emissions, the refugee problem or accidental nuclear explosions. These effects are mediated through a global nexus comprising:

- an international banking system which, though less corruption tolerant than it was, still offers many hiding places for black money;

- networks of international organized criminals;
- international organizations dispensing but inadequately auditing resources in aid, loans and subsidies;
- a global hegemony of economic liberalism;
- the technology of round-the-clock financial services.

To this extent, therefore, both cause and effect are international and transnational in scope and character. So, accordingly, must any solution be; and while the obstacles to achieving such a solution are daunting, the desirability of trying explains why the language of international relations has been used periodically throughout this book.

The international system retains the nation state structure formulated in the Treaty of Westphalia, 1648, although, with its emphasis on the sovereignty of nation states, it is not self-evidently well suited to deal with transnational problems. Nonetheless it would be defeatist to say that because the system is still recognizably post-Westphalian, lacking as it does a developed supranational framework to deal with transnational problems, nothing can be done. On the contrary, the system has in many ways proved both adaptive and resilient.

Historically sovereign states established rules, with different levels of formality, to govern their relations, leading to Hedley Bull's classic conceptualization of the anarchical society (Bull 1977). International society may have emerged from gentlemen's agreements among the various related European royal families, but as the class and cultural homogeneity necessary for this system to succeed diminished, and as international society became larger and more diverse, for the sovereignty system to continue new intermediary structures became necessary. In the light of this, structures have been created which work with and across states. This is the framework within which political corruption must be tackled, even though one has to proceed a little haltingly. But we have seen improved police collaboration through Interpol, Europol and other coordinating bodies. Interpol in particular, from its base in Lyon, has taken a coordinating role in relation both to transnational crime and to the international implications of domestic crime, collecting, maintaining and disseminating up-to-date information on rapidly changing developments in such activities as money laundering, terrorism and people smuggling. We have seen developments in international banking and anti-money-laundering protocols inconceivable even a decade ago. Since 1997 there has been greater determination by the World Bank and IMF to tighten the monitoring of loan expenditure and to set targets for health (as against military) spending, while the drive, spearheaded by OECD and FATF, to coordinate a transnational response to money laundering, has gained further momentum. Transaction costs have increased as a result of improved international coordination, and US leverage on some tax havens, notably Panama following its inclusion on the 'non-cooperating list' in 2000, is intense, though it is too soon to assess its effect. In fact in the case of Panama new legislation has expanded the list of crimes defined as financial, and the international sharing of certain forms of banking information is now permitted under Panamanian law. In a situation in which the short-term objective must be to enable the authorities to compete on equal terms with the criminals, but in which democratic governments have also to maintain a politically feasible balance between pursuing money launderers and acknowledging strong pressure for privacy, such modest developments are encouraging.

We have argued that the evidence is overwhelming that in the absence of firmer monitoring of aid and loans new influxes of money will simply perpetuate and expand political corruption. Equally, however, such an approach, unless sensitively handled, has undesirable side-effects and provokes sensitivities both about national sovereignty and about a range of historical grievances, mainly centred on colonialism. Of course for most high-corruption countries, using national sovereignty as a defence against international monitoring of aid and loan expenditure is no more than a very low trump card. After all, if one requires high levels of borrowing, debt relief or rescheduling, UN welfare aid, periodic disaster relief and entry to or influence on the World Trade Organization one must expect to swallow one's pride just a little. So the problem has less to do with the indignation of debtor countries, many of them post-colonial entities so weak as to be virtually paralysed, than with the fact that maintaining a strong form of sovereignty is in the interests of powerful countries including China, Russia and the United States. The fact that the very nations sufficiently powerful to exercise the leverage to challenge the negative consequences of national sovereignty are very unlikely to do so is a central dimension of contemporary international relations.

There is, of course, scope for more pressure to be applied on debtor countries by intermediary bodies such as the United Nations, the World Bank, IMF and the World Trade Organization. Indeed such bodies have, since the late 1990s, been increasingly willing to qualify the sovereignty principle. The UN Secretary-General, for example, has several times attempted to appeal to natural law in relation to the human rights agenda. Indeed such an agenda was deployed by the western powers as a justification for the Kosovo intervention in 1999 in the face of Russian opposition, and, prior to the 2001 attack on the World Trade Center and Washington, for leverage on Russia and China in respect of Chechnya and Xizang Zizhiqu (Tibet) respectively. The World Bank and IMF have, since 1997, espoused a more robust approach to enforcing conditionality clauses on loan expenditure, and OECD and FATF have shown signs of willingness to embarrass reluctant signatory countries in respect of their anti-money-laundering commitments. Robust carrot-and-stick diplomacy by such bodies, particularly if debt rescheduling and relief constitute the carrot, is clearly a feasible method of pressing countries to begin the lengthy process of bringing institutional corruption under control.

We have also argued that while, with the institution of international organizations as intermediary bodies, a global hegemony has emerged around
economic liberalization, and while the creation of a functioning liberal
economic system is antithetical to political corruption, it does not follow
that forced liberalization is wise. On the contrary, the evidence of the last
twenty years is that attempting this in respect of high-corruption societies
is fraught with danger. Certainly early experiments with this approach
were not encouraging, and it became increasingly apparent in the 1980s, as
the debt crisis loomed, that while the medicine may have been right, the
manner of administering it was making the patient worse. While it is true
that there is a strong correlation between the extent of governmental monopoly and corruption, the idea that liberalization necessarily offers a panacea
by opening up markets to the cleansing draught of competition is incorrect.
While a healthy functioning market economy is certainly as antithetical to
the conditions conducive to political corruption as is a healthy democracy,
both liberalism and democracy are *symptoms* of a low-corruption society
not, independently of other variables, its *causes*.

So imposing liberalization on a corrupt, monopolistic state is a high-risk
strategy, and increasingly recognized as such by the World Bank and IMF
in particular. *First*, where liberalization is premature only the already
corrupt will have the resources to buy privatized industries. *Second*, bureaucrats and politicians who envisage the end of rent-seeking will aim to maximize utility by increasing their demands. *Third*, the new competition to
which stable patron–client relations will be exposed will destabilize corruption's internal political economy, creating the chaos surrounding a Klondike
fever, as occurred in South Africa (Heymans and Lipietz 1999; Lodge 2002)
and, particularly, China.

While it is barely conceivable that debt rescheduling (never mind remission) could be countenanced without stringent conditions, these conditions
have in many cases been insufficient to stem the tide of internal corruption;
meanwhile the payments have themselves been subject to rent-seeking depredation. Only at the right political moment – towards the end of a corrupt
presidency, when a country faces internal political turmoil or when a
viable opposition can be identified and groomed – can a situation be
engineered in which a high-corruption recipient nation is likely to accept
stringent monitoring of internal expenditure. At present international organizations lack the unequivocal authority of, and adequate resources from,
their members to be able to undertake such an activity on a widespread
basis. In addition, however, problems typically arise from an aggressive
approach to enforcement. *First*, coercive measures almost always backfire.
Second, those who lose most from the inevitable stand-offs are the poor,
not the corrupt rich. *Third*, however intense the scrutiny, there are always
ways of evading it. *Fourth*, such a policy would lack legitimacy among
large sections of, in particular, the left-leaning continental European population. *Fifth*, the evidence of recent WTO and G7 meetings in particular is that

there currently exists the potential for globally coordinated forms of public disorder on the part of a wide range of humanitarian and environmental pressure groups.

We have also shown that the isolationist and competitive logic of national sovereignty has been moderated by the increasing willingness of nation states to trade aspects of sovereignty for the security and potential trade benefits of participating in supranational organizations. Hence it is clear that supranational regional groupings also play an increasingly important role. Here, however, it would be premature to assume that in the case of such bodies the whole is necessarily greater than the sum of its parts. The European Union has taken money laundering, drugs, illegal immigration and organized crime very seriously at a political and diplomatic level, but failures in policy execution have done little to enhance its popular legitimacy. For example, the Union failed to prevent a smuggling epidemic following the removal of internal border controls among the signatories to the Schengen agreement in 1995[3] by ensuring the tightening of external border controls – a problem which can only become worse following the Union's eastward extension in 2004. It has also consistently failed to prevent wholesale fraudulent use of agricultural subsidies (which account for almost half of total expenditure), up to 10 per cent of which has been fraudulently converted (Behan 1996: 133).[4] The Court of Auditors has repeatedly declined to affirm the legality and regularity of the accounts, reporting that cereal farmers have been overpaid by millions of pounds, that Mediterranean tobacco and olive growers have received subsidies for non-existent crops and that thousands of similarly non-existent cattle have been slaughtered. The preferential import scheme for non-EU member nations has also been widely abused. In one case the volume of orange juice imported from Israel under preferential arrangements was equivalent to almost three times that country's orange production. Scandals of this kind (for a fuller analysis of which see Peterson 1997), which are indicative of institutional corruption, contributed to the resignation of twenty Commissioners in 1999 in the discredited Santer administration.

Not only has the European Union failed to prevent corruption among its many millions of clients, however, it has also failed to resolve similar problems among its own staff and elected members. The mass resignation of Commissioners in 1999 was precipitated by an unauthorized book by an internal auditor which told of mismanagement and fraud running through many of the Union's areas of responsibility (van Buitenen 2000). The response of the new, reformed Commission was to set a tough reform agenda and to give one of its vice-presidents, Neil Kinnock, responsibility for delivering it. But the Kinnock reform plans encountered fierce opposition from EU staff, accustomed to being permitted considerable latitude in this area.[5] The position of Kinnock, who had, by early 2003, shown few signs of achieving the reforms to which he had committed himself in 1999, was further weakened by his dismissal of yet another whistle-blower, this time a chief accountant, Marta Andreasen. In this particular case Mrs Andreasen, appointed only five months earlier, had refused to sign off the Union's accounts, which she deemed non-compliant with basic and minimum accepted accounting standards.

As a case study in institutional corruption, the European Union has, like other bodies similarly afflicted, demonstrably failed to reform itself from within, all attempts to do so encountering fierce and well-informed resistance from those with a vested interest in the status quo. The European Union is a sprawling, weakly accountable, supranational organization lacking public legitimation and staff loyalty, and engaging in almost constant tussles with member states as to how much sovereignty should be surrendered. It has a large, well-educated and well-fed bureaucracy responsible for distributing vast sums in innumerable small grants and subsidies on the basis of poor, outdated or even non-existent assessments, while lacking the resources, energy, commitment or expertise to undertake more than token audit. Clearly the structural problems to be resolved if such an institution is to be radically reformed are immense, and the case of the European Union gives no reason for confidence that creating supranational bodies will do other than multiply rent-seeking opportunities. As a supranational organization the European Union is a club which no member can in practice afford to leave, and which is ultimately accountable only to itself. It generates no income, taking all its funds from member states. Justified by an anti-competitive redistributive ethos, it recycles almost half these funds into subsidizing inefficient agricultural producers, failing even to monitor its expenditure, never mind report fully on it or demonstrate added value. Why should anyone be surprised when such an organization generates a multitude of corrupt opportunities for employees, agents and clients alike?

The problem of political corruption and international relations can now be reformulated in the light of these considerations. Few debtor countries have successful liberal economies, and there is evidence, both from individual states and from the European Union, that monopoly state control over resources and major departures from market principles breed inefficiency, complacency and corruption. Conversely there is reason to believe the process of economic liberalism to be antithetical to political corruption. Such liberalism, however, is not an attainable short-term objective for some of the most corrupt countries in the world, and there is strong evidence that a coercive approach to premature liberalization is likely to be counterproductive. Nonetheless the status quo in such countries permits institutional corruption, and given the predatory tendencies of many ruling elites, loans and aid money are inevitably stolen with no realistic prospect of any significant internal impetus for reform. This in turn leads to aid withdrawals by donor countries. In consequence, the sum of western aid diminishes while the sum of human misery increases. So neither the status quo nor a coercive cure seems likely to break the deadlock.

It follows that it must be in all respects desirable to work towards achieving consensus between donor and recipient. This, however, is very hard to secure, since clearly significant and sometimes unbreachable structural differences exist between the interests of the two parties. Nonetheless, if we are correct in believing that at specific historical moments a convergence of interests is possible, it is just conceivable that, at least in parts of sub-Saharan Africa, the early twenty-first century may prove such a moment. On the face of it, and given our gloomy account of the failures in administration of the European Union, there is every reason to be sceptical about the capacity of the African Union[6] to address the problem of corruption in Africa. The failure of any African leader to denounce the violent and corrupt rule of Mugabe in Zimbabwe, for example, and the near-unanimous public view among African leaders that the blatantly corrupt Zimbabwean election in March 2002 was free and fair was not an auspicious start. One of the Union's first tasks was to draw up a Convention on Corruption, proposing that all public officials should declare their assets on taking office, that governments should take the power to seize bank documents and that those convicted of corruption should have their assets confiscated. It is frankly implausible to regard such a set of procedures, which would constitute a minimal response even in a low-corruption country, as likely to have any effect in the high-corruption African context.

Nonetheless it is just possible, if one is in optimistic mode, to read the Convention as signalling a genuine willingness (whether temporary or permanent remains to be seen) among at least some African countries to engage more constructively with donor nations and organizations. If so, this would be a significant shift from the traditionally counterproductive 'one for all and all for one' approach African leaders adopt in public to dealings with the west, associated as it is with the claim that aid, as a recompense for colonialism, should carry no reciprocal obligations. If such a shift were to occur it could create a foundation for a longer-term strategy, and it is in this context that the Convention has potential significance.

The formation of the African Union is one of a series of events occurring in 2001–2002 which together, in characteristically flamboyant, not to say extravagant, language, the UN Secretary-General described as 'a turning point in the history of Africa, and indeed, the world'. *First*, the New Partnership for Africa's Development (NEPAD), comprising fifteen member states[7] claiming to be ambitious to trade good governance and transparency for increased levels of aid, was inaugurated in Abuja, Nigeria, in October 2001. NEPAD is an African response to the pincer movement created by an increase in need (stemming mainly from crop failure and the spread of AIDS) and a diminution of supply (stemming from superpower withdrawal following the Cold War and the reluctance of donor countries to commit aid to corrupt regimes). Any longer-term significance NEPAD may have will lie in the willingness of the more progressive and reform-minded African nations to bid for support on their own merits to avoid facing the problem of most African nations being treated with equal suspicion. Given the corrupt and violent legacy of many African regimes, and in particular the festering sore of Zimbabwe's brutal response to its colonial experience – a response which can only damage African credibility in the eyes of western donors – partializing Africa for the purposes of aid, loans, debt relief and trade would be a significant step forward.

Second, in March 2002 a major International Conference on Financing for Development in Monterrey, Mexico, was attended by fifty-one world leaders, who pledged to increase aid, with the United States committing itself to a 50 per cent increase in its own percentage-poor but dollar-rich contribution. Addressing a NEPAD meeting a few months after this conference, in an indication of World Bank support the President, James Wolfensohn, pressed yet again for developed nations to lower tariff barriers against African imports and proposed that half the additional aid pledged in Monterrey should go to Africa. *Third*, the NEPAD proposals, whose progenitors tactically if implausibly declared them based on the Marshall Plan of 1948, were a central topic at a G-8 meeting in Kananaskis, Alberta, in June 2002. The outcome of this was a pledge to reduce the debt of twenty-two African countries by $19 billion in view of their 'sound economic policies and good governance'. When aggregated with other debt relief, this represents a reduction of around $30 billion, or two-thirds of African debt.

Though we should not expect the ensuing political process to be straightforward, even the possibility of the acceptance by some African countries of the western agenda offers medium- to long-term hope that the framework will yield some benefit. If it does, its impact on political corruption as against famine, AIDS and other more politically attractive targets is difficult to assess, albeit that failure to address it will inevitably impact severely on the achievement of these more obviously humanitarian goals. The idea that compliance can be secured only with a bigger carrot is, however, almost certainly correct; though without a commensurately bigger stick, however discreetly wielded, we should anticipate that increased rent-seeking by politicians, bureaucrats and businessmen will be the main outcome. If this occurs, neither the problems of Africa nor the problems Africa poses for the rest of the world will have moved towards resolution.

Of course whatever unfolds in Africa, even the improbable achievement of a state of pure liberalism on a global basis would not lead to the abolition of corruption and organized crime. On the contrary, we have stressed throughout that, like any fundamentally sound organization faced with a changed business environment, competent organized criminals will regroup and reform. Even with increasingly liberal legislation on drugs and prostitution there will always be products it is necessary to prohibit. Smuggling nuclear arms, succouring terrorists, springing prisoners, selling forged qualification certificates, violating intellectual property rights, dealing in stolen goods, propping up corrupt politicians and corrupting bankers and civil servants can never be legalized. In addition, new and currently unpredictable opportunities are always waiting to be found by enterprising businessmen. It is, however, reasonable to aim for a diminution in 'easy pickings' such that, by a principle of criminal Darwinism, a changing and where possible diminishing criminal market will force less efficient syndicates out of business, permitting more police time to be devoted to a smaller number of large operators. With stronger leverage attaching to debt rescheduling and new loan facilities it should also be possible to begin to reduce the number of hiding places available to such criminals. Making the targets more manageable may in turn lead to a higher probability of arrest, so enhancing the deterrent effect.

Political corruption as an interstitial activity

> Its [political corruption's] presence depends upon political and bureaucratic elites and power structures being intermeshed, upon politicians and party-politics intruding into the bureaucracy, upon the consequent availability of bureaucratic resources for party-political purposes, and upon an elite political culture that treats such deployment of bureaucratic resources as (at least unofficially) acceptable. Conversely, elimination of this sort of political corruption and the development of (in this sense) proper democratic procedures hinges upon a certain change in the political–bureaucratic rules of the game, upon the bureaucratic elites countervailing the power of political elites, upon bureaucratic structures gaining independence from the intrusion of politicians and party politics, and upon the consequent withdrawal of bureaucratic resources from the party-political contest.
>
> (Etzioni-Halevy 2002: 246)

The third limb of our theory is that political corruption is an interstitial activity. In the absence of mature, coherent or integrated bureau–political machinery, interstices between different parts of the machinery of state create conflicts and ambiguities exploited by corrupt politicians and officials. Where civil society is weak, corruption can appear in low standards of professional conduct and lack of safeguards for consumers; indeed the very notion of a consumer as a political entity with rights against providers is antithetical to a corrupt and centralized state. Naturally interstices of this kind are greater in high-corruption than in low-corruption countries. Cracks do not just appear, however, but are created and maintained, and the scope for entrepreneurial activity when, in particular, the legal and bureaucratic systems are subordinated to the political system, and when, within that system, the executive claims dominance over the legislature, is immense. Hence two of our four interstices – political–judicial and political–bureaucratic relationships – reflect this fact, while the further blurring of the interstice between politics and banking helps create the obfuscation which makes such banks attractive to international criminals. In the absence of constitutional checks and balances, some form of oligarchical tyranny is almost unavoidable.

These interstices make it difficult to distinguish the corrupt activities of politicians, bureaucrats, judicial officials and military leaders, obfuscation, secrecy and interdependence being the hallmarks of corruption networks. Equally it is difficult to distinguish corrupt politicians and bureaucrats from the corrupt businesspeople with whom they will come into contact during the contracting process and thereafter. These businesspeople, some of whom will have links with organized crime, will also serve as fixers or middlemen, conduits between domestic and international corruption, by facilitating the laundering of dirty money and effecting introductions to compliant bankers in tax havens around the world. During the economic liberalization process the power of the fixers may even be such as to enable them to seize substantial parts of the state by securing control of privatized industries. Hence, far from contributing to a liberal, open and competitive economy they prevent its emergence by creating new monopolies in the utilities or services they have bought.

Tackling corruption

> 98 . . . New arrivals in the Force are tested to see how strong is their sense of duty. The testing may take various forms – sums of money placed in their desks, etc. If an officer fails to report the first overture of this sort he is really 'hooked' for the rest of his service, and is afraid to report any corrupt activities which may thereafter come to his notice.
>
> 99 On a number of occasions during this inquiry I have been told that there is a saying in Hong Kong:
>
> 1   'Get on the bus,' i.e., if you wish to accept corruption, join us;
> 2   'Run alongside the bus,' i.e., if you do not wish to accept corruption, it matters not, but do not interfere;
> 3   'Never stand in front of the bus,' i.e., if you try to report corruption, the 'bus' will knock you down and you will be injured or even killed or your business will be ruined. We will get you, somehow.
>
> (Blair-Kerr 1973b)

In high-corruption countries the problem is how an institutionally corrupt political system which by definition lacks the capacity to reform itself is to be changed. In Chapter 3 we demonstrated the problems facing the Chinese economy, where the political structure lacks the internal dynamic necessary for self-reform. In Chapter 4 we showed how such a transformation occurred in nineteenth-century Britain through a conjunction of circumstances wherein non-corruption became in the interests of the ruling elite. The United Kingdom, it will be remembered, passed from high- to low-corruption in the first half of the nineteenth century, and a number of factors were associated with this. The main such factors were the striking social and economic changes at home stemming from industrialization and the frequent fear among the ruling elite of armed revolt. The transformations to the class system stemming from the collapse of agricultural land values and the emergence of a new and self-made bourgeoisie led the old aristocracy to make major concessions to avoid the *déluge* precipitated by the failure of their counterparts in France and elsewhere to make similar concessions. Meanwhile demographic changes led to electoral reform and the redundancy of the old methods of vote rigging. In central government the remarkable and happy attainment of a non-corrupt Civil Service created the framework for a polity in which, with few exceptions (of which local government was the most troubling and persistent), corruption could reasonably be considered as stemming from individual depredation, not structural flaw.

One possible problem with the British case study, however, is that the events which occurred seem to have been not so much engineered by reformers as historical facts which are not obviously replicable. On the other hand, it would be wrong to discount the possibility of a democratic movement in a state which is anyway strengthening its social structures having the capacity to scare its leaders into more radical reform than they intended. It is perfectly plausible to hypothesize that such a movement could at the very least speed up a process already underway, serving as a watchdog in the event of backtracking or deception; and that it might, indeed, be capable of more.

In contemporary politics, however, Hong Kong's Independent Commission Against Corruption (ICAC) is often cited as a case study in tackling corruption. Though it was indeed an important development we have mentioned it only in passing for three main reasons. *First*, it has been widely reported elsewhere;[8] *second*, its greatest triumphs have been against bureaucratic and private sector corruption rather than against political corruption per se;, and *third* its logic and structure are colonial, and hence no more replicable than the British case study. It is, however, relevant to this book in particular ways, and hence we outline aspects of it here.

The creation of ICAC was precipitated by the concern of a new Governor, Sir Murray MacLehose, at a specific corruption scandal in the Royal Hong Kong Police Force which involved a senior officer, Chief Superintendent Godber, fleeing to England to escape justice. This scandal had been detrimental to public confidence and had brought into political focus the extent of the systemic corruption operating within the Force, which had been tolerated for many years. The Governor appointed a judge, Sir Alastair Blair-Kerr, to investigate and make recommendations concerning improvements to existing anti-corruption arrangements. The Blair-Kerr Report (Blair-Kerr 1973a, b)[9] revealed sophisticated corruption syndicates operating throughout the Territory, involving not only the normal kick backs from illicit vice, gambling and licensing applications but straying into extortion of the public, intimidation of complainants and areas of internal organization including promotions. This latter finding was especially disturbing since the involvement of very senior officers showed the institutional nature of the corruption. Though Blair-Kerr stopped short of recommending a wholly independent investigative body, restricting himself to weighing the arguments on both sides, the Independent Commission Against Corruption (ICAC) was established only five months after publication of his Report. The Commission was indeed to be wholly independent of the Force with the first Head, Jack Cater, reporting directly to the Governor.

Though ICAC was never centrally concerned with political corruption, not a major problem in Hong Kong, in its context, organization and mandate it contains elements relevant to it. *First*, it was introduced as an external solution to a problem of institutional corruption which had proved internally insoluble. Previous Governors' attempts to create a credible anti-corruption unit with quasi-independent status within the Force had failed to bring corruption under control. Certainly the former Anti-Corruption Office's continued locus within the Force, which presented several subsidiary problems, contributed to these failures. Blair-Kerr reported on these problems, while giving varying weight to each. He noted that many members of the public were unwilling to report corruption to the police, whom they feared and did not trust, and that it had been claimed that the Force's *esprit de corps* might discourage officers from reporting on each other (though Blair-Kerr himself was unpersuaded about this). Certainly, however, information about the Office's inquiries periodically leaked to those under investigation, and officers also took their knowledge about anti-corruption procedures with them at the end of their secondments. Most tellingly, in relation to the Office's effectiveness Blair-Kerr wrote:

> I feel that this argument that the A.C. Office is 'ineffective' is simply a polite way of saying that the Office (as well as the Force) is corrupt from end to end and that one corrupt police officer will not diligently investigate alleged corruption on the part of another police officer – irrespective of the latter's rank.
>
> (Blair-Kerr 1973b: para 231.9)

Second, ICAC's formation was precipitated by extensive public clamour following the Godber case. More significant, however, may have been the fact that the legitimacy of colonial rule, already threatened by unprecedented popular demonstrations during the Cultural Revolution, was further shaken by the seemingly preferential treatment of expatriate officers.[10] Hence genuine concern mounted, both in Hong Kong and London, about the possibility of repetitions of the disorder of a few years earlier. *Third*, the Commission, being from the first divided into separate departments, Operations, Corruption Prevention and Community Relations, developed its strategy on three fronts. This tripartite approach was neatly encapsulated as 'raising the risk of being caught, restructuring government bureaucracies to reduce opportunities of corruption and changing people's attitudes about corruption' (Klitgaard 1988: 110). *Fourth*, the Commission was staffed by officers (including some imported from the United Kingdom) hand-picked by the Governor and given financially advantageous renewable short-term contracts, but liable to instant dismissal without stated cause. *Fifth*, the Commission was given draconian powers, including search without warrant, access to bank details, deployment of undercover agents in 'sting' operations, document seizure without prior notification, reporting restrictions and a reverse onus provision which required any civil servant in possession of undue wealth to prove honest acquisition. Between 1974 and 1977 proceedings were begun against 260 police officers, but the scale of police corruption became apparent in 1977 when a violent demonstration by 2,000 officers forced the Governor to concede an amnesty in respect of almost all corrupt acts investigated prior to that year.

Following the Bill of Rights Ordinance 1991, which in part reflected fears that a post-1997 government might act repressively, the more draconian provisions were reduced without loss of efficacy (Lo and Yu 2000). The Commission's structure and reporting line have thus far been unaffected by the retrocession to China (Moran 2000)[11] and the Commission is at pains to stress its close working relationship with China's People's Armed Police. Nonetheless it is clear that in criminal and civil matters affecting both China and the Hong Kong Special Administrative Region (SAR) the National People's Congress will claim interpretation rights. All in all, therefore, it would be surprising if ICAC were diverted away from the time-consuming task of investigating mainly private sector corruption in Hong Kong, and into addressing the alleged corrupt activities of Chinese officials in Hong Kong.

Moran outlines what are probably the two most awkward situations to have arisen thus far, though it might be added that what made them especially awkward was the fact that in both cases the weight of Hong Kong popular opinion was with the Chinese Government. *First*, in 1998 a jurisdictional dispute arose concerning the arrest, trial and execution in Guangdong Province of the flamboyant Hong Kong gangster Cheung Tze-keung, who liked to be known as 'The Big Spender'. Cheung's crimes, primarily committed in Hong Kong, included the (unreported) kidnapping of the son of the Hong Kong billionaire businessman and philanthropist Li Ka-shing, who was part of the Chinese leadership's *guanxi* network and who had paid a ransom for his son's release. The inference is that Li persuaded President Jiang to instruct Hong Kong's Chief Executive, Tung Chee-hwa, to ensure that Cheung and his numerous associates (the case was a complex multi-hander) were dealt with in China, where Cheung's conviction and speedy execution were certain. *Second*, in 1999, with the eventual support of Tung, the National People's Congress rejected the Hong Kong Court of Final Appeal's interpretation of a 'right of abode' provision in the Basic Law, claiming it was 'mistaken' – an impossible formulation for any political body where the rule of law was supreme. It seems clear in fact that drafters of the Basic Law, which gave the right of abode in Hong Kong to the offspring of Hong Kong citizens, had no idea of the numbers of PRC-domiciled potential claimants involved or how contentious status disputes could be. From Hong Kong's point of view the arrival of up to two million immigrants in a region with a population only slightly over six million could have put the SAR's economic, health and welfare provisions under intolerable strain. From the no less self-interested perspective of several thousand married Hong Kong men, the arrival of their illegitimate offspring from Mainland China, with or without their mistresses in tow, would have been a little embarrassing for them and quite a surprise for their wives. From China's political perspective the exercise of their 'right' by Chinese people would have meant that Chinese migration policy was being determined by the Hong Kong judiciary, an entirely unacceptable state of affairs.

Overall, an anti-corruption strategy conducted by a well-resourced, hand-picked, independent force unencumbered by any excessive regard for civil liberties, with full governmental backing, and which has successfully culti-vated and maintained widespread public support and involvement has a lot to be said for it. It is, however, only colonized states which have a *deus ex machina* in the form of a Governor able to produce such an organization; and maintaining such a body in a state lacking a mature society might be more than challenging. Nonetheless, negotiating to develop some such agency under international control would not be a foolish medium-term world objective for dealing with those aspects of debtor countries' cor-ruption which have international ramifications, such as money laundering, bribery and political involvement with organized crime. It would also consti-tute a logical extension of activities in international policing already under way. Of course no judicial body exists by which defendants can be tried internationally,[12] and the prospect of senior officials and politicians being tried by weak and corrupt judges in their own countries is not appealing. Nonetheless securing agreement to involve an independent element in the judicial process would be a plausible negotiating aim and might, indeed, be welcomed by the anti-corruption lobbying groups which, largely thanks to the global spread of Transparency International, now exist in many less-developed countries.

Afterword

> Philosophy comes too late to teach the world what it should be. When it paints its grey on grey, a form of life has already grown old, and in grey on grey it can never be made young again. The owl of Minerva takes its last flight when the shades of twilight have already fallen.
>
> (G.W.F. Hegel, Preface to *The Philosophy of Right*, 1821)

Klitgaard (1988) finishes his very readable book with practical tips; research-based works often end with topics for further study. This kind of book does not, however, so much promote change as reflect upon the changes occurring all around us, and is best seen as an attempt to broaden our understanding of corruption by setting it in the context of both day-to-day politics and international relations. Our philosophy, no more than Hegel's, can teach the world what it ought to be, or how to get there; and while, unlike Hegel, we make no claim to privileged access to the owl of Minerva, our task has been more analytic than predictive, more retrospective than prospective. While the book is not devoid of suggestions, those suggestions are, like the definition of corruption we adopted, better regarded as signposts indicating a general direction than as specific advice.

In a nutshell, small-scale corruption in low-corruption countries is to politics what fiddling one's expenses, making private phone calls from work or slipping home early is to private corporations. It exists, that is to say, rather low on a spectrum from shameful acts which would put one's future employment at risk down to semi-legitimate perks silently tolerated and which may even, by motivating staff, enhance productivity. Even where there is, theoretically, a clear line one should not cross – by no means always the case – when everybody does cross it the line changes its meaning. It then ceases to be a decisive prohibition, becoming instead a topic for light discussion and cheerful anecdote at dinner parties, and, more seriously, a touchstone for negotiating the space between right and wrong.

Heidenheimer's classic typology of black, white and grey corruption is relevant here. Black corruption is deemed bad both by the public and by political and bureaucratic elites (in Heidenheimer's paper this may vary in contrasting styles of community). White corruption, though wrong, is universally deemed to fall short of demanding sanction. Grey corruption, which one group but not the other considers serious, constitutes two sub-categories, containing acts repugnant to the people but not the elites and vice versa (Heidenheimer 1970b).

Of course where an absolute line does exist it is not without significance. In our analysis political corruption is best viewed not as Heidenheimer views it, on a scale of severity, but contingently. The seriousness of an act, that is to say, is dependent less on its intrinsic nature and character than on its political significance as judged by more powerful others – this is a dynamic not a static process. Hence it is perfectly possible for a politician's non-corrupt activity – an adulterous affair, say, or an act of betrayal – to carry more serious consequences than a minor incident of rent-seeking. Political significance may be judged on a range of criteria – who committed it, how close it is to an election, what impact the corruption is likely to have on party donations, what has been the press response, what the miscreants' colleagues are saying privately, what the fall-out from any given response is likely to be and so on. Clearly one is exposed to the risk of this judgement immediately one has crossed the line, for it is not only in high-corruption countries that attacks on corruption have more to do with politics than with justice. While some politicians consistently seem to get away with much more than others, the same politicians may be dealt with differently for the same crime committed at different times.

But if judging an act of political corruption is itself political, the question arises as to the proper role of law, or, rather, legal process – rational, consistent, transparent and appealable – in dealing with it. Here the introduction in the United Kingdom of the Parliamentary Commissioner for Standards is an interesting innovation. If our argument is correct it is necessary for the Commissioner, whose most difficult problems will almost all relate to grey corruption, to avoid being seen to respond to acts which concern the elites but not the general public, but to act in a manner commanding the support of both. Clearly if the system loses the confidence of those subject to its jurisdiction it will fall into desuetude; equally, if it comes to be popularly regarded as indifferent to the perceptions of voters and interest groups it will breed further cynicism, not only about politicians but about politics itself. In this sense even a legalistic response to a political act unavoidably contains political elements.

In high-corruption countries the situation is, naturally, much more difficult because the system lacks the necessary internal impetus for reform and there is no scope for whistle-blowing, independent investigation or the other trappings of democracy. This appears to be one situation (there may well be others) in which in the land of the blind the one-eyed man is decidedly not king. In such countries political corruption, certainly on the grand scale, is not a private or bounded matter, and the problem for others is whether, when, how and at what cost to tackle it. We have argued that a more sophisticated exploitation of the sticks and carrots associated with international aid and loans is a necessary though not sufficient act, and that defining the common ground necessary to achieving a partnership approach with recipient nations should remain a diplomatic priority.

Though the process of transition cannot be rushed, it can be helped along the way. Accordingly, possible signs emerging in 2003 of a potential agreement between donor and recipient countries seem, at least in the immediate aftermath of their appearance, to offer the possible promise of a future framework on which the donor–recipient relationship might be based. We should, however, remind ourselves what false dawns look like and proceed cautiously, and only with the most politically compliant and economically promising states; and we should certainly not permit ourselves to be deceived by United Nations' rhetoric into believing that the world will never be the same again. Too many intractable problems and too many vested interests perpetually encircle a political world in which the significant actors are not idealists from international organizations but hard-nosed realists, concerned, if they are not corrupt, to protect their country's interests, and, if they are, to defend their own rent-seeking opportunities.

Notes

1 Astonishingly, doctors, for all the tales of medical scandal and incompetence with which the papers regularly feed their readers, and in spite of the fact that the United Kingdom's highest-scoring mass murderer is himself a doctor, consistently enjoy an enviable degree of public confidence. For example, 91 per cent of respondents to a MORI poll conducted in February 2002 believe that doctors tell the truth against 6 per cent who believe they do not. The comparable figures for politicians, at 19 per cent against 73 per cent, are superior only to those for journalists (13 per cent against 79 per cent).

2 The fact that the parliamentary commissioner is appointed and can be removed by members of the body under investigation diminishes but does not eliminate the independence of the office. Hence while policy development was fully independent (albeit that, Parliament being a sovereign body, ratification was required), policy execution cannot be reasonably described as more than semi-independent.

3 Belgium, France, Germany, Luxembourg, the Netherlands, Portugal and Spain.

4 Though more recently the Court of Auditors put the figure at 5–8 per cent – still, however, a figure of some £3 billion a year.

5 The MEP charged with overseeing the Anti-Fraud Office (OLAF) set up by Commissioner Kinnock, claimed in 2002 that the department had always been too soft on fraud allegations, adding that OLAF had dealt with ninety-two cases of alleged fraud where there was evidence of criminal activity but had pursued only two prosecutions. In the same year Paul van Buitenen himself threatened the European Parliament with further publicity unless the Commission responded to a 235-page dossier of allegations (backed by 5,000 pages of documents) he had submitted to Commissioner Kinnock six months previously (White 2002).

6 The AU was formed out of the former Organization of African Unity in 2002. Its inaugural meeting was held in Durban in July of that year.

7 Algeria, Ethiopia, Gabon, Mali, Mozambique, Nigeria, Sao Tome and Principe, Senegal, South Africa, Egypt, Ghana, Tunisia, Rwanda, Tanzania and Tunisia.

8 Among numerous studies the following are especially helpful: Klitgaard (1988: Chapter 4); Lo (1993, 1999); Lee (1981); Lo and Yu (2000); Quah (2002). In addition the Blair-Kerr Report which led to the Commission's creation makes instructive reading (Blair-Kerr 1973a, b), while the Commission itself produces annual reports and has an informative website on ⟨http://www.icac.org.hk/⟩.

9 The First Report dealt with the Godber incident; the second, of more immediate relevance to us, with the functioning of the Prevention of Bribery Ordinance and making recommendations for reform.

10 Blair-Kerr recommended broadening the scope for disciplinary action against corrupt Government officials where the burden of proof was insufficient to justify criminal prosecution (Blair-Kerr 1973b: para 241 (e)).

11 At a formal level ICAC's continued independence is guaranteed for fifty years under the Basic Law.

12 The International Criminal Court tries only individuals accused of committing genocide, war crimes and crimes against humanity, and anyway does not enjoy universal recognition.

Bibliography

Adams, J. and Frantz, D. (1992) *A Full Service Bank: How BCCI Stole Billions Around the World.* New York: Pocket Books.

Agbese, P. (1998) 'Africa and the Dilemmas of Corruption'. In J. Mbaku *op. cit.*

Agnew, S. (1980) *Go Quietly . . . Or Else.* New York: Morrow.

Alatas, Syed Hussein (1990) *Corruption: Its Nature, Causes and Functions.* Aldershot: Avebury.

Altman, Y. (1989) 'Second Economy Activities in the USSR: Insights from the Southern Republics'. In Ward *op. cit.*

Anderson, A. (1979) *The Business of Organized Crime: A Cosa Nostra Family.* Stanford, CA: Hoover Foundation.

Anderson, A. (1995) 'Organised Crime, Mafia and Governments'. In Fiorentini and Peltzman *op. cit.*

Anderson, M. and den Boer, M. (eds) (1994) *Policing Across National Boundaries.* London: Pinter.

Anechiarico, F. and Jacobs, J. (1996) *The Pursuit of Absolute Integrity: How Corruption Control Makes Government Ineffective.* Chicago: University of Chicago Press.

Asad, A. and Harris, R. (2003) *The Politics and Economics of Drug Production on the Pakistan–Afghanistan Border.* Aldershot: Ashgate.

Baldwin, T. (2001) 'Creative Accountants Will Run Rings Round Paper Tiger'. *The Times.* 6 January.

Banfield, E. (1975) 'Corruption as a Feature of Governmental Organisation'. *Journal of Law and Economics.* 18: 587–605.

Bank for International Settlements (1988) *Basle Committee on Banking Regulations and Supervisory Practices – Prevention of Criminal Use of the Banking System for the Purpose of Money Laundering* (The Basel Statement of Principles). Basel: Bank for International Settlements.

Baran, Z. (2000) 'Corruption: The Turkish Challenge'. *Journal of International Affairs.* 54: 127–146.

Barnett, A. Doak (1964) *Communist China: The Early Years, 1949–1955.* London: Pall Mall Press.

Baston, L. (2000) *Sleaze: The State of Britain.* London: Channel 4 Books.

Baum, R. (1997) 'The Road to Tiananmen: Chinese Politics in the 1980s'. In MacFarquhar *op. cit.*

Baumol, W. (1990) 'Entrepreneurship: Productive, Unproductive, and Destructive'. *Journal of Political Economy.* 98: 893–921.

Baumol, W. (1995) 'Discussion'. In Fiorentini and Peltzman, *op. cit.*

Bayart, J.-F. (1999) 'The "Social Capital" or the Ruses of Political Intelligence of the Felonious State'. In Bayart, Ellis and Hibou *op. cit.*

Bayart, J.-F., Ellis, S. and Hibou, B. (eds) (1999) *The Criminalization of the State in Africa*. Oxford: James Currey.

Beare, M. (2000a) 'Russian (East European) Organized Crime Around the Globe'. Paper presented to the Transnational Crime Conference, Canberra, 9–10 March. ⟨http://www.yorku.ca/nathanson/nathanso.htm⟩.

Beare, M. (2000b) 'Structures, Strategies, and Tactics of Transnational Criminal Organizations: Critical Issues for Enforcement'. Paper presented to the Transnational Crime Conference, Canberra, 9–10 March. ⟨http://www.yorku.ca/nathanson/nathanso.htm⟩.

Beare, M. and Naylor, R. (1999) 'Major Issues Relating to Organized Crime within the Context of Economic Relationships'. Paper prepared for the Law Commission of Canada. York University, Ontario: Nathanson Centre for the Study of Organized Crime and Corruption

Becker, J. (1998) 'Testament to a Leader who Saved Millions'. *South China Morning Post*. 15 October.

Behan, T. (1996) *The Camorra*. London: Routledge.

Bentham, J. [1789] (1970) *Introduction to the Principles of Morals and Legislation*. Athlone: Athlone University Press.

Bhakti, I. (1998) 'Chronology of Events Leading to the Fall of President Soeharto'. In Forrester and May *op. cit.*

Bhargava, V. (1999) *Combating Corruption in the Philippines*. New York: World Bank.

Bicchieri, C. and Duffy, J. (1997) 'Corruption Cycles'. In Heywood *op. cit.*

Bigo, D. (2000) 'Liaison Officers in Europe: New Officers in the European Security Field'. In Sheptycki *op. cit.*

Bird, G. (1995) *IMF Lending to Developing Countries: Issues and Evidence*. London: Routledge.

Blair-Kerr, A. (1973a) *First Report of the Commission of Inquiry Under Sir Alastair Blair-Kerr*. Hong Kong: Government Printing Office.

Blair-Kerr, A. (1973b) *Second Report of the Commission of Inquiry Under Sir Alastair Blair-Kerr*. Hong Kong: Government Printing Office.

Blatt, J. (2000) 'County Chief Faces Quake Cash Charges'. *South China Morning Post*. 15 November.

Bosworth-Davies, R. and Saltmarsh, G. (1994) *Money Laundering: A Practical Guide to the New Legislation*. London: Chapman & Hall.

Boulton, D. (1978) *The Lockheed Papers*. London: Jonathan Cape.

Bowden, M. (2001) *Killing Pablo: The Hunt for the Richest, Most Powerful Criminal in History*. London: Atlantic Books.

Braithwaite, J. (1986) *Corporate Crime in the Pharmaceutical Industry*. London: Routledge & Kegan Paul.

Branford, S. and Kucinski, B. (1988) *The Debt Squads: The US, The Banks, and Latin America*. London: Zed Books.

Bretton, H. (1962) *Power and Stability in Nigeria*. New York: Praeger.

Brodeur, J.-P. (2000) 'Transnational Policing and Human Rights: A Case Study'. In Sheptycki *op. cit.*

Brugger, B. and Reglar, S. (1994) *Politics, Economy and Society in Contemporary China*. London: Macmillan.

van Buitenen, P. (2000) *Blowing the Whistle*. London: Politico's.

Bull, H. (1977) *The Anarchical Society: A Study of Order in World Politics*. New York: Columbia University Press.

Bureau for International Narcotics and Law Enforcement Affairs (1998) *International Narcotics Control Strategy Report, 1997*. Washington, DC: US Department of State.

Bureau for International Narcotics and Law Enforcement Affairs (2000) *International Narcotics Control Strategy Report, 1999*. Washington, DC: US Department of State.

Buscaglia, E. (1997) 'Corruption and Judicial Reform in Latin America'. *Policy Studies Journal*. 17: 273–295.

Buscaglia, E. (n.d.) 'Judicial Corruption in Developing Countries: Its Causes and Economic Consequences'. ⟨http://www.hoover.stanford.edu/publications/epp/95/95a.html⟩ *Essays in Public Policy*. Stanford, CA: Hoover Institution.

Cadot, O. (1987) 'Corruption as a Gamble'. *Journal of Public Economics*. 33: 223–244.

Caiden, G. and Caiden, N. (1977) 'Administrative Corruption'. *Public Administration Review*. 37: 301–309.

Campbell, H. (2001) 'Politics is at Root of Violence'. *Evening Standard* (London). 12 July.

Caputo, D. (1976) 'Organized Crime and American Politics'. In Ianni and Reuss-Ianni *op. cit.*

Carbonell-Catilo, A. (1986) 'The Philippines: The Politics of Plunder'. *Corruption and Reform*. 1: 235–243.

Cartier-Bresson, J. (1997) 'Corruption Networks, Transaction Security and Illegal Social Exchange'. In Heywood *op. cit.*

Catanzaro, R. (1992) *Men of Respect: A Social History of the Sicilian Mafia*. New York: The Free Press.

Cavender, G., Jurik, N. and Cohen, A.K. (1993) 'The Baffling Case of the Smoking Gun: The Social Ecology of Political Accounts in the Iran–Contra Affair'. *Social Problems*. 40: 152–166.

Cheung, S.N.S. (1996) 'A Simplistic General Equilibrium Theory of Corruption'. *Contemporary Economic Policy*. 14: 1–5.

Chu, Y.-K. (1994) 'The Triad Threat to Europe'. *Policing*. 10: 205–215.

Chu, Y.-K. (1996) 'International Triad Movements: The Threat of Chinese Organised Crime'. *Conflict Studies*. July/August.

Chubb, J. (1982) *Patronage, Power and Poverty in Southern Italy: A Tale of Two Cities*. Cambridge: Cambridge University Press.

Clarke, M. (ed.) (1983) *Corruption: Causes, Consequences and Control*. London: Frances Pinter.

Clarke, T. and Tigue, J., Jr. (1976) *Dirty Money: Swiss Banks, the Mafia, and White Collar Crime*. London: Millington Books.

Cohen, R. and Deng, F. (1998) *Masses in Flight: The Global Crisis of Internal Displacement*. Washington, DC: Brookings Institution Press.

Committee on the Civil Service (1968) *The Civil Service*. (The Fulton Report) Cmnd 3638. London: Her Majesty's Stationery Office.

Conachy, J. (2000) 'Thousands of Officials Punished in China's Anti-Corruption Purge'. World Socialist Website. ⟨www.wsws.org/articles/2000/feb2000/chin-f01.shtml⟩.

Conner, A. (2000) 'True Confessions? Chinese Confessions Then and Now'. In Turner, Feinerman and Guy *op. cit.*

Copher, P. (1997) 'Instant Analysis'. *Environmental News Network*. 24 February.

Coronel, S. (ed.) (1998) *Pork and Other Perks: Corruption and Governance in the Philippines*. Manila: Philippine Center for Investigative Journalism.

Council of Europe (1990) *Convention on Laundering, Search, Seizure and Confiscation of the Proceeds from Crime*. ETS No. 141. Strasbourg: Council of Europe.

Council of Europe (1996) 'Council of Europe's Fight against Corruption and Organised Crime: Working Group on Civil Law Matters (GMCC) of the Multi-disciplinary Group on Corruption (GMC)' ⟨http://www.coe.fr/corruption/eetudeb.htm⟩.

Council of Europe (1998) *Corruption in Public Procurement*. Proceedings of the 2nd European Conference of Specialised Services in the Fight against Corruption held at Tallinn (Estonia) 27–29 October 1997. Strasbourg: Council of Europe Publishing.

Council of the European Communities (1991a) *Council Directive on Prevention of the Use of the Financial System for the Purpose of Money Laundering*. (91/308/EEC). Brussels: Council of the European Communities.

Council of the European Communities (1991b) *Proposal for a European Parliament and Council Directive Amending Council Directive 91/308/EEC of 10 June 1991 on Prevention of the Use of the Financial System for the Purpose of Money Laundering*. Brussels: Council of the European Communities.

Curl, J. (1986) *The Londonderry Plantation, 1609–1914: The History, Architecture and Planning of the Estates of the City of London and its Livery Companies in Ulster*. Chichester: Phillimore.

Curl, J. (2000) *The Honourable the Irish Society and the Plantation of Ulster, 1608–2000: The City of London and the Colonization of County Londonderry: A History and Critique*. Chichester: Phillimore.

Cusimano, M. (ed.) (2000a) *Beyond Sovereignty: Issues for a Global Agenda*. Boston, MA: Bedford/St Martin's.

Cusimano, M. (2000b) 'Beyond Sovereignty: The Rise of Transsovereign Problems'. In Cusimano *op. cit.*

Cusimano, M. (2000c) 'Nuclear Smuggling'. In Cusimano *op. cit.*

Daily Sun (Hong Kong) (2002) 'PLA Declares Emergence of *Guanxi* Soldiers'. 23 February.

Danaher, K. (ed.) (1994) *Fifty Years is Enough: A Case Against the World Bank and the International Monetary Fund*. Boston, MA: South End Press.

Das, S. (2001) *Public Office, Private Interest: Bureaucracy and Corruption in India*. New Delhi: Oxford University Press.

della Porta, D. (1998) 'A Judges' Revolution? Political Corruption and the Judiciary in Italy'. Paper delivered to the European Consortium for Political Research. Warwick, March.

della Porta, D. and Pizzorno, A. (1996) 'The Business Politicians: Reflections from a Study of Political Corruption'. *Journal of Law and Society*. 23: 73–94.

della Porta, D. and Vannucci, A. (1997) 'The "Perverse Effects" of Political Corruption'. In Heywood *op. cit.*

della Porta, D. and Vannucci, A. (1999) *Corrupt Exchanges: Actors, Resources and Mechanisms of Political Corruption*. New York: Aldine de Gruyter.

Doig, A. (1983) '"You Publish at your Peril!" The Restraints on Investigatory Journalism'. In Clarke *op. cit.*

Doig, A. (1984) *Corruption and Misconduct in Contemporary British Politics.* Harmondsworth: Penguin Books.

Doig, A. (1996) 'From Lynskey to Nolan: The Corruption of British Politics and Public Service'. In Levi and Nelken *op. cit.*

Doig, A. and Theobald, R. (eds) (2000) *Corruption and Democratization.* London: Frank Cass.

Donovan, M. (1994) 'Political Corruption in Italy'. In Heywood, Donovan and Boswell *op. cit.*

Downs, A. (1957) *An Economic Theory of Democracy.* New York: Harper & Row.

Dynes, M. (2000) 'Nigeria May Be Under New Management, But It Is Still Paying for Decades of Corruption'. *The Times.* 4 March.

Efficiency Unit (1988) *Improving Management in Government: The Next Steps.* London: Her Majesty's Stationery Office.

Egmont Group of Financial Intelligence Units (1997) *Statement of Purpose.* Madrid: Egmont Group.

Emery, F. (1994) *Watergate: The Corruption and Fall of Richard Nixon.* London: Jonathan Cape.

Etzioni-Halevy, E. (2002) 'Exchanging Material Benefits for Political Support: A Comparative Analysis'. In Heidenheimer and Johnston *op. cit.*

Ewing, K. (2001) 'Corruption in Party Financing: The Case for Global Standards'. *Global Corruption Report 2001.* Berlin: Transparency International.

Fan, S. and Grossman, H. (2001) 'Incentives and Corruption in Chinese Economic Reform'. *Journal of Policy Reform.* 4: 195–206.

Feinerman, J. (2000) 'The Rule of Law Imposed from Outside: China's Foreign-Oriented Legal Regime Since 1978'. In Turner, Feinerman and Guy *op. cit.*

Fennell, P. (1983) 'Local Government Corruption in England and Wales'. In Clarke *op. cit.*

Fewsmith, J. (1997) 'Reaction, Resurgence and Recession: Chinese Politics Since Tiananmen'. In MacFarquhar *op. cit.*

Fijnaut, C. (ed.) (1993) *The Internationalization of Police Co-operation in Western Europe.* Deventer: Kluwer.

Findlay, M. (1999) *The Globalisation of Crime: Understanding Transitional Relationships in Context.* Cambridge: Cambridge University Press.

Fiorentini, G. and Peltzman, S. (eds) (1995) *The Economics of Organized Crime.* Cambridge: Cambridge University Press.

Flynn, S. (2000) 'The Global Drug Trade versus the Nation-State: Why the Thugs are Winning'. In Cusimano *op. cit.*

Fong, T.-H. (2002) 'Law to Root Out the Corrupt and Unfit who Sit in Judgment'. *South China Morning Post.* 2 January.

Forrester, G. and May, R. (eds) (1998) *The Fall of Soeharto.* Bathurst, NSW: Crawford House.

Fu, F. (ed.) (2001) *The Development of Social Sciences in the 21st Century.* Hong Kong: Faculty of Social Sciences, Hong Kong Baptist University.

Gallant, T. (1999) 'Brigandage, Piracy, Capitalism, and State-Formation: Transnational Crime from a Historical World-Systems Perspective'. In Heyman *op. cit.*

Gambetta, D. (1993) *The Sicilian Mafia: The Business of Protection.* Cambridge, MA: Harvard University Press.

Gambetta, D. and Reuter, P. (1995) 'Conspiracy Among the Many: The Mafia in Legitimate Industries'. In Fiorentini and Peltzman *op. cit.*

George, S. (1988) *A Fate Worse than Debt*. Harmondsworth: Penguin Books.

Gillard, M. (1974) *A Little Pot of Money*. London: *Private Eye* and Andre Deutsch.

Ginsborg, P. (2001) *Italy and Its Discontents, 1980–2001*. Harmondsworth: Penguin Books.

Goldstein, J. (2001) *International Relations*. 4th edn. New York: Longman.

Goldsworthy, C. (2001) *The Satyr: An Account of the Life and Work, Death and Salvation of John Wilmot, Second Earl of Rochester*. London: Weidenfeld & Nicolson.

Goldthorpe, J.E. (1975) *The Sociology of the Third World: Disparity and Involvement*. Cambridge: Cambridge University Press.

Gong, T. (1994) *The Politics of Corruption in Contemporary China: An Analysis of Policy Outcomes*. Westport, CT: Praeger.

Grossman, H. (1995) 'Rival Kleptocrats: The Mafia versus the State'. In Fiorentini and Peltzman *op. cit.*

Hall, D. and Ames, T. (1999) *The Democracy of the Dead: Dewey, Confucius, and the Hope for Democracy in China*. Chicago, IL: Open Court.

Hao, Y. (1999) 'From Rule of Man to Rule of Law: An Unintended Consequence of Corruption in China in the 1990s'. *Journal of Contemporary China*. 8: 405–423.

Hao, Y. and Johnston, M. (2002) 'Corruption and the Future of Economic Reform in China'. In Heidenheimer and Johnston *op. cit.*

Harding, H. (1997) 'The Chinese State in Crisis, 1966–9'. In MacFarquhar *op. cit.*

Harling, P. (1996) *The Waning of 'Old Corruption': The Politics of Economical Reform in Britain, 1779–1846*. Oxford: The Clarendon Press.

Harris, R. (2003) 'Social Welfare Policy'. In M. Kogan and M. Hawkesworth (eds) *The Routledge Encyclopaedia of Government and Politics*. 2nd edn. London: Routledge.

Hauri, K. (2000) 'Transnational Commercial Bribery and Corruption: A Challenge for the Financial Industry, Regulators and Supervisors'. Speech delivered to the 11th International Conference of Banking Supervisors, Basel, September.

Heidenheimer, A. (ed.) (1970a) *Political Corruption: Readings in Comparative Analysis*. New York: Holt, Rinehart & Winston.

Heidenheimer, A. (1970b) 'Perspectives on the Perception of Corruption'. In Heidenheimer *op. cit.* Reprinted in Heidenheimer and Johnston *op. cit.*

Heidenheimer, A. and Johnston, M. (eds) (2002) *Political Corruption: Concepts and Contexts*. 3rd edn. New Brunswick, NJ: Transaction.

Heidenheimer, A., Johnston, M. and LeVine, V. (eds) (1989) *Political Corruption: A Handbook*. 2nd edn. New Brunswick, NJ: Transaction.

Heilbuth, P. and Bülow, H. (1997) 'Corruption as a Lifestyle – a Ghost Passes Through Africa'. ⟨http://www.dr.dk/afrika/english/baggrund/hkor.htm⟩.

Held, D. (1991) 'Democracy and the Global System'. In Held, D. (ed.) *Political Theory Today*. Cambridge: Polity Press.

Heyman, J. (ed.) (1999) *States and Illegal Practices*. Oxford: Berg.

Heyman, J. and Smart, A. (1999) 'States and Illegal Practices: An Overview'. In Heyman *op. cit.*

Heymans, C. and Lipietz, B. (1999) *Corruption and Development: Some Perspectives*. ISS Monograph Series. No 40. Pretoria: Institute for Security Studies.

Heywood, P. (1994) 'Political Corruption in Modern Spain'. In Heywood, Donovan and Boswell *op. cit.*

Heywood, P. (ed.) (1997) *Political Corruption*. Oxford: Blackwell for the PSA.

Heywood, P., Donovan, M. and Boswell, D. (eds) (1994) *Distorting Democracy: Political Corruption in Spain, Italy, and Malta*. Bristol: Centre for Mediterranean Studies, University of Bristol. CMS Occasional Paper 10.

Hibou, B. (1999) 'The "Social Capital" of the State as an Agent of Deception or the Ruses of Economic Intelligence'. In Bayard, Ellis and Hibou *op.cit.*

Hill, H. (1998) 'The Indonesian Economy: The Strange and Sudden Death of a Tiger'. In Forrester and May *op. cit.*

Hillman, A. and Katz, E. (1987) 'Hierarchical Structure and the Social Costs of Bribes and Transfers'. *Journal of Public Economics*. 34: 129–142.

Hillman, A. and Schnytzer, A. (1986) 'Illegal Economic Activities and Purges in a Soviet-type Economy: A Rent-seeking Perspective'. *International Review of Law and Economics*. 6: 87–99.

Hilton, A. (2000) 'Laundry Rules Could Take Firms to Cleaners'. *Evening Standard* (London). 23 June.

Hilton, A. (2001) 'Laundry Service'. *Evening Standard* (London). 31 May.

Hinton, W. (1990) *The Great Reversal: The Privatization of China*. New York: Monthly Review Press.

Hope, K. (1987) 'Administrative Corruption and Administrative Reform in Developing States'. *Corruption and Reform*. 2: 127–147.

Hopkin, J. (1997) 'Political Parties, Political Corruption and the Economic Theory of Democracy'. *Crime, Law and Social Change*. 27: 255–274.

Hua, G.-F. (1977) 'Political Report to the Eleventh National Congress of the Communist Party of China'. In *The Eleventh National Congress of the Communist Party of China*. Beijing: Foreign Languages Press.

Humphrey, C. (1999) 'Russian Protection Rackets and the Appropriation of Law and Order'. In Heyman *op. cit.*

Huntington, S. (1968) *Political Order in Changing Societies*. New Haven, CT: Yale University Press.

Hurstfield, J. (1973) *Freedom, Corruption and Government in Elizabethan England*. London: Jonathan Cape.

Hutchcroft, P. (1998) *Booty Capitalism: The Politics of Banking in the Philippines*. Ithaca, NY: Cornell University Press.

Hutton, W. (1995) *The State We're In*. London: Jonathan Cape.

Ianni, F. and Reuss-Ianni, E. (eds) (1976) *The Crime Society: Organized Crime and Corruption in America*. New York: New American Library.

International Monetary Fund (2000) *Globalization: Threat or Opportunity?* IMF Issues Brief. Washington, DC: IMF.

International Monetary Fund (2001a) *A Brief Guide to Committees, Groups, and Clubs*. IMF Factsheet. Washington, DC: IMF.

International Monetary Fund (2001b) *Social Dimensions of the IMF's Policy Dialogue*. IMF Factsheet. Washington, DC: IMF.

International Monetary Fund (2001c) *Debt Relief for Poor Countries (HIPC): What Has Been Achieved?* IMF Factsheet. Washington, DC: IMF.

Johansen, E. (1990) *Political Corruption: Scope and Resources: An Annotated Bibliography*. New York: Garland.

Johnston, L. (2000) 'Transnational Private Policing: The Impact of Global Commercial Security'. In Sheptycki *op. cit.*

Johnston, M. (1993) 'Social Development as an Anti-Corruption Strategy'. Paper delivered to the VI International Anti-Corruption Conference, Cancun, Quintana Roo, Mexico, November.

Johnston, M. and Hao, Y. (1995) 'China's Surge of Corruption: Delayed Political Development, Markets, and Democratic Reform'. *Journal of Democracy*. 6: 80–94.

Kameir, E.-W. and Kursany, I. (1985) *Corruption as a 'Fifth' Factor of Production in the Sudan*. Uppsala: The Scandinavian Institute of African Studies.

Kane, H. (2000) 'Leaving Home: The Flow of Refugees'. In Cusimano *op. cit.*

Kang, D. (2002) *Crony Capitalism: Corruption and Development in South Korea and the Philippines*. Cambridge: Cambridge University Press.

Kefauver, E. (1952) *Crime in America*. London: Victor Gollancz.

van Kemenade, W. (1997) *China, Hong Kong, Taiwan, Inc.* New York: Knopf.

Keohane, R. and Nye, J. (1989) *Power and Interdependence*. 2nd edn. New York: HarperCollins.

Killick, T. (1995) *IMF Programmes in Developing Countries: Design and Impact*. London: Routledge.

van Klaveren, J. (1989) 'The Concept of Corruption'. In Heidenheimer, Johnston, and LeVine *op. cit.*

Klitgaard, R. (1988) *Controlling Corruption*. Berkeley, CA: University of California Press.

Klitgaard, R. (1991) *Adjusting to Reality: Beyond State versus Market in Economic Development*. San Francisco: ICS Press.

Klitgaard, R., MacLean-Abaroa, R. and Parris, H. (2000) *Corrupt Cities: A Practical Guide to Cure and Prevention*. Oakland, CA: ICS Press.

Korkhet, C. (1995) 'Special Army Force Tightens Noose on Khun Sa's Empire'. *The Nation* (Bangkok). 13 January.

Korner, P., Maass, G., Siebold, T. and Tetzlaff, R. (1986) *The IMF and the Debt Crisis: A Guide to the Third World's Dilemma*. Translated by P. Knight. London: Zed Books.

Kpundeh, S. (2002) 'The Institutional Framework for Corruption Control in Uganda'. In Heidenheimer and Johnston *op. cit.*

Kraar, L. (2000) 'The Corrupt Archipelago'. *Fortune*. 24 July. 200–204.

Krueger, J. (1974) 'The Political Economy of the Rent Seeking Society'. *The American Economic Review*. 64: 291–303.

Kwong, J. (1997) *The Political Economy of Corruption in China*. Armonk, NY: ME Sharpe.

Lancaster, T. and Montinola, G. (1997) 'Toward a Methodology for the Comparative Study of Political Corruption'. *Crime, Law & Social Change*. 27: 185–206.

LaPalombara, J. (1994) 'Structural and Institutional Aspects of Corruption'. *Social Research*. 61: 325–351.

Lau, C.-C. and Lee, R. (1978) *Bureaucratic Corruption in Nineteenth-Century China*. Occasional Paper No. 79. Hong Kong: Social Research Centre, Chinese University of Hong Kong.

Lawrance, A. (1998) *China under Communism*. London: Routledge.

Lawrence, S. (2000) 'A City Ruled by Crime'. *Far Eastern Economic Review*. November.

Lee, R. (1981) (ed.) *Corruption and its Control in Hong Kong*. Hong Kong: Chinese University Press.

Lee, R. and Ford, J. (2000) 'Nuclear Smuggling'. In Cusimano *op. cit.*

Leigh, D. (1993) *Betrayed: The Real Story of the Matrix Churchill Trial*. London: Bloomsbury.

Leiken, R. (1996) 'Controlling the Global Corruption Epidemic'. *Foreign Policy*. 5: 55–73.

Leonard, J. (2001) 'The Myth of the Qing State'. In Fu *op. cit.*

Levi, M. (1996) 'Equal Before the Law? Politics, Powers and Justice in Serious Fraud Prosecutions'. *Crime, Law and Social Change*. 24: 319–340.

Levi, M. and Nelken, D. (eds) (1996a) *The Corruption of Politics and the Politics of Corruption. Journal of Law and Society*. 23: 1. Special Issue.

Levi, M. and Nelken, D. (1996b) 'The Corruption of Politics and the Politics of Corruption: An Overview'. In Levi and Nelken *op. cit.*

Lieberthal, K. (1997) 'The Great Leap Forward and the Split in the Yan'an Leadership 1958–65'. In MacFarquhar *op. cit.*

Lloyd, H. (1975) 'Corruption and Sir John Trevor'. *Transactions of the Honourable Society of Cymmrodorion*. 77–102.

Lo, T.W. (1993) *Corruption and Politics in Hong Kong and China*. Buckingham: Open University Press.

Lo, T.W. (1999) 'The Political–Criminal Nexus: The Hong Kong Experience'. *Trends in Organized Crime*. Spring: 60–80.

Lo, T.W. and Yu, R. (2000) 'Curbing Draconian Powers: The Effects on Hong Kong's Graft-Fighter'. *International Journal of Human Rights*. 4: 54–73.

Lodge, T. (2002) 'Political Corruption in South Africa: From Apartheid to Multiracial State'. In Heidenheimer and Johnston *op. cit.*

Loescher, G. (1993) *Beyond Charity*. Oxford: Oxford University Press.

Loughlin, M. (1992) *Administrative Accountability in Local Government*. York: Joseph Rowntree Foundation.

Low, V. (2001) 'Political Sleaze: Lloyd George Knew How to Go Further'. *Evening Standard* (London). 30 January.

Lui, F. (1986) 'A Dynamic Model of Corruption Deterrence'. *Journal of Public Economics*. 31: 215–236.

Lupsha, P. (1996) 'Transnational Organized Crime Versus the Nation-State'. *Transnational Organized Crime*. 2: 21–48.

McCoy, A. (1991) *The Politics of Heroin: CIA Complicity in the Global Drug Trade*. New York: Lawrence Hill.

McCoy, A. (1999) 'Requiem for a Drug Lord: State and Commodity in the Career of Khun Sa'. In Heyman *op. cit.*

McCoy, A. and Block, A. (eds) (1992) *War on Drugs*. Boulder, CO: Westview Press.

MacDougall, T. (1988) 'The Lockheed Scandal and the High Costs of Politics in Japan'. In Markovits and Silverstein *op. cit.*

MacFarquhar, R. (ed.) (1997) *The Politics of China: The Eras of Mao and Deng*. 2nd edn. Cambridge: Cambridge University Press.

MacFarquhar, R. (1997b) 'The Succession to Mao and the End of Maoism, 1969–82'. In MacFarquhar *op. cit.*

Manning, P. (2000) 'Policing New Social Spaces'. In Sheptycki *op. cit.*

Markovits, A. and Silverstein, M. (eds) (1988) *The Politics of Scandal: Power and Process in Liberal Democracy*. New York: Holmes and Meier.

Masud-Piloto, F. (1996) *From Welcomed Exiles to Illegal Immigrants: Cuban Migration to the U.S., 1959–1995*. Lanham, MD: Rowman & Littlefield.

Maudling, R. (1978) *Memoirs*. London: Sidgwick & Jackson.

Mauro, P. (1995) 'Corruption and Growth'. *Quarterly Journal of Economics.* 110: 681–711.

Mbaku, J. (ed.) (1998) *Corruption and the Crisis of Institutional Reforms in Africa.* Lewiston, NY: The Edwin Mellen Press.

Merrill, T. (1993) *Nicaragua: A Country Study.* Washington, DC: Federal Research Division, Library of Congress. ⟨http://lcweb2.loc.gov/frd/cs/nitoc.html⟩.

Mohan, C. (1996) 'Countermeasures to the Abuse of Power and Corruption: Some Lessons from Singapore'. In UNAFEI *op. cit.*

Moran, J. (2000) 'The Changing Context of Corruption Control: The Hong Kong Special Administrative Region, 1997–99'. In Doig and Theobald *op. cit.*

Morris, N. and Hawkins, G. (1970) *The Honest Politician's Guide to Crime Control.* Chicago: Chicago University Press.

Mosley, P., Harrigan, J. and Toye, J. (1991) *Aid and Power: The World Bank and Policy-Based Lending.* Volume 1: *Analysis and Policy Proposals.* London: Routledge.

Murphy, K., Shleifer, A. and Vishny, R. (1991) 'The Allocation of Talent: Implications for Growth'. *Quarterly Journal of Economics.* 106: 503–530.

Myrdal, G. (1968) *Asian Drama: An Inquiry into the Poverty of Nations.* Volume II. New York: Pantheon.

Nadelmann, E. (1993) *Cops Across Borders: The Internationalization of US Criminal Law.* University Park, PA: Pennsylvania State University Press.

Narayan, K. (1989) *Storytellers, Saints, and Scoundrels.* Philadelphia: University of Pennsylvania Press.

Naylor, R. (1999) 'Follow-the-Money Methods in Crime Control Policy'. A study prepared for the Nathanson Centre for the Study of Organized Crime and Corruption, York University, Toronto. ⟨http://www.yorku.ca/nathanson/nathanso.htm⟩.

Neild, R. (2001) 'Scandals as Evidence of Corruption'. Paper presented to the conference Political Scandals Past and Present. University of Salford, 21–23 June.

Neill, P. (1998) (Chairman) *The Funding of Political Parties in the United Kingdom.* Fifth Report of the Committee on Standards in Public Life. 2 volumes. London: Her Majesty's Stationery Office.

Nelken, D. (ed.) (1994) *The Futures of Criminology.* London: Sage.

Nelken, D. (1996) 'The Judges and Political Corruption in Italy'. In Levi and Nelken *op. cit.*

Neville, D. (1999) 'State and Shadow State in Northern Peru circa 1900: Illegal Political Networks and the Problem of State Boundaries'. In Heyman *op. cit.*

Nolan, Lord (1995) (Chairman) *Conduct in Public Life.* First Report of the Committee on Standards in Public Life. 2 volumes. London: Her Majesty's Stationery Office.

Northcote, S. and Trevelyan, C. (1854) *Report on the Organization of the Permanent Civil Service.* London. Parliamentary Papers XXVII.

Nye, J. (1967) 'Corruption and Political Development: A Cost–Benefit Analysis'. *American Political Science Review.* 61: 417–427. Reprinted in Heidenheimer and Johnston *op. cit.*

Ocko, J. (2000) 'Using the Past to Make a Case for the Rule of Law'. In Turner, Feinerman and Guy *op. cit.*

Oliver, D. (1997) 'Regulating the Conduct of MPs. The British Experience of Combating Corruption'. In Heywood *op. cit.*

Olson, M. (1965) *The Logic of Collective Action.* Cambridge, MA: Harvard University Press.

Olson, M. (1982) *The Rise and Decline of Nations: Economic Growth, Stagflation, and Social Rigidities*. New Haven, CT: Yale University Press.

O'Neill, M. (2000) 'Illegal Fines Paid for Prosecutor's Lavish Offices'. *South China Morning Post*. 4 December.

Padhy, K.S. (1986) *Corruption in Politics (A Case Study)*. Delhi: BR Publishing Corporation.

Palmier, L. (1985) *The Control of Bureaucratic Corruption: Case Studies in Asia*. New Delhi: Allied Publishers Private Ltd.

Passas, N. (1993) 'Structural Sources of International Crime: Policy Lessons from the BCCI Affair'. *Crime, Law and Social Change*. 20: 293–309.

Pastor, M., Jr. (1987) 'The Effects of IMF Programs in the Third World: Debate and Evidence from Latin America'. *World Development*. 15: 249–262.

Pasuk, P. and Sungsidh, P. (1994) *Corruption and Democracy in Thailand*. Bangkok: Political Economy Centre, Chulalongkorn University.

Pavarini, M. (1994) 'Is Criminology Worth Saving?' In Nelken *op. cit.*

Payer, C. (1974) *The Debt Trap: The IMF and the Third World*. London: Monthly Review Press.

Pedrosa, C. (1987) *Imelda Marcos: The Rise and Fall of One of the World's Most Powerful Women*. New York: St. Martin's Press.

Peters, J. and Welch, S. (1978) 'Political Corruption in America. A Search for Definitions and a Theory. Or if Political Corruption Is in the Mainstream of American Politics, Why Is It Not in the Mainstream of American Politics Research?' *American Political Science Review*. 72: 974–984.

Peterson, J. (1997) 'The European Union: Pooled Sovereignty, Divided Accountability'. In Heywood *op. cit.*

Philp, M. (2002) 'Conceptualizing Political Corruption'. In Heidenheimer and Johnston *op. cit.*

President's Commission on Law Enforcement and the Administration of Justice (1967) *Task Force Report: Organized Crime*. Washington, DC: US Government Printing Office.

Pyper, R. (1995) *The British Civil Service*. Hemel Hempstead: Prentice Hall/Harvester Wheatsheaf.

Quah, J. (1999) 'Corruption in Asian Countries: Can It Be Minimized?' *Public Administration Review*. 59: 483–495.

Quah, J. (2002) 'Responses to Corruption in Asian Societies'. In Heidenheimer and Johnston *op. cit.*

Redcliffe-Maud, Lord (1974) (Chairman) *Conduct in Local Government: Report of the Prime Minister's Committee on Local Government Rules of Conduct*. 2 volumes. London: Her Majesty's Stationery Office.

Reuter, P. (1983) *Disorganized Crime: The Economics of the Invisible Hand*. Cambridge, MA: MIT Press.

Riddell, P. (2000) *Parliament Under Blair*. London: Politico's.

Riley, S. (1983) '"The Land of Waving Palms": Political Economy, Corruption Inquiries and Politics in Sierra Leone'. In Clarke *op. cit.*

Rogow, A. and Lasswell, H. (1963) *Power, Corruption and Rectitude*. Englewood Cliffs, NJ: Prentice-Hall.

Rose-Ackerman, S. (1975) 'The Economics of Corruption'. *Journal of Public Economics*. 4: 187–203.

Rose-Ackerman, S. (1978) *Corruption: A Study in Political Economy*. New York: Academic Press.

Rose-Ackerman, S. (1999) *Corruption and Government: Causes, Consequences, and Reform*. Cambridge: Cambridge University Press.

Rosenthal, E. (2000) 'China's Fierce War on Smuggling Uproots a Vast Hidden Economy'. *New York Times*. 6 March.

Saich, T. (1981) *China: Politics and Government*. London: Macmillan.

Salerno, R. and Tompkins, J. (1976) 'Protecting Organized Crime.' In Ianni and Reuss-Ianni *op. cit.*

Salmon, Lord (Chairman) (1976) *Report of the Royal Commission on Standards of Conduct in Public Life, 1974–1976*. Cmnd 6524. London: Her Majesty's Stationery Office.

Schneider, J. and Schneider, P. (1994) 'Mafia, Antimafia and the Question of Sicilian Culture'. *Politics and Society*. 22: 237–258.

Schneider, J. and Schneider, P. (1999) 'Is Transparency Possible? The Political–Economic and Epistemological Implications of Cold War Conspiracies and Subterfuge in Italy'. In Heyman *op. cit.*

Schneider, S., Beare, M. and Hill, J. (2000) 'Alternative Approaches to Combating Transnational Crime'. A report prepared for the Federal Transnational Crime Working Group. York, Ontario: Nathanson Centre for the Study of Organized Crime and Corruption.

Schram, S. (1966) *Mao Tse-Tung*. Harmondsworth: Penguin Books.

Scott, J.C. (1972) *Comparative Political Corruption*. Englewood Cliffs, NJ: Prentice-Hall.

Scott, Sir Richard (Chairman) (1996) *Report of the Inquiry into the Export of Defence Equipment and Dual-Use Goods to Iraq and Related Prosecutions*. (The Scott Report). London: Her Majesty's Stationery Office.

Searle, G. (1987) *Corruption in British Politics 1895–1930*. Oxford: The Clarendon Press.

Shelley, L. (1990) 'The Internationalization of Crime: The Changing Relationship Between Crime and Development'. In Zvekic *op. cit.*

Shelley, L. (1994) 'Post-Soviet Organized Crime: Implications for Economic, Political and Social Development'. *Demokratizatsiya*. 2: 341–358.

Sheptycki, J. (ed.) (2000a) *Issues in Transnational Policing*. London: Routledge.

Sheptycki, J. (2000b) 'Policing the Virtual Launderette: Money Laundering, New Technology and Global Governance'. In Sheptycki *op. cit.*

Silverstein, M. (1988) 'Watergate and the American Political System'. In Markovits and Silverstein *op. cit.*

Singh, G. (1997) 'Understanding Political Corruption in Contemporary Indian Politics'. In Heywood *op. cit.*

Skaperdas, S. and Syropolous, C. (1995) 'Gangs as Primitive States'. In Fiorentini and Peltzman *op. cit.*

Smart, A. (1988) 'The Informal Regulation of Illegal Economic Activities: Comparisons Between the Squatter Property Market and Organized Crime'. *International Journal of the Sociology of Law*. 16: 91–101.

Smart, A. (1999) 'Predatory Rule and Illegal Economic Practices'. In Heyman *op. cit.*

Smith, H. (1988) *The Power Game: How Washington Works*. New York: Random House.

Somerset, K. (2001) *What the Professionals Know: The Trafficking of Children Into and Through the UK for Sexual Purposes*. London: ECPAT (End Child Prostitution, Pornography and Trafficking) UK. ⟨http://www.antislavery.org/homepage/resources/Children.PDF⟩.

South China Morning Post (1999) 'The Reinterpretation by the Standing Committee of the National People's Congress'. Hong Kong. 25 October.

Stasavage, D. (2000) 'Causes and Consequences of Corruption: Mozambique in Transition'. In Doig and Theobald *op. cit.*

Sterling, C. (1993) *The Mafia: The Long Reach of the International Sicilian Mafia*. London: HarperCollins.

Summers, M. (1987) *The Plundering Generation: Corruption and the Crisis of the Union, 1849–1861*. New York: Oxford University Press.

Szeftel, M. (1983) 'Corruption and the Spoils System in Zambia'. In Clarke *op. cit.*

Tanzania, Presidential Commission of Inquiry Against Corruption (1996) *Report of the Commission Against Corruption* (The Warioba Report). Dar Es Salaam: Government of Tanzania.

Teiwes, F. (1997) 'The Establishment and Consolidation of the New Regime, 1949–57'. In MacFarquhar *op. cit.*

Theobald, R. (2000) 'Conclusion: Prospects for Reform in a Globalized Economy'. In Doig and Theobald *op. cit.*

Tilman, R. (1968) 'Emergence of Black-Market Bureaucracy: Administration, Development and Corruption in the New States'. *Political Administration Review*. XXVIII: 437–444.

Transparency International (n.d.) *National Integrity Systems: The TI Source Book*. ⟨http://www.transparency.de/documents/source-book/summary.html⟩.

Trouillot, M.-R. (1990) *Haiti: State Against Nation. The Origins and Legacy of Duvalierism*. New York: Monthly Review Press.

Tullock, G. (1989) *The Economics of Special Privilege and Rent Seeking*. Boston: Kluwer Academic.

Tullock, G. (1993) *Rent Seeking*. The Shaftesbury Papers, 2. Aldershot: Edward Elgar.

Turner, K., Feinerman, J. and Guy, R. Kent (eds) (2000) *The Limits of the Rule of Law in China*. Seattle: University of Washington Press.

United Nations Asia and Far East Institute for the Prevention of Crime and the Treatment of Offenders (UNAFEI) (1996) *Resource Material Series No. 48*. Fuchu City: UNAFEI.

United States Congress (1951) *Report of the Senate Special Committee to Investigate Organized Crime in Interstate Commerce* (Kefauver Report). Washington, DC: US Government Printing Office.

Varese, F. (1997) 'The Transition to the Market and Corruption in Post-Socialist Russia'. In Heywood *op. cit.*

Vásquez-León, M. (1999) 'Neoliberalism, Environmentalism, and Scientific Knowledge: Redefining Use Rights in the Gulf of California Fisheries'. In Heyman *op. cit.*

Wade, R. (1989) 'Politics and Graft: Recruitment, Appointment, and Promotions to Public Office in India'. In Ward *op. cit.*

Walsh, L. (1997) *Firewall: The Iran–Contra Conspiracy and Cover-up*. New York: Norton.

Walter, I. (1985) *Secret Money: The World of International Financial Secrecy.* London: Allen & Unwin.

Wang, H.-W. (1973) 'Report on the Revision of the Party Constitution'. In *The Tenth National Congress of the Communist Party of China (Documents)*. Beijing: Foreign Languages Press.

Ward, P. (ed.) (1989) *Corruption, Development and Inequality: Soft Touch or Hard Graft?* London: Routledge.

Watt, D., Flanary, R. and Theobald, R. (2000) 'Democratization or the Democratization of Corruption? The Case of Uganda'. In Doig and Theobald *op. cit.*

Weber, M. (1904) *The Protestant Ethic and the Spirit of Capitalism.* Trans. T. Parsons. New York: Charles Scribner's Sons.

White, C. (2002) 'EU Executive Charged with Ignoring Fraud'. *United Press International.* 27 February.

White, G. (1996) 'Corruption and the Transition from Socialism in China'. In Levi and Nelken *op. cit.*

Whitehead, L. (1983) 'On Presidential Graft: The Latin American Evidence'. In Clarke *op. cit.*

Williams, P. (1994) 'Transnational Criminal Organizations and International Security'. *Survival.* 36: 96–113.

Williams, R. (1987) *Political Corruption in Africa.* Aldershot: Gower.

Williams, R. (ed.) (2000a) *Explaining Corruption. The Politics of Corruption 1.* Cheltenham: Edward Elgar.

Williams, R. (2000b) 'Democracy, Development, and Anti-Corruption Strategies: Learning from the Australian Experience'. In Doig and Theobald *op. cit.*

Williams, R. and Doig, A. (eds) (2000) *Controlling Corruption. The Politics of Corruption 4.* Cheltenham: Edward Elgar.

Williams, R. and Theobald, R. (eds) (2000) *Corruption in the Developing World. The Politics of Corruption 2.* Cheltenham: Edward Elgar.

Williams, R., Moran, J. and Flanary, R. (eds) (2000) *Corruption in the Developed World. The Politics of Corruption 3.* Cheltenham: Edward Elgar.

Williamson, J. (1977) *The Failure of World Monetary Reform, 1971–74.* Sunbury-on-Thames: Thomas Nelson.

Woo, M. (2000) 'Law and Discretion in Contemporary Chinese Courts'. In Turner, Feinerman and Guy *op. cit.*

Woodworth, P. (2001) *Dirty War, Clean Hands: ETA, the GAL and Spanish Democracy.* Cork: Cork University Press.

World Bank (1997) *Helping Countries Combat Corruption.* Washington, DC: World Bank.

Wraith, R. and Simpkins, E. (1963) *Corruption in Developing Countries.* London: Allen & Unwin.

Wright, E. (1989) *The Chinese People Stand Up.* London: BBC Books.

Wrong, M. (2000) *In the Footsteps of Mr Kurtz: Living on the Brink of Disaster in the Congo.* London: Fourth Estate.

Yang, M. M-h. (1994) *Gifts, Favors and Banquets: The Art of Social Relationships in China.* Ithaca, NY: Cornell University Press.

Zhu, T. (1999) 'China's Corporatization Drive: An Evaluation and Policy Implications'. *Contemporary Economic Policy*, 17: 530–539.

Zvekic, U. (ed.) (1990) *Essays on Crime and Development.* Rome: United Nations Interregional Crime and Justice Research Institute.

Index